Heparin: Structure, Functions and Clinical Applications

Heparin: Structure, Functions and Clinical Applications

Editor: Alexandre Cunningham

MURPHY & MOORE
www.murphy-moorepublishing.com

www.murphy-moorepublishing.com

MURPHY & MOORE

Cataloging-in-Publication Data

Heparin : structure, functions and clinical applications / edited by Alexandre Cunningham.
p. cm.
Includes bibliographical references and index.
ISBN 978-1-63987-782-9
1. Heparin. 2. Heparin--Therapeutic use. I. Cunningham, Alexandre.
QP702.H4 H47 2023
612.115--dc23

Murphy & Moore Publishing
1 Rockefeller Plaza,
New York City,
NY 10020, USA

ISBN 978-1-63987-782-9

Contents

Preface

Heparin refers to a naturally occurring glycosaminoglycan which is used as a type of drug. These drugs are classified as anticoagulants since they rely on the activity of antithrombin. Heparin is primarily utilized to treat unstable angina and heart attacks. It is administered through injection into a vein under the skin. Its other applications include usage in kidney dialysis machines and inside test tubes. It is an unfractionated mixture of various partially sulfated polymers of different carbohydrates such as D-glucosamine, L-iduronic acid, 2-acetamido-2-deoxy-D-glucose, D-glucuronic acid, and 2-deoxy-2-sulfamino-D-glucose. Heparin chains are diverse in size and include both N- and O-sulfation and N-acetylation patterns, due to the complex biosynthesis process and unpredictability of animal species and tissues. This book provides comprehensive insights into the structure, functions and clinical applications of heparin. It aims to serve as a resource guide for students and experts alike.

After months of intensive research and writing, this book is the end result of all who devoted their time and efforts in the initiation and progress of this book. It will surely be a source of reference in enhancing the required knowledge of the new developments in the area. During the course of developing this book, certain measures such as accuracy, authenticity and research focused analytical studies were given preference in order to produce a comprehensive book in the area of study.

This book would not have been possible without the efforts of the authors and the publisher. I extend my sincere thanks to them. Secondly, I express my gratitude to my family and well-wishers. And most importantly, I thank my students for constantly expressing their willingness and curiosity in enhancing their knowledge in the field, which encourages me to take up further research projects for the advancement of the area.

Editor

1

Structural Features and PF4 Functions that Occur in Heparin-Induced Thrombocytopenia (HIT) Complicated by COVID-19

Zheng Cai, Mark I. Greene, Zhiqiang Zhu and Hongtao Zhang *

Departments of Pathology and Laboratory Medicine, Perelman School of Medicine, University of Pennsylvania, Philadelphia, PA 19301, USA; caizheng78@gmail.com (Z.C.); greenemarkirwin@gmail.com (M.I.G.); zhuzhuqiang@gmail.com (Z.Z.)

* Correspondence: zhanghon@pennmedicine.upenn.edu

Abstract: Platelet factor 4 (PF4, CXCL4) is a small chemokine protein released by activated platelets. Although a major physiological function of PF4 is to promote blood coagulation, this cytokine is involved in innate and adaptive immunity in events when platelets are activated in response to infections. Coronavirus disease 2019 (COVID-19) patients have abnormal coagulation activities, and severe patients develop higher D-dimer levels. D-dimers are small protein products present in the blood after blood clots are degraded by fibrinolysis. To prevent clotting, heparin is often clinically used in COVID-19 patients. Some clinical procedures for the management of COVID-19 patients may include extracorporeal membrane oxygenation (ECMO) and renal replacement therapy (CRRT), which also require the use of heparin. Anti-PF4 antibodies are frequently detected in severe patients and heparin-induced thrombocytopenia (HIT) can also be observed. PF4 and its role in HIT as well as in pathologies seen in COVID-19 patients define a potential therapeutic option of using blocking antibodies in the treatment of COVID-19.

Keywords: PF4; thrombin; COVID-19; Coronavirus

1. Introduction

Platelet factor 4 (PF4, CXCL4) is a small chemokine protein released by activated platelets [1]. The mature size of PF4 is 70-amino-acid protein, or 7.8 kDa. Its major physiological function is to promote blood coagulation. This function is related to PF4's affinity for heparin and other glycosaminoglycans (GAGs) [2,3], which are long linear polysaccharides consisting of repeating disaccharide units. By neutralizing the negatively charged heparan sulfate side chains of GAGs on the surface of platelets and endothelial cells, PF4 facilitates platelet aggregation to form a thrombus.

However, PF4 has additional activities beyond simply promoting blood coagulation, and the regulation of PF4 is very complex. PF4 expression is elevated following trauma. This is perfectly understandable, as coagulation is often needed to prevent blood loss from injury. Unexpectedly, a significant amount of PF4 is also released by activated platelets in response to infection. A systematic review of the functions of platelets in infectious diseases, especially in the current Coronavirus disease 2019 (COVID-19) pandemic, will be helpful in facilitating a better understanding of the role of PF4, as well as the potential use of a PF4-blocking antibody in the management of heparin-induced thrombocytopenia (HIT).

2. Platelets and Viral Infection of the Lung

Although platelets have an average life span of 8 to 12 days, this special class of anucleated cell fragments is critical for many important biological processes, such as hemostasis, thrombosis, wound healing, angiogenesis, immunity, and inflammatory responses [4–6]. The roles of platelets in innate immunity are relevant to viral infection of the lung, an important site for platelet biogenesis. By directly imaging the lung microcirculation in mice, Liu et al. demonstrated the circulation of a large number of megakaryocytes through the lungs and the release of platelets in this organ [7]. In fact, platelets released by megakaryocytes in the lungs account for approximately 50% of total platelet production, defining the lung as a major organ for platelet biogenesis. Patients with acute influenza infection possess activated platelets that engulf influenza A H1N1 virions and release antiviral molecules (e.g., α-granules) that can destroy the virus [8]. In response to bacterial or single-stranded viral infection, platelets also form heterotypic aggregates with neutrophils.

TLR7 is a Toll-like receptor (TLR) that is expressed on platelets. TLR7 is critical for viral- engulfment and subsequent neutrophil activation. TLR7 knockout (KO) mice display reduced neutrophil-DNA release. Engulfed influenza nucleic acids are sensed by platelet-TLR7. This interaction leads to complement C3 release, which is sufficient to mediate DNA release from neutrophils. In the presence of neutrophils, platelets also secrete GM-CSF, which acts as a negative regulator of the TLR7-dependent neutrophil-DNA release [8]. It is noteworthy that rare loss-of-function variants of the X-chromosomal *TLR7* gene have been identified in four young male patients with severe COVID-19 from two families [9]. One patient failed to survive due to concurrent secondary bacterial infection. Immunological defects in type I and II interferon production is found to be associated with this *TLR7* gene mutation.

The platelet response to respiratory viruses includes granule production and release. In general platelets contain three types of granule: α-granules, dense granules, and lysosomes. α-granules are the most abundant granule type. The α-granules are composed of various chemokines, cytokines, membrane proteins, and proteases, as well as proinflammatory and anti-inflammatory mediators [3,10].

Platelets are also involved in adaptive immunity. The Fcγ receptor, FcγRIIA, is expressed on the surface of activated platelets and is responsible for the endocytosis of immunoglobulin G (IgG) coated pathogens. This has been further demonstrated by the ability of platelets from FcγRIIA transgenic mice, but not wild-type mice (which are deficient for FcγRIIA expression in platelets), to bind and endocytose IgG complexes [11]. Manne and colleagues have studied platelet gene expression and function in COVID-19 patients [12]. Differential gene expression changes have been identified in pathways related to protein ubiquitination, antigen presentation and mitochondrial dysfunction. Platelets from COVID-19 patients tend to be hyperactive, and can form significantly more circulating platelet-neutrophil, -monocyte, and -T-cell aggregates compared to healthy donors.

P-selectin is an adhesion molecule on platelets. P-selectin can bind to its receptor P-selectin glycoprotein ligand 1 (PSGL1) on myeloid and a subset of lymphocytes. The interaction between P-selectin and PSGL1 thus becomes the driving force for the adhesion, immobilization, and recruitment of leukocytes [13,14] and lymphocytes during inflammation, tissue repair and thrombotic disorders [15]. By interacting with PSGL1 on monocytes, platelet P-selectin can also induce a cross-presentation program in peripheral blood monocytes and lead to dendritic cell differentiation [16]. In COVID-19 patients, platelets have higher P-selectin expression levels both at resting and after activation [12]. This feature may account for the hyperactivity of platelets and clotting risk in COVID-19 [17,18].

3. Role of PF4 in Infections

During infections, activated platelets release PF4 in response to microorganisms [19,20]. PF4 contributes to the recruitment of neutrophils and facilitates neutrophil exocytosis to release myeloperoxidase and lysozyme. After respiratory virus invasion, PF4 is capable of stimulating antigen-presenting cells (APCs) to induce the proliferation of lymphocytes and the cytotoxic activity of NK cells. PF4 plays a critical role in the clearance of viruses, as PF4 KO mice show diminished viral clearance from the lung as compared to wild-type mice [21]. This feature is consistent with the reduced innate immunity observed in the PF4 KO mice during early infections.

Plasmodium falciparum infection leads to malaria, an infection that kills ~half million people worldwide annually. During *Plasmodium falciparum* infection, platelets release PF4 to kill intraerythrocytic *P. falciparum* parasites via the Duffy-antigen receptor (Fy/DARC) on erythrocytes [22]. During HIV-1 infections, activated platelets also produce PF4, which acts as an anti-viral cytokine. The oligomeric status of PF4 influences whether PF4 inhibits or enhances HIV infection. When PF4 exists predominantly in a monomeric state, it binds to the HIV-1 envelope protein gp120 and inhibits HIV-1 attachment to the cell surface, thus reducing HIV-1 entry into CD4+ T cells [23]. HIV-1-infected patients with low serum levels of PF4 tend to have more advanced clinical outcomes. As its concentration increases, PF4 tends to form tetramers or higher-ordered forms, which enhance HIV-1 infection in vitro. Soluble glycosaminoglycans (GAGs) can prevent the tetrameric PF4 from enhancing virus infection [24], indicating that interacting with cell surface GAGs is required by the tetrameric PF4 to help HIV infection. PF4 may also be involved in host responses to coronavirus infection. Protein–protein interactions (PPI) and gene co-expression data indicate that PF4 is among cytokines produced by host innate immunity in response to the S-glycoprotein of MERS-CoV [25].

While there are clearly anti-infective activities of PF4, the PF4 species itself may also contribute to pathogenic infections. As a pro-inflammatory cytokine, PF4 is related to the pathogenesis of cerebral malaria (CM), a serious complication of *P. falciparum infection*. This may occur after the disruption of the blood–brain barrier [26].

4. Structural Basis for PF4 Function: Binding Activity of PF4 to Polysaccharides

Heparin is a naturally occurring GAG and has been clinically used as an anticoagulant in the treatment of heart attacks and unstable angina, and most recently in the clinical care of COVID-19 patients [27]. GAGs are long linear polysaccharides consisting of repeating disaccharide units. This feature is distinct from N- or O-linked glycans, which are branched polysaccharides. The repeating unit of GAGs typically consists of a uronic acid (or galactose) and an amino sugar (N-acetylglucosamine or N-acetylgalactosamine). The acidic sugar residues and sulphate groups account for the high negative charge of GAGs.

Based on core disaccharide structures, GAGs are classified into four groups (Figure 1):

- Heparin/heparan sulfate;
- Chondroitin sulfate/dermatan sulfate (CSGAGs);
- Keratan sulfate;
- Hyaluronic acid.

The difference between heparin and heparan sulfate moieties relates to cellular location. Heparan sulfate polysaccharides exist ubiquitously on the cell surface and extracellular matrix, whereas heparin is present within mast cells and can be considered as a more sulfated variant of heparan sulfate. Heparin/heparan sulfates are synthesized in the Golgi apparatus and attached by glycosyltransferases to protein cores via O-linked glycosylations. Proteins carrying GAGs are called Proteoglycans (PGs). One of the platelet proteins that heparin/heparin are abundantly attached to is serglycin, an intracellular proteoglycan found in platelet and other hematopoietic cells, as well as endothelial cells. Differences exist in the GAG attachment on serglycin in different tissues, with heparin and chondroitin sulfate as the preferred GAGs in connective tissue mast cells and mucosal mast cells/activated macrophages, respectively. Chondroitin sulfate/dermatan sulfate are also synthesized in the Golgi apparatus and attached to protein cores via O-linked glycosylations.

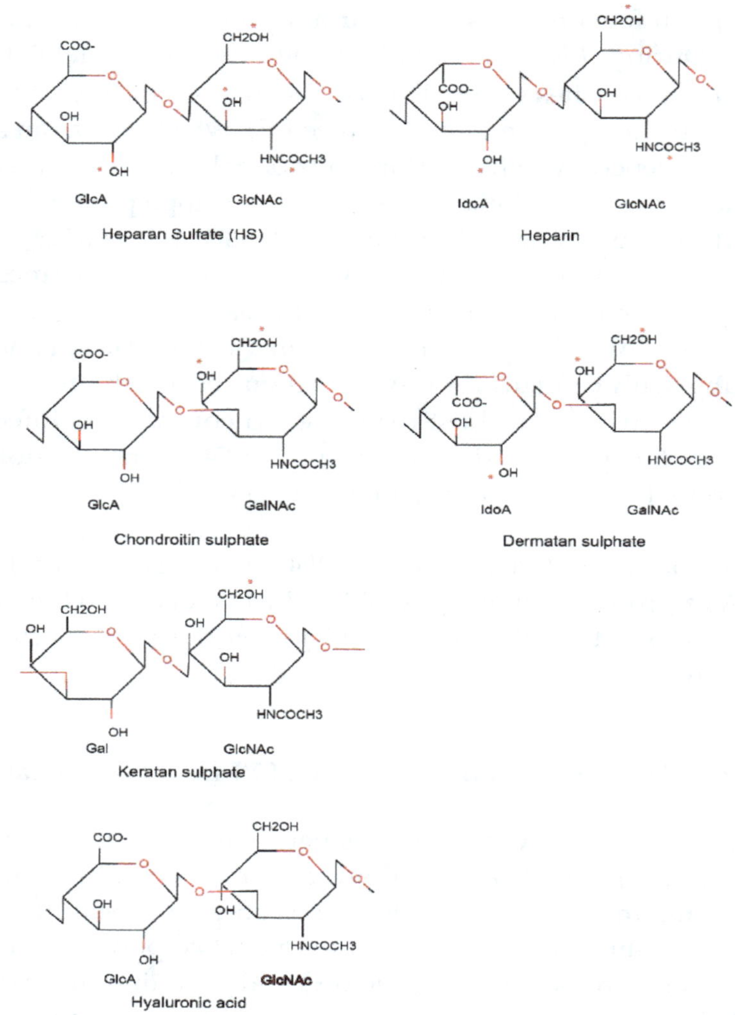

Figure 1. Structure of glycosaminoglycan chains. The repeating disaccharides in different types of glycosaminoglycan chains are presented. The different sulphation positions in each glycosaminoglycan (GAG) are marked by * in red.

As reported by Kolset et al., the multimeric forms of PF4 are the major platelet-derived proteins that are bound to serglycin [28]. PF4 has a very high affinity for heparin (K_D: ~30 nM), while its affinity for heparin sulfate and serglycin is about 10-fold less. Like other platelet-derived chemokines, such as RANTES and pro-platelet basic protein (PPBP), PF4 has a positively charged antimicrobial peptide (AMP) domain. With its positively charged surface, PF4 is also able to bind to heparin, which has the highest negative charge density of all known natural molecules due to its heavily sulfated glycosaminoglycans.

5. Heparin-Induced Thrombocytopenia (HIT)

As a widely used anti-coagulant during invasive vascular surgery, heparin therapy (in 1–5% of individuals so treated) can cause a complication termed heparin-induced thrombocytopenia (HIT) [29,30]. In patients with HIT, antibodies against PF4/heparin complexes induce thrombocytopenia and thrombosis, even under situations when the platelet counts are low [31]. This is a life- threatening immune-mediated disorder that typically occurs 4–10 days after exposure to heparin, and is different from so called "Type 1 HIT", in which thrombocytopenia occurs within the first 2 days after exposure to heparin, but platelet count returns to normal with continued heparin therapy.

To identify the risk for HIT in patients who are currently or were recently treated with heparin-derived agents, a 4 T's -scoring system has been used [32,33]. This scoring system evaluates the following clinical features: the degree of Thrombocytopenia, the Timing of platelet count fall, the associated Thrombosis, and the concurrent presence of other potential etiologies of Thrombocytopenia. For patients with intermediate or high-risk 4T scores, further laboratory evaluation for HIT or switching to a non-heparin derived anti-coagulant is recommended. The diagnosis can be essentially confirmed if the 4 T's score is ≥4 and the HIT IgG-specific antibody is positive.

To reduce the risk of HIT, the use of low-molecular weight heparin (LMWH) instead of unfractionated heparin is suggested [34]. However, there are still reports of HIT after the use of LMWH, such as Enoxaparin [35]. Alternative, a homogenous synthetic anticoagulant fondaparinux, which is a modified pentasaccharide heparin, can also be used. Although fondaparinux can still form complexes with PF4 [36], the complexes are poorly recognized by HIT antibodies [37]. Therefore, fondaparinux renders lower risk for HIT. Because of this, fondaparinux has been used in HIT patients complicated with or without thrombosis [38–41]. However, fondaparinux is not an ideal treatment for HIT. Low-dose fondaparinux does not necessarily prevent thrombotic complications of HIT [42]. Furthermore, it is reported that a patient who underwent aortic stent graft placement developed thrombocytopenia after fondaparinux was used for anticoagulation [43]. In stroke patients, administration of fondaparinux led to further reduction in platelet counts. Heparin-induced platetet activation assay (HIPA) showed platelet activation in the presence of both heparin and fondaparinux, although IgG-PF4/heparin antibodies were not detected [44]. To rescue patients from fondaparinux-cross reactive or fondaparinux-refractory HIT, high-dose intravenous immunoglobulin (IVIG) was clinically used [45]. Switching blood thinners to rivaroxaban is considered safe and effective for the management of clinically suspected HIT [46].

Heparin, PF4, and the PF4 antibody forms HIT immune complexes that induce the crosslinking of Fc-receptors on platelets, neutrophils and monocytes and lead to the production of pro-inflammatory and procoagulant cytokines, such as PF4, tissue factor (TF) and thrombin [47,48]. For example, binding of the HIT immune complexes to human monocytes induces TF expression on peripheral blood mononuclear cells (PBMCs) and monocytes [49]. TF is the high-affinity receptor and cofactor for Factor VII/VIIa (FVII/F VIIa), and the TF-FVIIa complex is the primary initiator of blood coagulation cascade that generates coagulation proteases, such as FXa, and thrombin [50]. Although the FcγRIIA on monocytes is critical for the HIT immune complexes to bind monocytes [51], Cines and colleagues have recently pointed out that FcRn, which is commonly involved in the recycling of IgGs, augments the induction of TF activity by the HIT immune complexes [52].

Since HIT is an immune disease, and patients may have elevated pro-inflammatory cytokines, cyclophosphamide may help overcome certain features of cytokine storm during HIT. For example, a patient with severe lupus nephritis (SLE) developed HIT during treatment and the thrombin inhibitor argatroban was used for thrombosis prophylaxis. Due to decreases in oxygen saturation and blood pressure, the patient with congestive heart failure was admitted to the intensive care unit (ICU). The patient received medical support for his circulation and was treated with antibiotics for microbial infection. The patient's myocardial damage, however, was believed to be caused by cytokine storm. After treatment with methylprednisolone (mPSL) pulse therapy, the patient showed stable vital signs and was discharged from ICU. His thrombocytopenia persisted and hemoptysis occurred two days later. The patient was found to have alveolar hemorrhage. He was admitted to the ICU again due to decreased oxygen saturation, and started on ventilator management with endotracheal intubation. Eventually the patient responded to cyclophosphamide, an inhibitor to suppress the immune system in general to control SLE activity. In three days, the patient displayed increased platelet count, and was released from mechanical ventilation and discharged from the ICU [53].

6. Structural Basis for Heparin-Induced Thrombocytopenia (HIT)

PF4 is a cationic monomeric protein with a propensity to form tetramers that assemble into oligomers in the presence of polyanions [54–56]. To form the immune complex that induces HIT, PF4 first binds heparin or other polyanions to obtain a structure that has much higher affinity and avidity for a set of HIT antibodies [57]. Through the Fc of recruited HIT antibodies, the micron-sized immune complex can cross-link cell-surface Fc receptors and activate platelets and other types of immune cells. The activated platelets have procoagulant activity, which leads to a pathology contrary to the expected activity of the anti-coagulant activity of heparin [58].

Not all PF4 antibodies are pathogenic and lead to HIT [59–62]. Pathogenic HIT antibodies are known to bind PF4 in the presence of heparin. However, current clinical tests are not effective to determine whether the PF4 antibodies are pathogenic or non-pathogenic. Arepally and colleagues identified that the murine monoclonal antibody KKO forms PF4/heparin complexes and causes heparin-induced thrombosis and thrombocytopenia in a murine model, thus classifying KKO as a pathogenic antibody [59]. Human HIT antibodies compete with KKO for binding to PF4/heparin, and KKO augments the formation of pathogenic immune complexes [63].

To understand how PF4 structurally interacts with heparin and pathogenic HIT antibodies, our laboratory successfully crystallized PF4 in complex with fondaparinux [64]. More importantly, we also obtained the crystal structure of PF4 tetramer with the pathogenic antibody KKO [64]. These two structures enabled our laboratory to understand the structure of the HIT immune complex (Figure 2, [64]) and, along with the solution of other crystal complexes, determine the atomic pathway that leads to HIT in vivo. PF4 tetramers cluster around a semi-rigid linear heparin chain that resides in the middle of the complex. Multiple HIT antibodies KKO (blue) bind to the outer surface of PF4 tetramers, ultimately assembling into the ultra-large immune complexes (ULICs) that mediate cell activation. Heparin and HIT antibodies operate in a collaborative manner to stabilize the PF4 tetramers and the resultant ULICs [64].

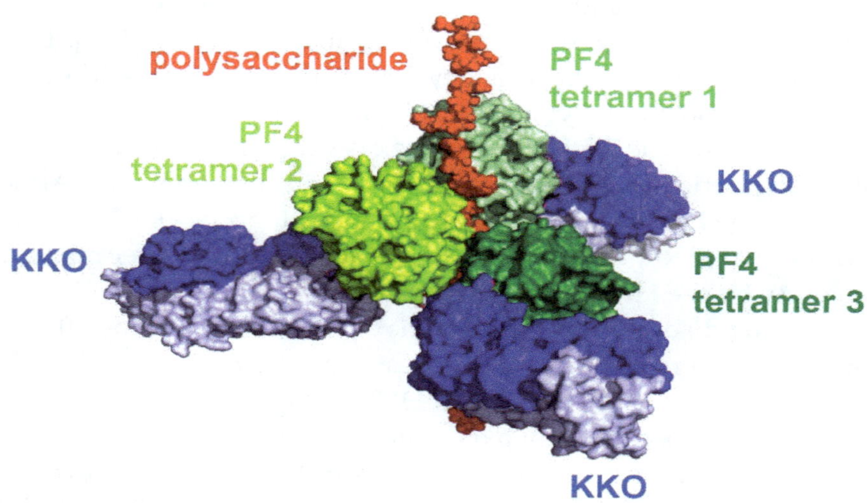

Figure 2. Current understanding of the structure of the HIT immune complex.

7. Coagulation Dysfnction in COVID-19 and the Risk of HIT

Thrombocytopenia is a common clinical feature of viral infections, especially for RNA viruses (e.g., HIV-1, HCV, dengue) [65,66]. The occurrence of thrombocytopenia can be caused by platelet activation and platelet-monocyte aggregate formation after viral infection [67]. In COVID-19 patients, elevated concentrations of inflammatory cytokines have been observed [68]. The release of excessive cytokines damages endothelial cells and disturbs their function, leading to problems with coagulation dysfunction and microvascular disease [69,70]. Thrombosis within the brain can lead to strokes, and clots in the lungs can reduce blood flow into the lungs and limit the usefulness of ventilators.

Being caused by the infection of severe acute respiratory syndrome coronavirus 2 (SARS-CoV-2), COVID-19 was initially defined as a lung disease. However, due to the inflammatory cytokine storms induced by SARS-CoV-2 infection [71–73], the coagulation pathway can be activated in severe COVID-19 patients and cause excessive consumption of coagulation factors and platelets. Subsequently, coagulation dysfunction can occur in a certain percentage of patients, and thrombosis is one of the major causes of death in patients with severe COVID-19 [74–77]. In one study from China involving 183 COVID-19 patients, non-survivors had significantly higher D-dimer and fibrin degradation product (FDP) levels. The normal range of D-dimer is under 0.5 μg/mL, but the average D-dimer levels in survivors and non-survivors were 0.61 and 2.12 μg/mL, respectively. During their hospital stay, 71.4% of non-survivors, vs. 0.6% of survivors met the criteria of disseminated intravascular coagulation [75]. In French studies, 23~30% of COVID-19 patients were found by computed tomography (CT) to have pulmonary embolisms [78,79]. These patients also had higher D-dimer levels and were more likely to be in the intensive care unit.

In a prospective study of hospitalized COVID-19 patients in non-intensive care units, 156 patients with D-dimer > 1 μg/mL were screened for asymptomatic DVT with complete compression doppler ultrasound (CCUS). A total of 23 patients (14.7%) were identified to have DVT. Patients with DVT had higher median D-dimer levels: 4.527 μg/mL vs. 2.05 μg/mL ($p < 0.001$). D-dimer levels > 1.57 μg/mL were associated with asymptomatic DVT (OR 9.1; CI 95% 1.1–70.1) [80]. When autopsies were performed in a German hospital on the first 12 consecutive COVID-19-positive deaths, deep venous thrombosis was found in seven patients (58%). None of these patients were suspected to have venous thromboembolism before death. In addition, pulmonary embolism was identified as the direct cause of death in four patients [81]. In another autopsy study of 11 deceased COVID-19 patients, thrombosis of small and mid-sized pulmonary arteries was found in various degrees in all these patients and was associated with infarction in eight patients and bronchopneumonia in six patients [74]. Again, none of these patients had clinical evidence of venous thromboembolism before death, although 10 of the 11 patients had already received prophylactic anticoagulant therapy.

Since elevated D-dimer levels are often found in patients with clotting problems, severe COVID-19 patients with elevated D-dimer levels are treated with unfractionated heparin or LMWH as an anticoagulation to reduce mortality (Table 1) [82–87]. However, the current anticoagulation options have limited effect on thrombosis in general COVID-19 patients, and some of the observed effects were not significant [88–91]. In a Dutch study of COVID-19 patients, all 184 ICU patients received at least standard doses thromboprophylaxis, but thrombosis still occured in 31% patients, including 27% venous thromboembolism (VTE) and 3.7% arterial thrombotic events [92]. Pulmonary embolism was the most frequent thrombotic complication (81%). The dosage of anticoagulation agents is also important for the management of COVID-19 patients. It is possible that some patients benefited most from the use of anti-coagulants. In a retrospective review of 245 COVID-19 patients admitted to the ICU requiring mechanical ventilation at Mount Sinai Hospital, patients treated with therapeutic anticoagulation for a minimum of 5 days had a 79% reduction in death when compared with those treated with prophylactic dose [27]. Although a slight trend towards increased bleeding complications was observed in the therapeutic anticoagulation group, the effect was not statistically significant. It is thought that the benefit of initiating therapeutic anticoagulation in intubated COVID19 patients outweighs the risk of bleeding.

Table 1. Use of anticoagulants and outcomes in COVID-19 patients. CHD: chronic heart disease; aRR: adjust risk ratio; HR: Hazard ratio; OR: odd ration; LMWH: Low molecule weight heparin.

Patient Number	Patient Condition	Anti-Coagulation	Outcome	Ref.
2773	hospitalized	therapeutic anticoagulation	For patients who required mechanical ventilation (n = 395), in-hospital mortality was lower in those treated with anticoagulation (29.1% vs. 62.7%); no difference in general population	[84]
2075	hospitalized	Heparin	Lower mortality in patients who used Heparin (OR 0.55, 95% CI 0.37–0.82, p = 0.003)	[85]
1716		therapeutic anticoagulation	Subjects receiving new therapeutic anticoagulation, especially for those in the absence of other indications, were more likely to die (OR 5.93; 95% CI 3.71–9.47). Continuation of outpatient prescribed anticoagulant was not associated with improved clinical outcomes.	[91]
449	severe	mainly LMWH	In patients with D-dimer >6-fold of upper limit of normal, 28-day mortality was lower in heparin users than nonusers (32.8% vs. 52.4%, p = 0.017).	[83]
374	hospitalized	therapeutic vs. prophylatic	higher in-hospital mortality in patients receiving preemptive therapeutic anticoagulation (aRR: 2.3, 95% CI = 1.0, 4.9; p = 0.04)	[90]
245	ICU	therapeutic vs. prophylatic	79% reduction in death with therapeutic dose	[27]
184	ICU	thromboprophylaxis	thrombosis rate: 31%	[92]
115	hospitalized	therapeutic anticoagulation	Lower mortality in patients with anticoagulation (OR 0.055, 95% Cl 0.008–0.386, p = 0.03)	[87]
101	Nursing Home Residents		Only a trend of lower mortality in patients with anticoagulation (OR 0.89, 95% Cl 0.41–1.95)	[89]
70	elderly patients with interstitial pneumonia and CHD	direct oral anticoagulants	Lower mortality in patients with anticoagulation (HR 0.38, 95% Cl 0.17–0.58, p = 0.01)	[86]

Thrombocytopenia is another problem in COVID-19 patients [93,94]. In one study from China, which involved 1099 COVID-19 patients, thrombocytopenia was present in 31.6% of non-severe patients, but was observed in 57.7% of patients with severe disease [93]. While the coagulation in COVID-19 is related to the host response to SARS-CoV-2 infection, thrombocytopenia can be HIT, caused by the use of heparin [95]. In a retrospective cohort analysis of 652 hospitalized patients with COVID-19 at Beth Israel Deaconess Medical Center, 88 patients who received at least 5 days of UFH were selected to check if HIT occurred. Eight patients had suspected HIT, and five patients tested positive for HIT by latex immunoassay. All five patients were treated with direct thrombin inhibitors after HIT antibody test (four with argatroban, one with bivalirudin). While three patients developed major hemorrhagic events and died after progressive respiratory failure, only one patient suffered acute cerebrovascular infarct as well as extensive areas of splenic infarction [96].

There are abundant reports of thrombocytopenia in severe COVID-19 patients. In a study of 61 critical COVID-19 patients admitted into intensive care unit (ICU) and 93 severe non-ICU patients in the Huoshenshan Hospital (Wuhan, China), 41% of ICU patients (25/61) had severe thrombocytopenia with a platelet count less than 50×10^9/L. All except one (24/25) had a fatal outcome. 52.2% of non-survivors (24/46) had severe thrombocytopenia, compared to 6.7% (1/15) in survivors. High levels of anti-Heparin-PF4 antibodies were observed in most of ICU patients [95]. Riker et al. reported the cases of thrombocytopenia with anti-PF4 antibodies among 16 intubated COVID-19 patients with ARDS. All three patients had evidence of thrombosis (pulmonary embolism, upper extremity venous thromboses, and skin necrosis, respectively). One case was confirmed as HIT by the serotonin release assay [97].

In addition to the use of anticoagulation agents for potential coagulation dysfunction in COVID-19, some medical care procedures also require the use of heparin. For critically ill COVID-19 patients, extracorporeal membrane oxygenation (ECMO) is used to replace the function of the lungs and heart. ECMO pumps and oxygenates the patient's blood outside the body, for which unfractionated heparin is frequently administered to patients to prevent coagulation. This also exposes these severe or critically ill patients to a high risk of HIT. In a study of patients with severe heart failure, out of 57 adult patients who underwent an ECMO for at least 5 days, 29 patients (50%) were positive for PF4-specific Abs. HIT was suspected in two patients with ECMO dysfunction and unexpected platelet count decrease after day 5. These two patients also had high levels of PF4-specific IgG levels. Eventually, HIT was confirmed in both individuals by a serotonin release assay [98].

Much more frequent thrombocytopenia episodes are also observed among those who underwent continuous renal replacement therapy (CRRT), a procedure commonly used in the intensive care unit for correction of metabolic acidosis and removal of cytokines in critically ill COVID-19 patients. Unfractionated heparin is the most commonly used anticoagulant to maintain circuit patency during CRRT [99]. In one study, most of the 16 CRRT patients (13/16) experienced a sharp decrease in platelets to less than 50×10^9/L. In comparison, only 26.7% of non-CRRT ICU patients (12/45), and 1.1% of non-ICU patients (1/93) showed such a decrease in platelets [95]. The high risk of thrombocytopenia in CRRT patients suggests that heparin use in CRRT might contribute to the high mortality of critically ill COVID-19 patients.

Thus, for a severe case of COVID-19, if the platelet count is decreased by >50% from the basal value and there are signs of arteriovenous thrombosis after an administration of heparin, patients should be evaluated for HIT. For COVID-19 patients using ECMO support, it is recommended that patients are monitored for HIT. If the ECMO circuit is frequently abnormal and platelets progressively decrease, and if there are high levels of PF4-specific IgG antibodies, HIT should be considered.

It was also noticed that HIT antibodies and a progressive decrease in platelets occurred in heparin-naïve patients (i.e., before CRRT or other heparin exposure), and even in non-ICU patients, suggesting that a spontaneous HIT might occur in COVID-19 patients, probably related to the formation of PF4 tetrameric complexes during viral or secondary bacterial infection. In COVID-19 patients, the serum concentrations of HIT antibodies are largely correlated to C3a levels. Since complement activation can induce the release of heparin from master cells, spontaneous HIT in COVID-19 may be related to the complement activation that was reported for IgM [100].

8. Potential Use of a Humanized PF4 Antibody to Prevent HIT

As we mentioned before, not all PF4 antibodies are pathogenic, and this actually creates problems in HIT diagnosis. While KKO can cause HIT, an isotype matched anti-PF4 antibody RTO binds PF4 but does not generate pathogenic complexes [101]. KKO promotes the oligomerization of PF4, while RTO only binds to the PF4 monomer and prevents it from oligomerization [63]. We have also solved the crystal structure of the PF4 monomer in complex with RTO [64]. Our data indicated that RTO binds to the PF4 monomer and prevents it from forming tetramers (Figure 3), a critical structure that is required for HIT antibody binding and HIT immune complex formation. Since PF4 exists in a dynamic equilibrium between monomers and tetramers, stabilizing monomer populations of PF4 proteins will promote the dissociation of PF4 tetramers, thereby preventing the subsequent development of PF4 tetramer-based pathogenic immune complexes [64].

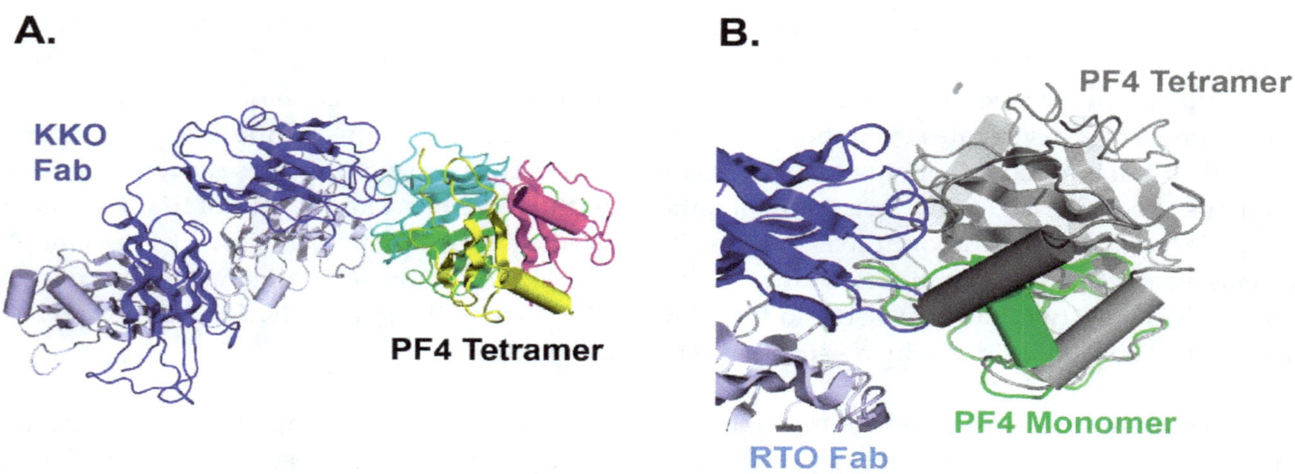

Figure 3. RTO binding to PF4 monomer impedes PF4 from forming tetramers, thus prevent PF4 tetramer-based immune complex formation, which underlies the pathogenesis of HIT. (**A**) HIT-like antibody KKO (blue) binds to PF4 tetramers (green, yellow, cyan and magenta; (**B**) blocking antibody RTO (blue) binds to PF4 monomer (green) and prevents tetramer (gray) formation.

KKO and RTO have shared but not identical epitopes [61,102] (Figure 4). To verify that RTO can block the pathogenic activity of KKO, we performed both in vitro and in vivo assays [64]. When platelet-rich plasma is incubated with PF4 and KKO, platelet activation and aggregation can be observed by measuring light transmission using a dual-channel lumi-aggregometer. However, when platelet-rich plasma is pre-incubated with RTO, KKO-induced platelet aggregation is prevented. The in vivo activity is demonstrated with the cremaster laser injury model performed on transgenic male C57BL mice that are deficient in mouse PF4 but express human PF4 and human FcγRIIA26 [103,104]. After focal arterial injury, circulating platelets can be observed with a fluorescently labeled CD41 antibody. In the presence of KKO, the formation of thrombus is observed. If mice are pre-treated with RTO, the effect of KKO-induced thrombosis is completely inhibited [64]. Our data have shown that RTO is a blocking antibody, as it blocks the in vitro and in vivo platelet-activating capacity of KKO.

```
hPF4  1    MSSAAGFCASRPG--LLFLGLLLLPLVVAFASAEAEE-DGDLQCLCVKT-TSQVRPRHIT  56
           MS AA F   RP   LL LGLL LP VVA  SA  EE DGDL C+CVKT +S +   +HIT
mPF4  1    MSVAAVFRGLRPSPELLLLGLLFLPAVVAVTSAGPEESDGDLSCVCVKTISSGIHLKHIT  60

hPF4  57   SLEVIKAGPHCPTAQLIATLKNGRKICLDLQAPLYKKIIKKLLES  101
           SLEVIKAG HC   QLIATLKNGRKICLD QAPLYKK+I+K+LES
mPF4  61   SLEVIKAGRHCAVPQLIATLKNGRKICLDRQAPLYKKVIEKILES  105
```

KKO epitope
RTO epitope

Figure 4. Comparison of human PF4 (hPF4) and mouse PF4 (mPF4) sequences, showing the overlap of KKO and RTO epitopes. Since KKO preferentially binds to PF4 tetramer, its epitopes are contributed by amino acid residues from different chains within a PF4 tetramer. Dash lines depict the internal disulfide bonds.

RTO is a mouse monoclonal antibody. With current data suggesting that RTO, as an HIT-blocking antibody, can be developed as a non-anticoagulant intervention in HIT, RTO needs to be humanized first before the antibody can be tested in clinical trial [105,106]. Recently, we have humanized the RTO antibody and are planning for pre-clinical testing and, ultimately, clinical application.

9. Conclusions

COVID-19 is not just a lung disease, but also a vascular and coagulation disease that is related to immune response to virus infection. Therapies targeting overreactive immune response and cytokine release storm are under clinical trials [68,107]. As coagulation abnormalities occur frequently in COVID-19 patients, the clinical use of heparin to prevent coagulation may lead to HIT. HIT symptoms and clinical signs should be monitored, especially in patients prone to developing this problem.

Although anticoagulants such as argatroban/bivalirudin may be administered instead of heparin to avoid HIT, they are not perfect solutions and issues with reversing the activity of argatroban/bivalirudin should be considered [108]. HIT-blocking antibodies should be investigated for potential clinical use to prevent fatal outcomes after HIT in COVID-19-infected individuals.

Author Contributions: Conceptualization, H.Z.; software, Z.C. and Z.Z.; writing—original draft preparation, H.Z.; writing—review and editing, M.I.G.; visualization, Z.C.; funding acquisition, H.Z., M.I.G. and Z.C. All authors have read and agreed to the published version of the manuscript.

Acknowledgments: We acknowledge the administrative and technical supports from Gail Massey and Angelica Patterson.

References

1. Poncz, M.; Surrey, S.; LaRocco, P.; Weiss, M.J.; Rappaport, E.F.; Conway, T.M.; Schwartz, E. Cloning and characterization of platelet factor 4 cDNA derived from a human erythroleukemic cell line. *Blood* **1987**, *69*, 219–223. [CrossRef]
2. Barber, A.J.; Kaser-Glanzmann, R.; Jakabova, M.; Luscher, E.F. Characterization of a chondroitin 4 -sulfate proteoglycan carrier for heparin neutralizing activity (platelet factor 4) released from human blood platelets. *Biochim. Biophys. Acta* **1972**, *286*, 312–329. [CrossRef]
3. Holt, J.C.; Niewiarowski, S. Biochemistry of alpha granule proteins. *Semin. Hematol.* **1985**, *22*, 151–163.
4. Qiu, J.; Ma, J.; Zhang, S.; Han, J.; Liu, S. Promoting platelets is a therapeutic option to combat severe viral infection of the lung. *Blood Adv.* **2020**, *4*, 1640–1642. [CrossRef]
5. Salamanna, F.; Maglio, M.; Landini, M.P.; Fini, M. Platelet functions and activities as potential hematologic parameters related to Coronavirus Disease 2019 (COVID-19). *Platelets* **2020**, *31*, 627–632. [CrossRef]
6. Schrottmaier, W.C.; Mussbacher, M.; Salzmann, M.; Assinger, A. Platelet-leukocyte interplay during vascular disease. *Atherosclerosis* **2020**. [CrossRef]
7. Lefrancais, E.; Ortiz-Munoz, G.; Caudrillier, A.; Mallavia, B.; Liu, F.; Sayah, D.M.; Thornton, E.E.; Headley, M.B.; David, T.; Coughlin, S.R.; et al. The lung is a site of platelet biogenesis and a reservoir for haematopoietic progenitors. *Nature* **2017**. [CrossRef]
8. Koupenova, M.; Corkrey, H.A.; Vitseva, O.; Manni, G.; Pang, C.J.; Clancy, L.; Yao, C.; Rade, J.; Levy, D.; Wang, J.P.; et al. The role of platelets in mediating a response to human influenza infection. *Nat. Commun.* **2019**, *10*, 1780. [CrossRef]
9. van der Made, C.I.; Simons, A.; Schuurs-Hoeijmakers, J.; van den Heuvel, G.; Mantere, T.; Kersten, S.; van Deuren, R.C.; Steehouwer, M.; van Reijmersdal, S.V.; Jaeger, M.; et al. Presence of Genetic Variants among Young Men With Severe COVID-19. *JAMA* **2020**. [CrossRef]
10. Rosowski, E.E.; Huttenlocher, A. Motile Collectors: Platelets Promote Innate Immunity. *Immunity* **2018**, *48*, 16–18. [CrossRef]
11. Worth, R.G.; Chien, C.D.; Chien, P.; Reilly, M.P.; McKenzie, S.E.; Schreiber, A.D. Platelet FcgammaRIIA binds and internalizes IgG-containing complexes. *Exp. Hematol.* **2006**, *34*, 1490–1495. [CrossRef]
12. Manne, B.K.; Denorme, F.; Middleton, E.A.; Portier, I.; Rowley, J.W.; Stubben, C.J.; Petrey, A.C.; Tolley, N.D.; Guo, L.; Cody, M.J.; et al. Platelet Gene Expression and Function in COVID-19 Patients. *Blood* **2020**. [CrossRef]
13. Zuchtriegel, G.; Uhl, B.; Puhr-Westerheide, D.; Pörnbacher, M.; Lauber, K.; Krombach, F.; Reichel, C.A. Platelets Guide Leukocytes to Their Sites of Extravasation. *PLoS Biol.* **2016**, *14*, e1002459. [CrossRef]

14. Kuckleburg, C.J.; Yates, C.M.; Kalia, N.; Zhao, Y.; Nash, G.B.; Watson, S.P.; Rainger, G.E. Endothelial cell-borne platelet bridges selectively recruit monocytes in human and mouse models of vascular inflammation. *Cardiovasc. Res.* **2011**, *91*, 134–141. [CrossRef]
15. Carlow, D.A.; Tra, M.C.; Ziltener, H.J. A cell-extrinsic ligand acquired by activated T cells in lymph node can bridge L-selectin and P-selectin. *PLoS ONE* **2018**, *13*, e0205685. [CrossRef]
16. Han, P.; Hanlon, D.; Arshad, N.; Lee, J.S.; Tatsuno, K.; Robinson, E.; Filler, R.; Sobolev, O.; Cote, C.; Rivera-Molina, F.; et al. Platelet P-selectin initiates cross-presentation and dendritic cell differentiation in blood monocytes. *Sci. Adv.* **2020**, *6*, eaaz1580. [CrossRef]
17. Di Micco, P.; Russo, V.; Carannante, N.; Imparato, M.; Rodolfi, S.; Cardillo, G.; Lodigiani, C. Clotting Factors in COVID-19: Epidemiological Association and Prognostic Values in Different Clinical Presentations in an Italian Cohort. *J. Clin. Med.* **2020**, *9*, 1371. [CrossRef]
18. Zaid, Y.; Puhm, F.; Allaeys, I.; Naya, A.; Oudghiri, M.; Khalki, L.; Limami, Y.; Zaid, N.; Sadki, K.; El Haj, R.B. Platelets can contain SARS-CoV-2 RNA and are hyperactivated in COVID-19. *medRxiv* **2020**. [CrossRef]
19. Kullaya, V.; van der Ven, A.; Mpagama, S.; Mmbaga, B.T.; de Groot, P.; Kibiki, G.; de Mast, Q. Platelet-monocyte interaction in Mycobacterium tuberculosis infection. *Tuberculosis (Edinb.)* **2018**, *111*, 86–93. [CrossRef]
20. Wilkinson, J.M.; Ladinig, A.; Bao, H.; Kommadath, A.; Stothard, P.; Lunney, J.K.; Harding, J.C.; Plastow, G.S. Differences in Whole Blood Gene Expression Associated with Infection Time-Course and Extent of Fetal Mortality in a Reproductive Model of Type 2 Porcine Reproductive and Respiratory Syndrome Virus (PRRSV) Infection. *PLoS ONE* **2016**, *11*, e0153615. [CrossRef]
21. Guo, L.; Feng, K.; Wang, Y.C.; Mei, J.J.; Ning, R.T.; Zheng, H.W.; Wang, J.J.; Worthen, G.S.; Wang, X.; Song, J.; et al. Critical role of CXCL4 in the lung pathogenesis of influenza (H1N1) respiratory infection. *Mucosal Immunol.* **2017**, *10*, 1529–1541. [CrossRef]
22. McMorran, B.J.; Wieczorski, L.; Drysdale, K.E.; Chan, J.A.; Huang, H.M.; Smith, C.; Mitiku, C.; Beeson, J.G.; Burgio, G.; Foote, S.J. Platelet factor 4 and Duffy antigen required for platelet killing of Plasmodium falciparum. *Science* **2012**, *338*, 1348–1351. [CrossRef]
23. Auerbach, D.J.; Lin, Y.; Miao, H.; Cimbro, R.; Difiore, M.J.; Gianolini, M.E.; Furci, L.; Biswas, P.; Fauci, A.S.; Lusso, P. Identification of the platelet-derived chemokine CXCL4/PF-4 as a broad-spectrum HIV-1 inhibitor. *Proc. Natl. Acad. Sci. USA* **2012**, *109*, 9569–9574. [CrossRef]
24. Parker, Z.F.; Rux, A.H.; Riblett, A.M.; Lee, F.H.; Rauova, L.; Cines, D.B.; Poncz, M.; Sachais, B.S.; Doms, R.W. Platelet Factor 4 Inhibits and Enhances HIV-1 Infection in a Concentration-Dependent Manner by Modulating Viral Attachment. *AIDS Res. Hum. Retrovir.* **2016**, *32*, 705–717. [CrossRef]
25. Messina, F.; Giombini, E.; Agrati, C.; Vairo, F.; Bartoli, T.A.; Moghazi, S.A.; Piacentini, M.; Locatelli, F.; Kobinger, G.; Maeurer, M.; et al. COVID-19: Viral-host interactome analyzed by network based-approach model to study pathogenesis of SARS-CoV-2 infection. *bioRxiv* **2020**. [CrossRef]
26. Wilson, N.O.; Jain, V.; Roberts, C.E.; Lucchi, N.; Joel, P.K.; Singh, M.P.; Nagpal, A.C.; Dash, A.P.; Udhayakumar, V.; Singh, N.; et al. CXCL4 and CXCL10 predict risk of fatal cerebral malaria. *Dis. Markers* **2011**, *30*, 39–49. [CrossRef]
27. Trinh, M.; Chang, D.R.; Govindarajulu, U.S.; Kane, E.; Fuster, V.; Kohli-Seth, R.; Ahmed, S.; Levin, M.A.; Chen, M.D. Therapeutic Anticoagulation Is Associated with Decreased Mortality in Mechanically Ventilated COVID-19 Patients. *medRxiv* **2020**. [CrossRef]
28. Kolset, S.O.; Mann, D.M.; Uhlin-Hansen, L.; Winberg, J.O.; Ruoslahti, E. Serglycin-binding proteins in activated macrophages and platelets. *J. Leukoc. Biol.* **1996**, *59*, 545–554. [CrossRef]
29. Chong, B.H. Evolving concepts of pathogenesis of heparin-induced thrombocytopenia: Diagnostic and therapeutic implications. *Int. J. Lab. Hematol.* **2020**, *42* (Suppl. S1), 25–32. [CrossRef]
30. Arepally, G.M.; Cines, D.B. Pathogenesis of heparin-induced thrombocytopenia. *Transl. Res. J. Lab. Clin. Med.* **2020**. [CrossRef]
31. Rauova, L.; Hirsch, J.D.; Greene, T.K.; Zhai, L.; Hayes, V.M.; Kowalska, M.A.; Cines, D.B.; Poncz, M. Monocyte-bound PF4 in the pathogenesis of heparin-induced thrombocytopenia. *Blood* **2010**, *116*, 5021–5031. [CrossRef]
32. Joseph, J.; Rabbolini, D.; Enjeti, A.K.; Favaloro, E.; Kopp, M.C.; McRae, S.; Pasalic, L.; Tan, C.W.; Ward, C.M.; Chong, B.H. Diagnosis and management of heparin-induced thrombocytopenia: A consensus statement from the Thrombosis and Haemostasis Society of Australia and New Zealand HIT Writing Group. *Med. J. Aust.* **2019**, *210*, 509–516. [CrossRef]

33. Althaus, K.; Straub, A.; Haberle, H.; Rosenberger, P.; Hidiatov, O.; Hammer, S.; Nowak-Harnau, S.; Enkel, S.; Riessen, R.; Bakchoul, T. Heparin-induced thrombocytopenia: Diagnostic challenges in intensive care patients especially with extracorporeal circulation. *Thromb. Res.* **2020**, *188*, 52–60. [CrossRef]
34. Warkentin, T.E. Clinical picture of heparin-induced thrombocytopenia (HIT) and its differentiation from non-HIT thrombocytopenia. *Thromb. Haemost.* **2016**, *116*, 813–822. [CrossRef]
35. Barcellona, D.; Melis, M.; Floris, G.; Mameli, A.; Muroni, A.; Defazio, G.; Marongiu, F. A "Catastrophic" Heparin-Induced Thrombocytopenia. *Case Rep. Med.* **2020**, *2020*. [CrossRef]
36. Greinacher, A.; Gopinadhan, M.; Gunther, J.U.; Omer-Adam, M.A.; Strobel, U.; Warkentin, T.E.; Papastavrou, G.; Weitschies, W.; Helm, C.A. Close approximation of two platelet factor 4 tetramers by charge neutralization forms the antigens recognized by HIT antibodies. *Arterioscler. Thromb. Vasc. Biol.* **2006**, *26*, 2386–2393. [CrossRef]
37. Warkentin, T.E.; Cook, R.J.; Marder, V.J.; Sheppard, J.A.; Moore, J.C.; Eriksson, B.I.; Greinacher, A.; Kelton, J.G. Anti-platelet factor 4/heparin antibodies in orthopedic surgery patients receiving antithrombotic prophylaxis with fondaparinux or enoxaparin. *Blood* **2005**, *106*, 3791–3796. [CrossRef]
38. Grouzi, E.; Kyriakou, E.; Panagou, I.; Spiliotopoulou, I. Fondaparinux for the treatment of acute heparin-induced thrombocytopenia: A single-center experience. *Clin. Appl. Thromb. Hemost.* **2010**, *16*, 663–667. [CrossRef]
39. Warkentin, T.E.; Pai, M.; Sheppard, J.I.; Schulman, S.; Spyropoulos, A.C.; Eikelboom, J.W. Fondaparinux treatment of acute heparin-induced thrombocytopenia confirmed by the serotonin-release assay: A 30-month, 16-patient case series. *J. Thromb. Haemost.* **2011**, *9*, 2389–2396. [CrossRef]
40. Dulicek, P.; Ivanova, E.; Kostal, M.; Fiedlerova, Z.; Sadilek, P.; Hirmerova, J. Heparin-induced thrombocytopenia treated with fondaparinux: Single center experience. *Int. Angiol.* **2020**, *39*, 76–81. [CrossRef]
41. D'Angelo, A.; Valle, P.D.; Fattorini, A.; Luciano, C. Disappearance of anti-PF4/heparin antibodies under prolonged fondaparinux administration in a patient with DVT associated with LMWH-induced thrombocytopenia. *Thromb. Haemost.* **2006**, *95*, 573–575. [CrossRef]
42. Alsaleh, K.A.; Al-Nasser, S.M.; Bates, S.M.; Patel, A.; Warkentin, T.E.; Arnold, D.M. Delayed-onset HIT caused by low-molecular-weight heparin manifesting during fondaparinux prophylaxis. *Am. J. Hematol.* **2008**, *83*, 876–878. [CrossRef] [PubMed]
43. Vadi, S.; Peshattiwar, V. The Fondaparinux Paradox: Fondaparinux-Related Heparin-induced Thrombocytopenia. *Indian J. Crit. Care Med.* **2018**, *22*, 116–118. [CrossRef] [PubMed]
44. Krecak, I.; Tomac, G.; Skugor, J.; Gveric-Krecak, V.; Pulanic, D. In vivo and in vitro cross-reactivity to fondaparinux in a stroke patient with IgG-PF4/heparin antibody-negative delayed-onset heparin-induced thrombocytopenia. *Blood Transfus.* **2020**. [CrossRef]
45. Manji, F.; Warkentin, T.E.; Sheppard, J.I.; Lee, A. Fondaparinux cross-reactivity in heparin-induced thrombocytopenia successfully treated with high-dose intravenous immunoglobulin and rivaroxaban. *Platelets* **2020**, *31*, 124–127. [CrossRef]
46. Farasatinasab, M.; Zarei, B.; Moghtadaei, M.; Nasiripour, S.; Ansarinejad, N.; Zarei, M. Rivaroxaban as an Alternative Agent for Heparin-Induced Thrombocytopenia. *J. Clin. Pharmacol.* **2020**. [CrossRef] [PubMed]
47. Kerendi, F.; Thourani, V.H.; Puskas, J.D.; Kilgo, P.D.; Osgood, M.; Guyton, R.A.; Lattouf, O.M. Impact of Heparin-Induced Thrombocytopenia on Postoperative Outcomes After Cardiac Surgery. *Ann. Thorac. Surg.* **2007**, *84*, 1548–1555. [CrossRef]
48. Haile, L.A.; Rao, R.; Polumuri, S.K.; Arepally, G.M.; Keire, D.A.; Verthelyi, D.; Sommers, C.D. PF4-HIT antibody (KKO) complexes activate broad innate immune and inflammatory responses. *Thromb. Res.* **2017**, *159*, 39–47. [CrossRef]
49. Kasthuri, R.S.; Glover, S.L.; Jonas, W.; McEachron, T.; Pawlinski, R.; Arepally, G.M.; Key, N.S.; Mackman, N. PF4/heparin-antibody complex induces monocyte tissue factor expression and release of tissue factor positive microparticles by activation of FcγRI. *Blood* **2012**, *119*, 5285–5293. [CrossRef]
50. Grover, S.P.; Mackman, N. Tissue Factor: An Essential Mediator of Hemostasis and Trigger of Thrombosis. *Arterioscler. Thromb. Vasc. Biol.* **2018**, *38*, 709–725. [CrossRef]
51. Tutwiler, V.; Madeeva, D.; Ahn, H.S.; Andrianova, I.; Hayes, V.; Zheng, X.L.; Cines, D.B.; McKenzie, S.E.; Poncz, M.; Rauova, L. Platelet transactivation by monocytes promotes thrombosis in heparin-induced thrombocytopenia. *Blood* **2016**, *127*, 464–472. [CrossRef] [PubMed]

52. Cines, D.B.; Zaitsev, S.; Rauova, L.; Rux, A.H.; Stepanova, V.; Krishnaswamy, S.; Sarkar, A.; Kowalska, M.A.; Zhao, G.; Mast, A.E.; et al. FcRn augments induction of tissue factor activity by IgG-containing immune complexes. *Blood* **2020**, *135*, 2085–2093. [CrossRef] [PubMed]
53. Suzuki, S.; Nakajima, S.; Ando, T.; Oda, K.; Sugita, M.; Maeda, K.; Nakiri, Y.; Takasaki, Y. Heparin-Related Thrombocytopenia Triggered by Severe Status of Systemic Lupus Erythematosus and Bacterial Infection. *Case Rep. Rheumatol.* **2016**, *2016*. [CrossRef] [PubMed]
54. Zhang, X.; Chen, L.; Bancroft, D.P.; Lai, C.K.; Maione, T.E. Crystal structure of recombinant human platelet factor 4. *Biochemistry* **1994**, *33*, 8361–8366. [CrossRef] [PubMed]
55. Cines, D.B.; Rauova, L.; Arepally, G.; Reilly, M.P.; McKenzie, S.E.; Sachais, B.S.; Poncz, M. Heparin-induced thrombocytopenia: An autoimmune disorder regulated through dynamic autoantigen assembly/disassembly. *J. Clin. Apher.* **2007**, *22*, 31–36. [CrossRef] [PubMed]
56. Rauova, L.; Poncz, M.; McKenzie, S.E.; Reilly, M.P.; Arepally, G.; Weisel, J.W.; Nagaswami, C.; Cines, D.B.; Sachais, B.S. Ultralarge complexes of PF4 and heparin are central to the pathogenesis of heparin-induced thrombocytopenia. *Blood* **2005**, *105*, 131–138. [CrossRef] [PubMed]
57. Lee, G.M.; Arepally, G.M. Heparin-induced thrombocytopenia. *Hematol. Am. Soc. Hematol. Educ. Program* **2013**, *2013*, 668–674. [CrossRef] [PubMed]
58. Poncz, M.; Rauova, L.; Cines, D.B. The role of surface PF4: Glycosaminoglycan complexes in the pathogenesis of heparin-induced thrombocytopenia (HIT). *Pathophysiol. Haemost. Thromb.* **2006**, *35*, 46–49. [CrossRef]
59. Arepally, G.M.; Kamei, S.; Park, K.S.; Kamei, K.; Li, Z.Q.; Liu, W.; Siegel, D.L.; Kisiel, W.; Cines, D.B.; Poncz, M. Characterization of a murine monoclonal antibody that mimics heparin-induced thrombocytopenia antibodies. *Blood* **2000**, *95*, 1533–1540. [CrossRef]
60. Kizlik-Masson, C.; Vayne, C.; McKenzie, S.E.; Poupon, A.; Zhou, Y.; Champier, G.; Pouplard, C.; Gruel, Y.; Rollin, J. 5B9, a monoclonal antiplatelet factor 4/heparin IgG with a human Fc fragment that mimics heparin-induced thrombocytopenia antibodies. *J. Thromb. Haemost.* **2017**, *15*, 2065–2075. [CrossRef]
61. Huynh, A.; Arnold, D.M.; Kelton, J.G.; Smith, J.W.; Horsewood, P.; Clare, R.; Guarne, A.; Nazy, I. Characterization of platelet factor 4 amino acids that bind pathogenic antibodies in heparin-induced thrombocytopenia. *J. Thromb. Haemost.* **2019**, *17*, 389–399. [CrossRef] [PubMed]
62. Yusuf, A.M.; Warkentin, T.E.; Arsenault, K.A.; Whitlock, R.; Eikelboom, J.W. Prognostic importance of preoperative anti-PF4/heparin antibodies in patients undergoing cardiac surgery. A systematic review. *Thromb. Haemost.* **2012**, *107*, 8–14. [CrossRef] [PubMed]
63. Sachais, B.S.; Litvinov, R.I.; Yarovoi, S.V.; Rauova, L.; Hinds, J.L.; Rux, A.H.; Arepally, G.M.; Poncz, M.; Cuker, A.; Weisel, J.W.; et al. Dynamic antibody-binding properties in the pathogenesis of HIT. *Blood* **2012**, *120*, 1137–1142. [CrossRef]
64. Cai, Z.; Yarovoi, S.V.; Zhu, Z.; Rauova, L.; Hayes, V.; Lebedeva, T.; Liu, Q.; Poncz, M.; Arepally, G.; Cines, D.B.; et al. Atomic description of the immune complex involved in heparin-induced thrombocytopenia. *Nat. Commun.* **2015**, *6*, 8277. [CrossRef] [PubMed]
65. Niyas, V.K.M.; Keri, V.C.; Ahuja, J.; Anand, A.; Nischal, N.; Wig, N. Severe Immune Thrombocytopenia in a Patient with HIV-HCV Co-infection: Challenges in Management. *J. Assoc. Phys. India* **2020**, *68*, 77–79.
66. Abeysuriya, V.; Choong, C.S.H.; Thilakawardana, B.U.; de Mel, P.; Shalindi, M.; de Mel, C.; Chandrasena, L.; Seneviratne, S.L.; Yip, C.; Yap, E.S.; et al. The atypical lymphocyte count: A novel predictive factor for severe thrombocytopenia related to dengue. *Trans. R. Soc. Trop. Med. Hyg.* **2020**, *114*, 424–432. [CrossRef]
67. Metcalf Pate, K.A.; Lyons, C.E.; Dorsey, J.L.; Shirk, E.N.; Queen, S.E.; Adams, R.J.; Gama, L.; Morrell, C.N.; Mankowski, J.L. Platelet activation and platelet-monocyte aggregate formation contribute to decreased platelet count during acute simian immunodeficiency virus infection in pig-tailed macaques. *J. Infect. Dis.* **2013**, *208*, 874–883. [CrossRef]
68. Cao, Y.; Wei, J.; Zou, L.; Jiang, T.; Wang, G.; Chen, L.; Huang, L.; Meng, F.; Huang, L.; Wang, N.; et al. Ruxolitinib in treatment of severe coronavirus disease 2019 (COVID-19): A multicenter, single-blind, randomized controlled trial. *J. Allergy Clin. Immunol.* **2020**. [CrossRef]
69. Sinha, A.; Ma, Y.; Scherzer, R.; Hur, S.; Li, D.; Ganz, P.; Deeks, S.G.; Hsue, P.Y. Role of T-Cell Dysfunction, Inflammation, and Coagulation in Microvascular Disease in HIV. *J. Am. Heart Assoc.* **2016**, *5*. [CrossRef]

70. Bikdeli, B.; Madhavan, M.V.; Jimenez, D.; Chuich, T.; Dreyfus, I.; Driggin, E.; Nigoghossian, C.; Ageno, W.; Madjid, M.; Guo, Y.; et al. COVID-19 and Thrombotic or Thromboembolic Disease: Implications for Prevention, Antithrombotic Therapy, and Follow-up: JACC State-of-the-Art Review. *J. Am. Coll. Cardiol.* **2020**, *75*, 2950–2973. [CrossRef]

71. Zhou, P.; Yang, X.L.; Wang, X.G.; Hu, B.; Zhang, L.; Zhang, W.; Si, H.R.; Zhu, Y.; Li, B.; Huang, C.L.; et al. A pneumonia outbreak associated with a new coronavirus of probable bat origin. *Nature* **2020**, *579*, 270–273. [CrossRef] [PubMed]

72. Li, X.; Xu, S.; Yu, M.; Wang, K.; Tao, Y.; Zhou, Y.; Shi, J.; Zhou, M.; Wu, B.; Yang, Z.; et al. Risk factors for severity and mortality in adult COVID-19 inpatients in Wuhan. *J. Allergy Clin. Immunol.* **2020**, *146*, 110–118. [CrossRef] [PubMed]

73. Zhou, Y.; Fu, B.; Zheng, X.; Wang, D.; Zhao, C.; Qi, Y.; Sun, R.; Tian, Z.; Xu, X.; Wei, H. Pathogenic T-cells and inflammatory monocytes incite inflammatory storms in severe COVID-19 patients. *Natl. Sci. Rev.* **2020**, *7*, 998–1002. [CrossRef]

74. Lax, S.F.; Skok, K.; Zechner, P.; Kessler, H.H.; Kaufmann, N.; Koelblinger, C.; Vander, K.; Bargfrieder, U.; Trauner, M. Pulmonary Arterial Thrombosis in COVID-19 With Fatal Outcome: Results From a Prospective, Single-Center, Clinicopathologic Case Series. *Ann. Intern. Med.* **2020**. [CrossRef] [PubMed]

75. Tang, N.; Li, D.; Wang, X.; Sun, Z. Abnormal coagulation parameters are associated with poor prognosis in patients with novel coronavirus pneumonia. *J. Thromb. Haemost.* **2020**, *18*, 844–847. [CrossRef]

76. Levi, M.; Thachil, J.; Iba, T.; Levy, J.H. Coagulation abnormalities and thrombosis in patients with COVID-19. *Lancet Haematol.* **2020**, *7*, e438–e440. [CrossRef]

77. McFadyen James, D.; Stevens, H.; Peter, K. The Emerging Threat of (Micro)Thrombosis in COVID-19 and Its Therapeutic Implications. *Circ. Res.* **2020**. [CrossRef]

78. Leonard-Lorant, I.; Delabranche, X.; Severac, F.; Helms, J.; Pauzet, C.; Collange, O.; Schneider, F.; Labani, A.; Bilbault, P.; Moliere, S.; et al. Acute Pulmonary Embolism in COVID-19 Patients on CT Angiography and Relationship to D-Dimer Levels. *Radiology* **2020**. [CrossRef]

79. Grillet, F.; Behr, J.; Calame, P.; Aubry, S.; Delabrousse, E. Acute Pulmonary Embolism Associated with COVID-19 Pneumonia Detected by Pulmonary CT Angiography. *Radiology* **2020**. [CrossRef]

80. Demelo-Rodríguez, P.; Cervilla-Muñoz, E.; Ordieres-Ortega, L.; Parra-Virto, A.; Toledano-Macías, M.; Toledo-Samaniego, N.; García-García, A.; García-Fernández-Bravo, I.; Ji, Z.; de-Miguel-Diez, J.; et al. Incidence of asymptomatic deep vein thrombosis in patients with COVID-19 pneumonia and elevated D-dimer levels. *Thromb. Res.* **2020**, *192*, 23–26. [CrossRef]

81. Wichmann, D.; Sperhake, J.P.; Lutgehetmann, M.; Steurer, S.; Edler, C.; Heinemann, A.; Heinrich, F.; Mushumba, H.; Kniep, I.; Schroder, A.S.; et al. Autopsy Findings and Venous Thromboembolism in Patients With COVID-19. *Ann. Intern. Med.* **2020**. [CrossRef]

82. Song, J.-C.; Wang, G.; Zhang, W.; Zhang, Y.; Li, W.-Q.; Zhou, Z.; People's Liberation Army Professional Committee of Critical Care Medicine, Chinese Society on Thrombosis and Haemostasis. Chinese expert consensus on diagnosis and treatment of coagulation dysfunction in COVID-19. *Mil. Med. Res.* **2020**, *7*, 19.

83. Tang, N.; Bai, H.; Chen, X.; Gong, J.; Li, D.; Sun, Z. Anticoagulant treatment is associated with decreased mortality in severe coronavirus disease 2019 patients with coagulopathy. *J. Thromb. Haemost.* **2020**, *18*, 1094–1099. [CrossRef] [PubMed]

84. Paranjpe, I.; Fuster, V.; Lala, A.; Russak, A.J.; Glicksberg, B.S.; Levin, M.A.; Charney, A.W.; Narula, J.; Fayad, Z.A.; Bagiella, E. Association of treatment dose anticoagulation with in-hospital survival among hospitalized patients with COVID-19. *J. Am. Coll. Cardiol.* **2020**, *76*, 122–124. [CrossRef]

85. Ayerbe, L.; Risco, C.; Ayis, S. The association between treatment with heparin and survival in patients with Covid-19. *J. Thromb. Thrombolysis* **2020**, *50*, 298–301. [CrossRef]

86. Rossi, R.; Coppi, F.; Talarico, M.; Boriani, G. Protective role of chronic treatment with direct oral anticoagulants in elderly patients affected by interstitial pneumonia in COVID-19 era. *Eur. J. Intern. Med.* **2020**, *77*, 158–160. [CrossRef]

87. Secco, E.; Pasqualetto, M.C.; Bombardini, T.; Picano, E.; Rigo, F. A possible benefit from therapeutic anticoagulation in COVID-19: The Dolo hospital experience in Veneto, Italy. *Kardiol. Pol.* **2020**. [CrossRef] [PubMed]

88. Poggiali, E.; Bastoni, D.; Ioannilli, E.; Vercelli, A.; Magnacavallo, A. Deep Vein Thrombosis and Pulmonary Embolism: Two Complications of COVID-19 Pneumonia? *Eur. J. Case Rep. Intern. Med.* **2020**, *7*, 001646. [CrossRef]
89. Brouns, S.H.; Brüggemann, R.; Linkens, A.E.; Magdelijns, F.J.; Joosten, H.; Heijnen, R.; ten Cate-Hoek, A.J.; Schols, J.M.G.A.; Ten Cate, H.; Spaetgens, B. Mortality and the use of Antithrombotic Therapies among Nursing Home Residents with COVID-19. *J. Am. Geriatr. Soc.* **2020**, *68*, 1647–1652. [CrossRef]
90. Motta, J.K.; Ogunnaike, R.O.; Shah, R.; Stroever, S.; Cedeno, H.V.; Thapa, S.K.; Chronakos, J.J.; Jimenez, E.J.; Petrini, J.; Hegde, A. Clinical Outcomes With the Use of Prophylactic Versus Therapeutic Anticoagulation in COVID-19. *medRxiv* **2020**. [CrossRef]
91. Patel, N.G.; Bhasin, A.; Feinglass, J.M.; Belknap, S.M.; Angarone, M.P.; Cohen, E.R.; Barsuk, J.H. Clinical Outcomes of Hospitalized Patients with COVID-19 on Therapeutic Anticoagulants. *medRxiv* **2020**. [CrossRef]
92. Klok, F.A.; Kruip, M.; Van der Meer, N.J.M.; Arbous, M.S.; Gommers, D.; Kant, K.M.; Kaptein, F.H.J.; van Paassen, J.; Stals, M.A.M.; Huisman, M.V. Incidence of thrombotic complications in critically ill ICU patients with COVID-19. *Thromb. Res.* **2020**, *191*, 145–147. [CrossRef] [PubMed]
93. Guan, W.-J.; Ni, Z.-Y.; Hu, Y.; Liang, W.-H.; Ou, C.-Q.; He, J.-X.; Liu, L.; Shan, H.; Lei, C.-L.; Hui, D.S.C.; et al. Clinical Characteristics of Coronavirus Disease 2019 in China. *N. Engl. J. Med.* **2020**, *382*, 1708–1720. [CrossRef] [PubMed]
94. Bao, C.; Tao, X.; Cui, W.; Yi, B.; Pan, T.; Young, K.H.; Qian, W. SARS-CoV-2 induced thrombocytopenia as an important biomarker significantly correlated with abnormal coagulation function, increased intravascular blood clot risk and mortality in COVID-19 patients. *Exp. Hematol. Oncol.* **2020**, *9*, 16. [CrossRef] [PubMed]
95. Liu, X.; Zhang, X.; Xiao, Y.; Gao, T.; Wang, G.; Wang, Z.; Zhang, Z.; Hu, Y.; Dong, Q.; Zhao, S. Heparin-induced thrombocytopenia is associated with a high risk of mortality in critical COVID-19 patients receiving heparin-involved treatment. *medRxiv* **2020**. [CrossRef]
96. Patell, R.; Khan, A.; Bogue, T.; Merrill, M.; Koshy, A.; Bindal, P.; Joyce, R.; Aird, W.C.; Neuberg, D.; Bauer, K.A. Heparin induced thrombocytopenia antibodies in COVID-19. *Am. J. Hematol.* **2020**. [CrossRef]
97. Riker, R.R.; May, T.L.; Fraser, G.L.; Gagnon, D.J.; Bandara, M.; Zemrak, W.R.; Seder, D.B. Heparin-induced thrombocytopenia with thrombosis in COVID-19 adult respiratory distress syndrome. *Res. Pract. Thromb. Haemost.* **2020**, *4*, 936–941. [CrossRef]
98. Vayne, C.; May, M.A.; Bourguignon, T.; Lemoine, E.; Guery, E.A.; Rollin, J.; Gruel, Y.; Pouplard, C. Frequency and Clinical Impact of Platelet Factor 4-Specific Antibodies in Patients Undergoing Extracorporeal Membrane Oxygenation. *Thromb. Haemost.* **2019**, *119*, 1138–1146. [CrossRef]
99. Dickie, H.; Tovey, L.; Berry, W.; Ostermann, M. Revised algorithm for heparin anticoagulation during continuous renal replacement therapy. *Crit. Care* **2015**, *19*, 376. [CrossRef]
100. Khandelwal, S.; Ravi, J.; Rauova, L.; Johnson, A.; Lee, G.M.; Gilner, J.B.; Gunti, S.; Notkins, A.L.; Kuchibhatla, M.; Frank, M.; et al. Polyreactive IgM initiates complement activation by PF4/heparin complexes through the classical pathway. *Blood* **2018**, *132*, 2431–2440. [CrossRef]
101. Cuker, A.; Rux, A.H.; Hinds, J.L.; Dela Cruz, M.; Yarovoi, S.V.; Brown, I.A.; Yang, W.; Konkle, B.A.; Arepally, G.M.; Watson, S.P.; et al. Novel diagnostic assays for heparin-induced thrombocytopenia. *Blood* **2013**, *121*, 3727–3732. [CrossRef]
102. Li, Z.Q.; Liu, W.; Park, K.S.; Sachais, B.S.; Arepally, G.M.; Cines, D.B.; Poncz, M. Defining a second epitope for heparin-induced thrombocytopenia/thrombosis antibodies using KKO, a murine HIT-like monoclonal antibody. *Blood* **2002**, *99*, 1230–1236. [CrossRef]
103. Rauova, L.; Zhai, L.; Kowalska, M.A.; Arepally, G.M.; Cines, D.B.; Poncz, M. Role of platelet surface PF4 antigenic complexes in heparin-induced thrombocytopenia pathogenesis: Diagnostic and therapeutic implications. *Blood* **2006**, *107*, 2346–2353. [CrossRef]
104. Falati, S.; Gross, P.; Merrill-Skoloff, G.; Furie, B.C.; Furie, B. Real-time in vivo imaging of platelets, tissue factor and fibrin during arterial thrombus formation in the mouse. *Nat. Med.* **2002**, *8*, 1175–1181. [CrossRef] [PubMed]
105. Kuramochi, T.; Igawa, T.; Tsunoda, H.; Hattori, K. Humanization and Simultaneous Optimization of Monoclonal Antibody. *Methods Mol. Biol.* **2019**, *1904*, 213–230. [CrossRef] [PubMed]
106. Ministro, J.; Manuel, A.M.; Goncalves, J. Therapeutic Antibody Engineering and Selection Strategies. *Adv. Biochem. Eng. Biotechnol.* **2020**, *171*, 55–86. [CrossRef] [PubMed]
107. Xu, X.; Han, M.; Li, T.; Sun, W.; Wang, D.; Fu, B.; Zhou, Y.; Zheng, X.; Yang, Y.; Li, X.; et al. Effective treatment of severe COVID-19 patients with tocilizumab. *Proc. Natl. Acad. Sci. USA* **2020**, *117*, 10970–10975. [CrossRef]

2

Heparin Blocks the Inhibition of Tissue Kallikrein 1 by Kallistatin through Electrostatic Repulsion

Lina Ma [1,†], Jiawei Wu [1,†], Ying Zheng [1,*], Zimei Shu [1], Zhenquan Wei [1], Yinbiao Sun [2], Robin W. Carrell [3] and Aiwu Zhou [1,*]

1 Department of Pathophysiology, Shanghai Jiao Tong University School of Medicine, Shanghai 200025, China; malina-china@foxmail.com (L.M.); wujiaweiyes@live.cn (J.W.); 15805197619@163.com (Z.S.); weizhq@gmail.com (Z.W.)

2 Randall Division of Cell & Molecular Biophysics, Faculty of Life Sciences & Medicine, King's College London, New Hunt's House, Guy's Campus, London SE1 1UL, UK; yin-biao.sun@kcl.ac.uk

3 Department of Haematology, University of Cambridge, Cambridge CB2 0XY, UK; rwc1000@cam.ac.uk

* Correspondence: zhengying@shsmu.edu.cn (Y.Z.); awz20@shsmu.edu.cn (A.Z.)

† These authors contributed equally to this work.

Abstract: Kallistatin, also known as SERPINA4, has been implicated in the regulation of blood pressure and angiogenesis, due to its specific inhibition of tissue kallikrein 1 (KLK1) and/or by its heparin binding ability. The binding of heparin on kallistatin has been shown to block the inhibition of KLK1 by kallistatin but the detailed molecular mechanism underlying this blockade is unclear. Here we solved the crystal structures of human kallistatin and its complex with heparin at 1.9 and 1.8 Å resolution, respectively. The structures show that kallistatin has a conserved serpin fold and undergoes typical stressed-to-relaxed conformational changes upon reactive loop cleavage. Structural analysis and mutagenesis studies show that the heparin binding site of kallistatin is located on a surface with positive electrostatic potential near a unique protruded 3^{10} helix between helix H and strand 2 of β-sheet C. Heparin binding on this site would prevent KLK1 from docking onto kallistatin due to the electrostatic repulsion between heparin and the negatively charged surface of KLK1, thus blocking the inhibition of KLK1 by kallistatin. Replacement of the acidic exosite 1 residues of KLK1 with basic amino acids as in thrombin resulted in accelerated inhibition. Taken together, these data indicate that heparin controls the specificity of kallistatin, such that kinin generation by KLK1 within the microcirculation will be locally protected by the binding of kallistatin to the heparin-like glycosaminoglycans of the endothelium.

Keywords: serpins; tissue kallikrein; heparin; serine protease; electrostatic repulsion

---

1. Introduction

Human kallistatin was first identified and characterized as a kallikrein binding protein [1,2]. Subsequent molecular cloning of its full-length cDNA showed that kallistatin is a glycoprotein with 401 residues and is expressed by many tissues such as liver, stomach, pancreas, kidney, and prostate [3]. Extensive studies have shown that kallistatin exerts a wide spectrum of biological activities in angiogenesis, apoptosis, and oxidative stress [4]. Kallistatin is a member of the serine protease inhibitor (serpin) superfamily and shares about 45% sequence identity with other serpins such as α_1-antitrypsin and protein C inhibitor (PCI) [5,6]. Serpins share a conserved mouse-trap mechanism in inhibiting their target proteases [5,7]. The protease binds and attacks the scissile bond (P1-P1′, nomenclature of Schechter and Berger [8] in the reactive center loop of the native serpin (Figure S1A). At the acyl-enzyme intermediate stage the serpin undergoes a rapid stressed-to-relaxed (S-to-R) conformational change where the reactive center loop is fully inserted into the central beta-sheet of the serpin resulting in translocation of the protease and distortion in the catalytic triad of the protease [7,9]. This leads to the formation of an SDS-stable covalent linkage and consequent inactivation of the protease complex [7]. Kallistatin was initially characterized as a specific inhibitor of tissue kallikrein 1 (KLK1), but it also inhibited other serine proteases such as KLK7 [10]. The protease specificity of a serpin is largely determined by its reactive loop sequence, especially the P1 residue, although in some cases, residues which do not belong to the reactive center loop can also critically affect specificity [9,11]. This appears to be so with kallistatin which unusually has a P2-P1-P1′ sequence of Phe-Phe-Ser targeting P1 Arg-preferred KLK1 [12,13].

Kallikreins are serine proteases which are widely expressed in various tissues and share the same conserved serine protease domain [14]. Human kallikreins can be divided into two categories: plasma kallikrein and tissue kallikreins (also called kallikrein-related peptidases, KLKs) [15,16]. Plasma kallikrein releases the vasoactive peptide bradykinin from high molecular weight kininogen [17]. KLKs have 15 members named from KLK1 to KLK15. In the human KLKs family, only KLK1 could release kinin from low molecular weight kininogen, while the other KLKs possess greatly reduced or no kininogen cleavage activity [16]. KLK1 is a key member of the kallikrein-kinin system that initiates and maintains vasodilation in mammalian system and its deficits are associated with cardiovascular and end-organ pathology [18]. KLK1 replenishment therapy is widely used in Asia for the treatment of diseases such as acute ischemic stroke [18].

Kallistatin belongs to a subclass of serpins known as the heparin binding serpins. In most cases, heparin binds to residues of the serpin helix D as with antithrombin [19–23], heparin cofactor II (HCII) [24–26], protease nexin 1 (PN1) [27,28], plasminogen activator inhibitor type 1 (PAI-1) [29], protein Z-dependent protease inhibitor (ZPI) [30,31], and lamprey angiotensinogen [32]. The binding of heparin promotes the interaction between serpin and protease either by an allosteric mechanism where heparin induces conformational changes in the serpin (Figure S1B), or by a bridging mechanism where heparin links serpin and protease together forming a transient ternary complex [9,33,34] (Figure S1C). However, it was proposed that the heparin biding site on kallistatin differed in being located near hH, similar to that of PCI [35,36]. It was also found that heparin blocked the interaction between kallistatin and KLK1, as compared to the acceleration of protease inhibition seen in other heparin binding serpins [37]. The detailed molecular mechanisms underlying these unique features of kallistatin are unclear.

Here we prepared and crystalized recombinant kallistatin and solved the crystal structures of the reactive loop cleaved kallistatin and its complex with heparin. The detailed characterization of its properties in heparin binding and protease inhibition shows that the heparin binding site of kallistatin is located around a unique 3^{10} helix between helix H and strand 2 of β-sheet C of kallistatin, and that heparin binding on kallistatin blocks the docking of KLK1 onto kallistatin through electrostatic repulsion.

2. Materials and Methods

2.1. Materials

The cDNA for human kallistatin, human kallikrein-related peptidase 1 (KLK1) was purchased from GENECHEM. Fluorescent substrate H-D-Val-Leu-Arg-AMC for KLK1 was synthesized by BankPeptide. Low molecular weight (LMW) heparin with an average molecular weight of ≈5 kDa and high molecular weight (HMW) heparin with an average molecular weight of 17–19 kDa were purchased from Sigma. Heparin oligosaccharides with 4, 6, 8, 10, and 12 saccharide units (DP4, DP6, DP8, DP10, and DP12) were from Iduron (Manchester, UK). Columns for protein purification were purchased from GE Healthcare. All reagents and kits for crystallization were purchased from Hampton Research. Precast 12% SDS-PAGE gels were purchased from Genscript (Nanjing, China) and run at 150 volts for ≈ 45 min using MOPS buffer. Protein samples were treated with reducing SDS loading buffer at 95 °C for 5 min before electrophoresis.

2.2. Cloning, Mutagenesis, Expression, and Purification of Recombinant Proteins

Recombinant kallistatin was prepared from *Escherichia coli* as previously described [38]. Briefly, the coding sequence covering residues 45–427 of human kallistatin was cloned in *E. coli* expression vector pE-SUMO3. All mutants were constructed by PCR mutagenesis using the KOD Plus mutagenesis kit (TYOBO). The expression plasmid construct was transformed into BL21 (DE3) cells and grown in 2 × YT at 37 °C until optical density at 600 nm reached 0.8. Then isopropyl-β-D-1-thiogalactopyranoside (IPTG) was added to a final concentration of 0.2 mM, and the culture was transferred to a 20 °C shaker for a further 12 h. The cells were collected by centrifugation and resuspended in ice cold buffer A (20 mM Tris-HCl, pH 7.4, 0.5 M NaCl, and 20 mM imidazole) and disrupted by a high-pressure cell breaker. The supernatant of the cell lysate was loaded onto a 5 mL HisTrap FF crude column and eluted by a 0.02–0.2 M imidazole gradient. The peak fractions were collected. Then the SUMO3-fusion protein was digested by protease SENP2 to release the SUMO3 tag. Kallistatin was further purified by a 5 mL HiTrap SP column and eluted by a NaCl gradient (0.05–1 M in 10 mM MES pH 6.0). Notably, during storage or crystallization, recombinant kallistatin was cleaved between P2 and P1 residues by an unknown protease and migrated as a doublet band on SDS-PAGE.

Recombinant tissue kallikrein KLK1, and its variants KLK1-99Lm, where nine residues from its 99 loop were deleted, and KLK1-70Lm with residues D75, D76 and E77 replaced by arginines, were prepared from *E. coli* expression system through refolding [39,40]. The sequence coding resides 25-262 were cloned in expression vector pE-SUMO3. KLK-70Lm and KLK1-99Lm mutants were constructed by PCR mutagenesis using the KOD Plus mutagenesis kit (TYOBO). Expression plasmids were transformed into BL21 (DE3) cells and grown in 2 × YT at 37 °C until optical density at 600 nm reached 0.8. Then IPTG was added to a final concentration of 0.2 mM and shaker for a further 12 h. The cells were collected by centrifugation and resuspended in 20 mM Tris-HCl, pH 7.4, 1% (v/v) Triton X-100, 20 mM EDTA and disrupted by a high-pressure cell breaker. The cell lysate was then centrifuged and the pellet containing inclusion bodies was collected and washed twice with 20 mM Tris-HCl, pH 7.4, 20 mM EDTA, and 1.0 M NaCl. Finally, the inclusion bodies were washed with 20 mM Tris-HCl, pH 7.4, 20 mM EDTA and dissolved in 6.0 M guanidinium chloride, 20 mM Tris-HCl, pH 8.0, 0.5 mM EDTA, and 10 mM DTT. Protein refolding was initiated by rapid dilution of dissolved inclusion bodies into refolding buffer containing 50 mM Tris-HCl, pH 8.0, 0.6 M arginine, 20 mM $CaCl_2$, 10% (v/v) glycerol, 10 mM reduced glutathione, and 1 mM oxidized glutathione with a final protein concentration less than 0.3 mg/mL. The refolding solution was kept at 4 °C for 16 h and then dialyzed against 20 mM Tris-HCl, pH 7.4, 0.5 M NaCl, and 20 mM imidazole. The refolded KLK1 fusion protein was purified by a 5 mL HiTrap FF column. KLK1 was activated by protease SENP2 which releases the SUMO3 tag from the fusion protein. Activated KLK1 was loaded onto a 5 mL Hitrap SP HP column and eluted by a NaCl gradient (0.05–1 M). The peak fractions were collected, concentrated, and buffer exchanged into 10 mM Tris-HCl, pH 7.4, 0.1 M NaCl.

2.3. Crystallization, Data Collection, and Structure Determination

The initial conditions for crystallization were screened at 22 °C by the sitting-drop vapor-diffusion method using screening kits from Hampton Research in MRC2 plates. Crystals were initially grown from a mixture of 200 nL protein solution (10 mg/mL in 10 mM Tris-HCl, pH 7.4, 0.1 M NaCl) and 200 nL precipitant solution (40% tert-butanol) equilibrated against 80 μL reservoir solution. A cryosolution consisting of 10% glycerol and 10% ethylene glycol was directly added to the drop and the crystals were quickly picked up using a micro-loop and flash-cooled in liquid nitrogen. Owing to rapid evaporation of *tert*-butanol, the crystals float around in the drop and crack once the well is opened. Therefore, for the heparin soaking experiment, 100 μM heparin pentasaccharide in the cryo-solution was similarly directly added to the drop and a small piece of cracked crystal was immediately picked up using a micro-loop and flash-cooled in liquid nitrogen. This synthetic heparin pentasaccharide was used previously in obtaining antithrombin-heparin crystal structure [22]. Diffraction data were collected on beamline BL17U at SSRF (Shanghai, China). The data set was indexed and processed with iMosflm [41] and scaled with AIMLESS from the CCP4 suite [42,43] A random choice of 5% of the data was selected as the R-free set. The structures were solved by molecular replacement with Phaser [44] using reactive loop cleaved PCI structure (PDB 3DY0) as search model. Notably, a phenix polder map for the kallistatin-heaprin complex structure was calculated (Figure S2). This confirmed that heparin is present in the crystal structure and the ligand was refine to have a partial occupancy of 0.69 by phenix.refine. The structure was built in COOT [45] and refined using Refmac and Phenix.refine [46] to good geometry (Table 1). Figures were produced with PyMOL software. The surface electrostatic representation was analyzed by APBS (Adaptive Poisson-Boltzmann Solver) [47].

Table 1. Data processing, refinement, and model statistics.

Crystal	PDB 6F4U	PDB 6F4V
	Kallistatin	Kallistatin-heparin
Space group	$P6_1$	$P6_1$
Cell dimensions		
a, b, c (Å)	113.51, 113.51, 76.17	113.77, 113.77, 76.56
α, β, γ (°)	90.00, 90.00, 120.00	90.00, 90.00, 120.00
Solvent content (%)	44	44
Data processing statistics		
Wavelength (Å)	1.196	1.196
Resolution (Å)	35.67–1.9; 2.0–1.9	56.88–1.80; 1.84–1.8
Total reflections	185,915; 26,532	366,297; 13,230
Unique reflections	44,414; 6433	52,290; 3094
Multiplicity	4.2; 4.1	7.0; 4.3
Mean I/sd(I)	14; 2.5	15.3; 1.5
Completeness (%)	99.9; 99.7	99.9; 99.3
R_{merge}	0.043; 0.326	0.061; 0.648
R_{meas}	0.049; 0.374	0.071; 0.832
Model		
Number of atoms modeled	3293	3364
Protein	3058	3067
Water	185	230
Refinement statistics (Å)		
Reflections in working/free set	42,206/2208	49,688/2602
R-factor/R-free (%)	0.168/0.193	0.173/0.196
[a] r.m.s. deviation of bonds (Å)/angles (°) from ideality	0.0068/1.12	0.0114/1.46
Ramachandran plot (favored/outliers, %)	98.40/0	95.89/0
Wilson B-factor (Å^2)	30.1	28.1
MolProbity score	0.98, [b] 100th percentile (n = 12,147, 1.9 ± 0.25 Å)	1.04, [b] 100th percentile (n = 11,444, 1.80 ± 0.25 Å)

[a] r.m.s., root mean square; PDB, Protein Data Bank. [b] 100th percentile is the best among structures of comparable resolution; 0th percentile is the worst.

2.4. *Stoichiometries of Inhibition and Rates of Inhibition*

Stoichiometries of inhibition (SI) were measured using similar procedures as previously described [32] by incubating KLK1, KLK1-70Lm, and KLK1-90Lm (1 μM) with increasing concentrations of kallistatin variants in phosphate buffered saline (PBS) with 0.1% PEG 8000 for 2 h at 37 °C. Residual protease activity was determined by diluting the reaction mixture into 0.2 mM H-D-Val-Leu-Arg-AMC for KLK1. Linear regression analysis of the decrease in protease activity with an increasing concentration of kallistatin yielded the estimates for the stoichiometry of inhibition as the intercept on the abscissa. Each measurement was repeated three times with the mean SI value ± SD calculated.

The rates of inhibition by recombinant kallistatin variants were determined at room temperature (22 ± 1 °C) by a discontinuous assay procedure as previously described [32]. Briefly, under pseudo–first-order conditions, 10 μL of 10 nM proteases was mixed with 10 μL of 100–500 nM kallistatin variants in PBS with 0.1% PEG 8000. The residual protease activity was determined at timed intervals by diluting the reaction mixture into 200 μL of the assay buffer containing substrate. The observed rate constant, k_{obs}, for the reaction was obtained from the slope of a semilog plot of the residual protease activity against time, and the apparent second-order rate constant, k_{app}, was calculated by dividing k_{obs} with the initial serpin concentration. The measurement for each kallistatin variant was repeated three times with the mean k_{app} value ± SD calculated. The product of $k_{app} \times$ SI represents the second order rate constant (k_2).

The effect of low molecular weight heparin (LMWH) on the interactions between kallistatin and KLK1-70Lm was similarly assessed as previously described [10,48]. A total of 1 μM rKAL was incubated with different concentrations of LMWH (0, 0.005, 0.025, 0.05, 0.25, 0.5, 1, and 2.5 mg/mL) for 5 min at room temperature, and then admixed with 10 nM KLK1-70Lm and the residual KLK1-70Lm activity was measured using 0.2 mM fluorescent substrate H-D-Val-Leu-Arg-AMC at different time intervals. The observed rate constants, k_{obs}, were then plotted with the concentrations of LMWH.

2.5. *Heparin Affinity Chromatography of Kallistatin Variants*

The relative heparin binding affinities of recombinant kallistatin variants were assessed by a heparin-Sepharose column [32]. About 200–400 μg of protein was loaded onto a 1 mL HiTrap heparin column pre-equilibrated with 10 mM Tris-HCl, pH 7.4, and eluted with a 20-column volume of 0–500 mM NaCl gradient using the AKTA system (GE Healthcare). The protein absorbance at 280 nm was recorded with the salt concentration of peak identified and the fractions analyzed by SDS-PAGE.

2.6. *Model of the Kallistatin-KLK1-Heparin Ternary Complex*

There are about a dozen different serpin-proteases Michaelis complex crystal structures in the Protein Data Bank. Although the relative positions of serpin and protease are somewhat different, it is apparent that all the proteases docked on top of the serpin are very close to the hH of the corresponding serpins. To illustrate the relative positions of KLK1 and kallistatin in their Michaelis complex without extensive optimization of the surface loop conformations of both proteins, a model of KLK1 and kallistatin Michaelis complex was prepared from the thrombin/antithrombin complex structure (PDB 1SR5) with KLK1 and kallistatin superposed onto thrombin and antithrombin, respectively. This resulted in minimum clashes between the two molecules. The heparin tetra-saccharide was docked onto kallistatin using ClusPro web server [49] and one of the top five output coordinates with the heparin chain in an optimal orientation forming interactions with key residues R259, R300, K307, and R394 was selected and further extended for presentation.

3. Results

3.1. *The Overall Structures of Kallistatin and Its Complex with Heparin*

Recombinant human kallistatin (rKAL) was prepared from an *Escherichia coli* expression system. SDS-PAGE was used to visualize the purity of rKAL and its interaction with proteases. As shown in Figure 1, the purified rKAL readily formed SDS-stable covalently linked rKAL-KLK1 complex with a molecular weight of ≈ 70 kDa, however in the presence of low molecular weight heparin (LMWH), little complex could be seen from the gel (Figure 1A). The closely migrated doublet bands of kallistatin in lane 2 reflects some of the rKAL being cleaved by KLK1 during inhibition, which is consistent with the stoichiometry of inhibition (SI) measurement (Table 2). The inhibition of KLK1 by rKAL was also quantitatively assessed by an enzymatic assay using a KLK1's fluorescent substrate. rKAL almost completely inhibited the KLK1 activity in the absence of heparin, but this inhibition is significantly reduced by the presence of 0.5 mg/mL of high or low molecular weight heparins with ≈ 60%–80% of KLK1's activity remaining after 30 min incubation (Figure 1B). Notably, as the formation of the covalently linked rKAL-KLK1 complex is irreversible and heparin binding of rKAL is reversible, prolonged incubation of rKAL and KLK1 even in the presence of high concentrations of heparin would lead to a gradual increase of rKAL-KLK1 complex formation and the loss of KLK1 activity. Subsequent second-order association rate constant measurement showed that rKAL inhibited KLK1 with a k_2 of 3.4×10^3 M^{-1} s^{-1} (Table 2). These results are consistent with previous findings that kallistatin is an inhibitor of KLK1 and their interaction can be blocked by heparin [10,48].

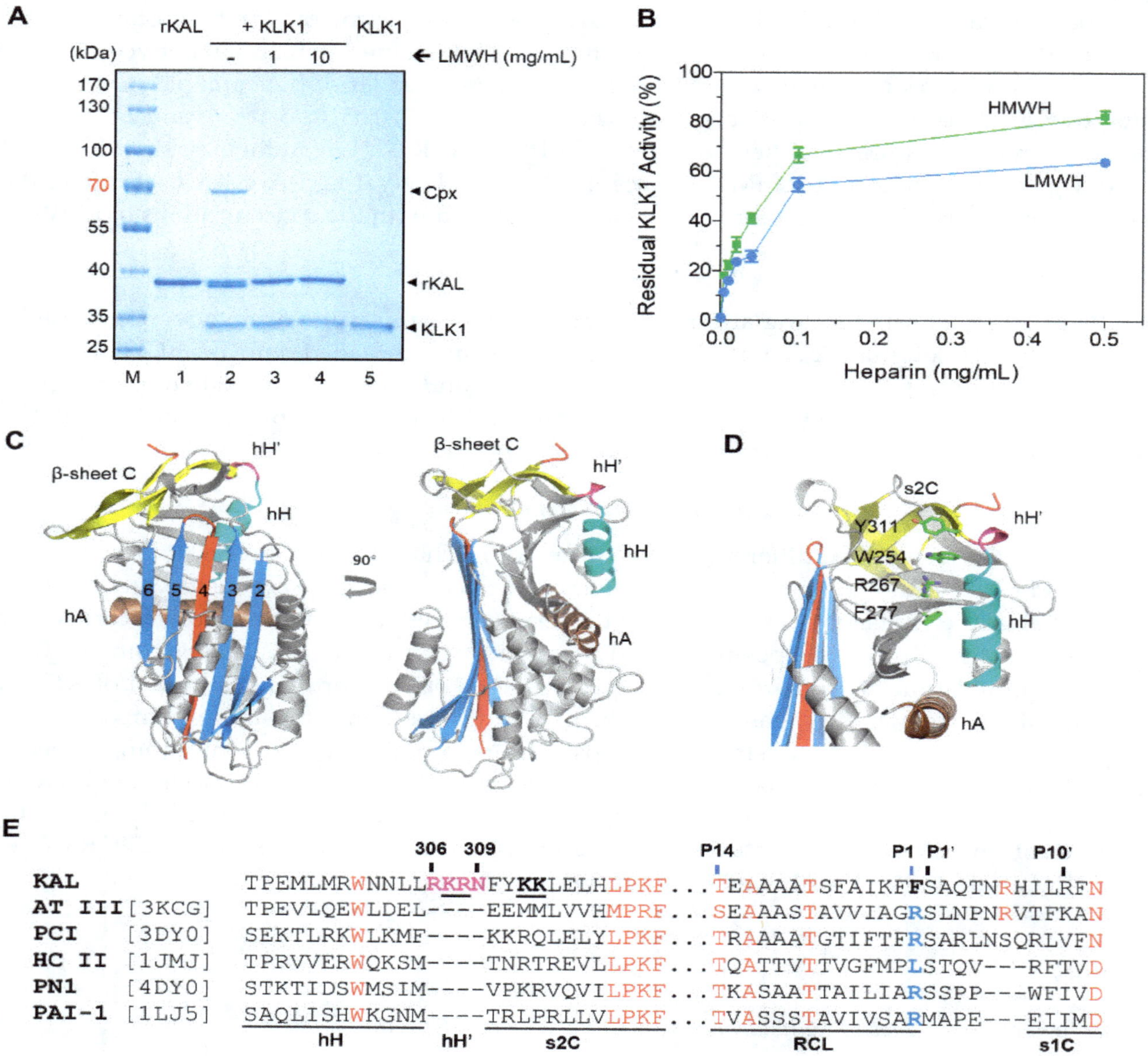

Figure 1. Characterization of recombinant Kallistatin. (**A**) A total of 2 µg of rKAL was incubated with 1 µg tissue kallikrein 1 (KLK1) for 2 min at room temperature in the absence or presence of LMWH and then analyzed by reducing SDS-PAGE. M, molecular weight marker. (**B**) Inhibition of KLK1 was also assessed by an activity assay where 500 nM of rKAL was mixed with different concentrations (0, 0.004, 0.01, 0.02, 0.04, 0.1, 0.5 mg/mL) of LMW (blue) or HMW (green) heparin and then incubated with 10 nM KLK1 at 37 °C for 30 min. The remaining activity of KLK1 was then measured using 0.2 mM fluorescent substrate H-D-Val-Leu-Arg-AMC. The normalized residual KLK1 activity (±SD, n = 3) was plotted against the concentration of heparin. (**C**) The structure of reactive loop cleaved kallistatin. The cleaved reactive center loop (RCL) (red) is completely inserted into the central β-sheet A (blue) as a middle strand. Residues R^{306}KRN^{309} between helix H (cyan) and strand 2 of β-sheet C (yellow) form an extra 3^{10} helix (hH', pink). (**D**) W254 from the 'hormone-binding pocket' is stabilized by R267, F277, and Y311. (**E**) Partial amino acid sequence alignment of kallistatin with other heparin binding serpins. The unique four-residue insertion is located between hH and strand 2 of β-sheet C (s2C). The RCL of kallistatin has the same length as those of antithrombin (ATIII) and protein C inhibitor (PCI), but it is four residues longer than those of HCII, PN1, and PAI-1. Highly conserved residues are shown in red and residues R^{306}KRN^{309} of hH' are shown in pink. Key residues K307, R308, K312, and K313 involved in heparin binding are underlined.

Table 2. Second order association rate constants for the interaction between kallistatin and tissue kallikrein 1 (KLK1). The apparent second order rate constant (k_{app}) was determined from the slope of the linear plot of k_{obs} versus the inhibitor concentration. KLK1 was mixed with different amounts of kallistatin and linear regression analysis of the decrease in protease activity with the concentration of kallistatin yielded the stoichiometry of inhibition (SI) as the intercept on the abscissa. The product of k_{app} × SI represents the second order rate constant (k_2). Each experiment was repeated three times with mean ± SD calculated.

Protein	k_{app} ($M^{-1}s^{-1}$)	SI	k_{app} × SI ($M^{-1}s^{-1}$)
rKAL-WT	$2.4 \pm 0.1 \times 10^3$	1.4 ± 0.1	3.4×10^3
rKAL-R259D	$2.2 \pm 0.\ 1 \times 10^3$	1.6 ± 0.1	3.5×10^3
rKAL-R300D	$1.6 \pm 0.1 \times 10^3$	1.8 ± 0.1	2.9×10^3
rKAL-R394D	$1.0 \pm 0.1 \times 10^3$	1.8 ± 0.1	1.8×10^3
rKAL-307/308D	$1.3 \pm 0.1 \times 10^3$	1.5 ± 0.1	2.0×10^3
rKAL-312/313D	$1.0 \pm 0.1 \times 10^3$	1.5 ± 0.1	1.5×10^3

To further characterize kallistatin, we firstly crystallized recombinant kallistatin and then soaked its crystals with a synthetic heparin pentasaccharide [22]. The crystal structures of rKAL and its complex with heparin pentasaccharide were then solved at 1.9 and 1.8 Å resolution, respectively (Table 1), using reactive loop cleaved PCI (PDB 3DY0) as the searching model [35]. The N-terminal amino acid sequencing of kallistatin from the crystallization drop indicated that it was cleaved between residues F387 and F388 (P2-P1 position) of the reactive center loop by an unknown protease during crystallization, which commonly occurs with many serpins [50]. One copy of reactive loop cleaved kallistatin was found in the asymmetric unit. Two heparin saccharide units were built in the rKAL-heparin structure. No significant structural difference in kallistatin was apparent between the two crystal structures. Overall, kallistatin showed a typical serpin fold in a relaxed conformation, with the cleaved reactive center loop completely inserted into the central β-sheet A as a middle strand (Figure 1C). When compared with other relaxed serpin structures, such as cleaved α_1-antitrypsin (PDB 3NDD), or cleaved PCI (PDB 3DY0), the root-mean-square-deviations of atomic positions were less than 1.5 Å indicating a remarkably conserved tertiary structure. Nevertheless, there are some differences. Sequence alignment of kallistatin with other human serpins (Figure 1E) indicated that kallistatin has a unique four-residue insertion ($R^{306}KRN^{309}$) between helix H and strand 2 of β-sheet C (s2C). In the kallistatin crystal structure, this four-residue insertion forms an extra 3^{10} helix (termed hH′) and it is packed against a bulky W254 from what is the hormone binding pocket in some other serpins [51]. The sidechain of W254 is further stabilized by cation-Pi and Pi-Pi interactions from nearby residues R267, F277, and Y311 (Figure 1D). R267 also forms salt bridges with D269 of s5B. Therefore, the tight packing within the 'hormone binding pocket' of kallistatin effectively forces the inserted four residues to stay as a protruded 3^{10} helix on the top of kallistatin. There are three potential glycosylation sites in kallistatin (Figure S3), which are far away from the protease docking position on kallistatin.

3.2. *Heparin Binding Site of Kallistatin*

In the crystal structure of kallistatin complexed with heparin pentasaccharide, there is clear electron density for two terminal saccharide units G and H with four sulfonate groups (Figure 2A). A phenix polder map calculated for the ligand further supported the presence of heparin pentasaccharide in the crystal structure. The stereoview of the electron density map around the heparin saccharides shows the detailed interactions of both saccharides (Figure 2B). The ring of saccharide unit H is sandwiched by the sidechains of R259 and Y260 with 6-O-sulfonate dipping into a shallow surface pocket (Figure 2B,C). R259 of s6B forms three salt bridges with two sulfonate groups from the two saccharides, and R300 of hH forms two salt bridges with the 6-O-sulfonate of saccharide unit H. The fourth sulphate, 3-O-sulfonate of saccharide H, has no direct interaction with kallistatin. The other three saccharides including saccharide unit F which harbored the key 3-O-sulfonate critical for antithrombin activation [40] were not built due to poor electron density. Notably residues K307 and R308 are involved in crystal packing which likely hinders direct heparin binding to these residues during soaking. Similarly, the soaked heparin pentasaccharide forms salt bridges with K150 of a symmetry-related kallistatin molecule. As K150 is located between hE and s2A at the bottom of kallistatin, this interaction is unlikely to play a significant role in the heparin binding of kallistatin.

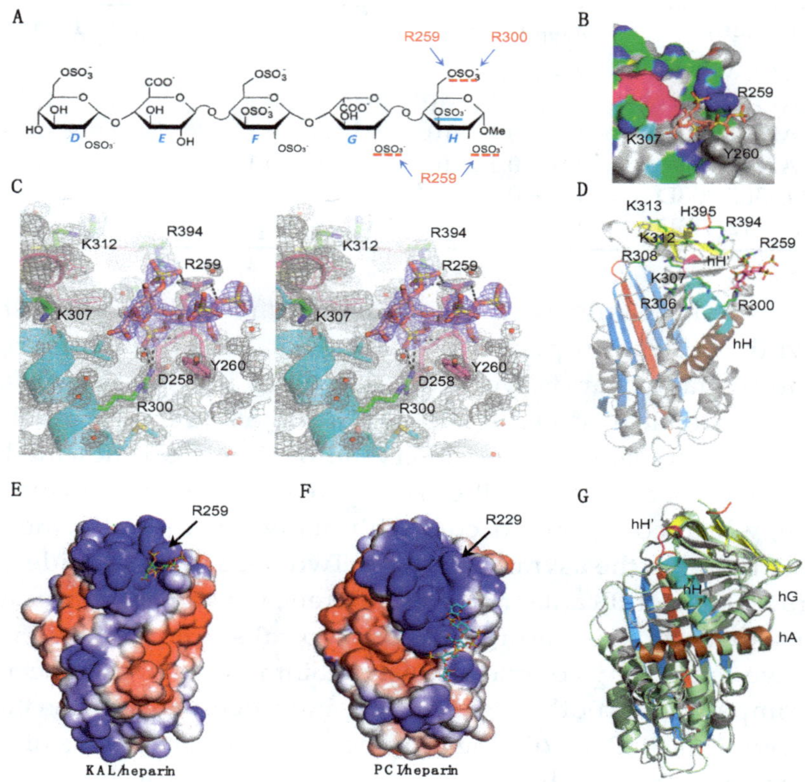

Figure 2. Crystal structure of kallistatin complexed with heparin. (**A**) Diagram showing the structure of heparin pentasaccharide. Three sulfonate groups (highlighted with red underlines) from saccharide unit *G* and *H* formed key interactions with R259 and R300 of kallistatin while the 3-*O*-sulfonate group (blue underline) from saccharide unit *H* has no direct interaction with the protein. (**B**) Stereoview of the electron density map covering the heparin saccharides and surrounding area with saccharide *G* and *H* built in the electron density. The $2F_0$-F_c electron density is contoured at 1σ. R300, stabilized by ionic interactions with D258, forms two salt bridges with 6-*O*-sulfonate from saccharide unit *H*. R259 forms two salt bridges with 2-*O*-sulfonate group of saccharide *G* and one salt bridge with 2-*O*-sulfonate group from saccharide *H*. Notably, 6-*O*-sulfonate from saccharide *H* also forms a hydrogen bond with the main chain amino group of R259. (**C**) Surface presentation showing saccharide unit *H* (sticks) is sandwiched between R259 and Y260 with its 6-*O*-sulfonate dipping into a shallow pocket forming interactions with R300 and R259 as seen above. The 3^{10} helix hH′ is colored pink and carbon atoms from surrounding residues are coloured in green with nitrogen atoms in blue. (**D**) The positively charged residues R259, R300, R306, K307, R308, K312, K313, R394, and H395 (green) near hH′ and the heparin saccharides (pink) are shown in sticks. (**E**) Surface electrostatic analysis shows that kallistatin has an area with extensive positive electrostatic potential on top of hH involving surrounding residues from hH′. (**F**) The heparin binding site of PCI (PDB 3DYO) is located to the lower part of hH with the extension of the heparin pentasaccharide expected to form interaction with R229. The orientations of KAL in (**D**,**E**) are same as PCI in (**F**). The electrostatic surface potential was calculated by APBS (red is negative and blue is positive, −3 to +3 kT/e). (**G**) The overlaid structures of PCI and rKAL showing an overall similar configuration. Helices G and H have slightly different positions and orientations. PCI is colored light green and kallistatin is color coded as in Figure 1C.

To further elucidate the property of this area, we identified all the basic residues around the heparin saccharide binding site (Figure 2D) and calculated the surface electrostatic potentials of kallistatin (Figure 2E). This clearly showed that kallistatin has an area with extensive positive electrostatic potential around the 3^{10} helix involving residues K307, R308, K312, and K313 as proposed previously [37], and other residues from helix H (R300), s6B (R259), and s1C (R394 and H395). Overall, the kallistatin-heparin complex structure shown here indicates that the surface with positive electrostatic potential is the likely heparin binding site of kallistatin.

PCI is another heparin binding serpin with a heparin binding site located close to helix H [35]. R229 of PCI, which corresponds to R259 in kallistatin, has also been implicated in heparin mediated inhibition of activated protein C (APC) by PCI (Figure 2F). However, there are differences in the exact locations of the heparin binding sites on these two serpins. The heparin binding site of PCI is located near the lower half of hH, while the heparin binding site of kallistatin is near the top of hH (Figure 2E,F). There are also minor changes in the positions of helix H and G when superposed (Figure 2G).

To elucidate the contribution of this surface with positive electrostatic potential of kallistatin towards heparin binding, we systematically mutated the positively charged residues from this area to Asp individually and assessed the heparin-binding affinities of these mutants by a heparin-Sepharose column (Figure 3). Wild type kallistatin was eluted from the heparin-Sepharose column at about 300 mM NaCl, while R259D, R308D, and R394D mutants were eluted earlier at ≈160 mM NaCl indicating substantial decrease in their heparin-binding affinity (Figure 3). Other mutations on R300, K307, K312, K313, and H395 also resulted in decreased heparin-binding. The binding affinity of the double mutant of 307/308D or 312/313D decreased even further with these two mutants being eluted from the heparin column at 95 and 125 mM NaCl, respectively (Figure 3), which is consistent with previous findings [37]. Therefore, this confirms that the surface positive electrostatic potential area is the heparin binding site of kallistatin.

A

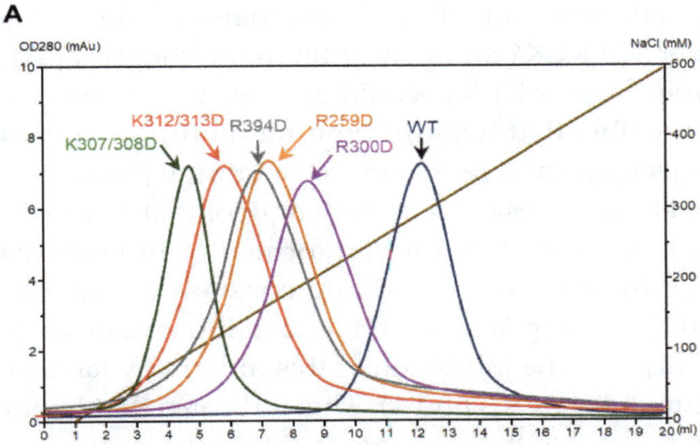

B

rKAL	NaCl(mM)
WT	300
R259D	162
R300D	200
K307D	210
R308D	160
K312D	205
K313D	205
R394D	160
H395D	197
K307/308D	95
K312/313D	125

Figure 3. Heparin binding affinity of kallistatin variants assessed by a heparin-Sepharose column. (**A**) Kallistatin variants were loaded onto a heparin-Sepharose column (1 mL bed volume) and then eluted with a gradient of NaCl solution. The elution profile is shown in (**A**) with the absorbances at 280 nm wavelength and salt gradient as Y axes. (**B**) The peak positions identified from the absorbance were confirmed by SDS-PAGE analysis of the eluted fractions and listed in a table. Wild-type rKAL (blue line), rKAL-K307/308D (green line) and rKAL-K312/313D (red line) were eluted from the column at about 300, 95, and 125 mM NaCl concentration, respectively. R259D, R308D, and R394D were eluted from the column at around 160 mM NaCl concentration.

We also tested if these mutations on kallistatin would affect the inhibitory activity of kallistatin towards KLK1 by measuring the association rate constants of these mutants (Table 2). This showed that the inhibition of KLK1 by rKAL-R394D, rKAL-K312/313D, and rKAL-K307/308D mutants decreased only by about 2-fold. Other residues such as R259 and R300 seemed to have a very limited effect on the KLK1 inhibition by kallistatin. This indicates that the heparin binding site residues of kallistatin are involved in KLK1 inhibition possibly through exosite interactions between the bodies of the KLK1 and kallikrein, but play a relatively minor role.

3.3. The Mechanism of Heparin in Blocking KLK1/Kallistatin Interaction

In general, heparin is considered as a cofactor in promoting the inhibition by serpins of their target proteases, however it functions as a blocker in the interaction between kallistatin and KLK1 (Figure 1). KLK1 shares a typical serine protease domain with other members of the KLKs family, but its kallikrein loop (also called 99 loop) is about nine residues longer than those of other KLKs (Figure 4A). During KLK1 inhibition by kallistatin, it is expected that the reactive center loop of kallistatin will dock into the substrate binding pocket of KLK1 forming the initial encounter complex, also called Michaelis complex as seen in many serpin-protease Michaelis complex crystal structures [34,51,52]. There are about eight serpin-protease Michaelis complex structures deposited in Protein Data Bank from the five serpins listed in Figure 1E [21,34,51–54]. The relative positions of protease and serpin amongst these complexes are slightly different and the proteases often utilize different surface loops to form different exosite interactions with different parts of the serpin molecules [34]. As the reactive loop of kallistatin has the same length as those of antithrombin and PCI (Figure 1E), two different antithrombin-thrombin-heparin ternary Michaelis complex structures (PDB 1SR5 and 1TB6) reflecting different stages of the Michaelis complex formation between antithrombin and thrombin [21,54], and one PCI-thrombin complex structure [55] were selected for initial evaluation. Superposition of these structures together (Figure S4) showed that thrombin docked differently on top of the serpins forming different exosite interactions. Molecular modelling of the KLK1-kallistatin Michaelis complex by substitution of the protease and serpin in the structure with KLK1 and kallistatin, respectively, showed that minimum clashes between the bodies of the protease and serpin would occur if based on PDB 1S5R. Notably, kallistatin has similarly positively charged residues at P5′ and P10′ positions of the reactive loop as those antithrombin. Therefore, the model of kallistatin and KLK1 Michaelis complex was subsequently generated by simply overlaying KLK1 and kallistatin onto the antithrombin-thrombin complex structure (PDB 1SR5) to indicate the relative positions of KLK1 and kallistatin in the complex [21].

This model showed that the kallikrein loop of KLK1 would be close to the heparin binding site of kallistatin (Figure 4B). It would be plausible that heparin binding on this area would block the docking of KLK1 onto kallistatin due to this long kallikrein loop. To test this, we made a KLK1 mutant (KLK1-99Lm) where this loop is shortened by nine residues to the length of that of KLK7 and assessed the effect of heparin on its inhibition by kallistatin. This mutant formed complexes with kallistatin slowly (Figure 4A, lane 2) and the second-order association rate constant of this reaction is only $\approx 200\ M^{-1}s^{-1}$. This confirms that the kallikrein loop is involved in forming exosite interactions with the body of kallistatin. However, to our surprise, the inhibition of this mutant by kallistatin remained blocked by the presence of heparin (Figure 4A, lanes 3 and 4). This indicates that heparin mediated inhibition of KLK1-kallistatin interaction is not due to the longer kallikrein loop of KLK1.

Subsequent molecular surface electrostatic potential analysis shows that KLK1 is an acidic protease with a highly negatively charged surface (Figure 4C). It is apparent that in the Michaelis complex of kallistatin with KLK1 this negatively charged surface is spatially very close to the positively charged heparin binding site of kallistatin. Any extension of the heparin chain bound on kallistatin, modeled with six heparin saccharides in Figure 4C would potentially cause electrostatic repulsion between the negative charged KLK1 surface and the heparin chain, which is also negatively charged. To further confirm this, we tested on SDS-PAGE the blocking effect of heparin oligosaccharides of different length. As seen in Figure 4D, rKAL readily formed a complex with KLK1 in the absence of heparin (lane 2) and little blocking effect was seen with 1 mM heparin containing four saccharides (DP4, lane 3). A substantial reduction of complex formation was observed with 1 mM DP6 (lane 4) while a near complete loss of complex formation was observed in the presence of 1 mM DP8 or DP10 or DP12 (Figure 4D, lanes 5–7). This further emphasizes that the heparin binding site of kallistatin is within close proximity to the docked KLK1 in the Michaelis complex, which makes this heparin mediated blocking possible. As 3-*O*-sulfonate is very rare in these normal heparin oligosaccharides and it is not involved in forming interactions with kallistatin in the crystal structure (Figure 2), it is unlikely that it would play an essential role in blocking the interaction between KLK1 and kallistatin.

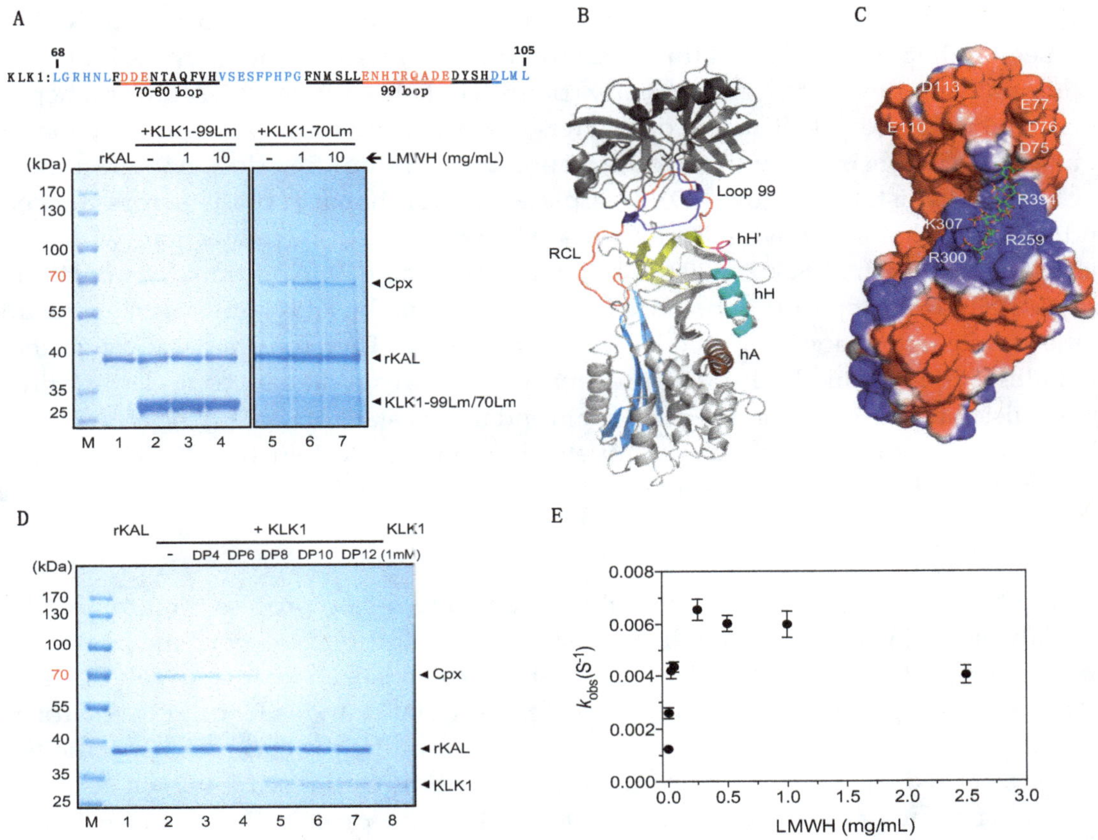

Figure 4. Effect of heparin on the interaction between KLK1 variants and kallistatin. (**A**) Amino acid sequence showing the KLK1 70–80 loop and 99 loop (kallikrein loop) with the negatively charged residues of 70–80 loop highlighted in red. A total of 2 µg of rKAL were mixed with 5 µg of KLK1-99Lm (nine residues highlighted in red from KLK1's 99 loop were deleted) for 20 min or 0.5 µg of KLK1-70Lm (residues D75, D76 and E77 replaced by arginines) for 2 min in the absence or presence of LMWH at room temperature. (**B**) A model of the KLK1 and kallistatin Michaelis complex was prepared from the thrombin/antithrombin complex structure (PDB 1SR5) with the reactive loop of kallistatin modeled in the active site of KLK1. The long 99 loop of KLK1 is colored blue. (**C**) Electrostatic presentation of the surface charges of the KLK1 and kallistatin Michaelis complex. A heparin chain with six saccharides was modeled along a groove involving R259, K307, R308, and R394 for binding. Further extension of this oligosaccharide would reach the negatively charged surface of KLK1. The electrostatic surface potential was calculated by APBS (red is negative and blue is positive, −1 to +1 kT/e). (**D**) Heparin length effect on the blocking of KLK1 inhibition by kallistatin. A total of 2 µg of rKAL were incubated with 0.5 µg KLK1 protease for 3 min at room temperature in 20 µL PBS, in the absence or presence 1 mM DP4, DP6, DP8, DP10, DP12. All samples were analyzed by reducing SDS-PAGE and stained by Coomassie Blue. (**E**) Effect of LMWH on the inhibition of KLK-70Lm by kallistatin. The observed inhibition rate constants, k_{obs}, of KLK-70Lm by kallistatin in the presence of different concentrations of LMWH were plotted.

As the exosite 1 of KLK1, the so called 70–80 loop of the serine protease, is likely to interact with the extension of a linear heparin chain bound on kallistatin, here we mutated the negatively charged residues of the exosite with basic residues present in thrombin and assessed the inhibition of this mutant (KLK1-70Lm) by kallistatin. As shown in Figure 4A (lane 5), the mutant formed SDS-stable complexes with kallistatin in the absence of heparin, but in contrast to wild type KLK1, more complexes between kallistatin and KLK1-70Lm were formed in the presence of heparin (Figure 4A, lanes 6 and 7). The second-order rate constant measurement showed that rKAL inhibited KLK1-70Lm with a k_2 of 1.8×10^3 M^{-1} s^{-1}, similar to that of wild type KLK1 (Table S1), but its reaction with rKAL could be accelerated by ≈ 5-fold in a heparin dose-dependent manner (Figure 4E). This indicates that heparin could function through a similar bridging mechanism in promoting inhibition of KLK1-70Lm by kallistatin as seen in heparin mediated thrombin inhibition by many other serpins [34].

More informatively, the existence of a ternary complex of kallistatin, KLK1-70Lm and heparin implies that the heparin binding site of kallistatin could engage heparin and form exosite interactions with KLK1 simultaneously. This is consistent with the observation that DP4 binding does not affect the interaction between KLK1 and kallistatin (Figure 4D). It is plausible that heparin binds across the center of the heparin binding area of kallistatin while KLK1 surface loops form exosite interactions with the rim of this area involving residues such as K307, R308, K312, and K313 (Table 2). Additionally, this finding directly excludes the possibility that heparin bound on kallistatin would inhibit KLK1-kallistatin interaction through preventing the exosite interactions between KLK1 and kallistatin. Therefore, heparin blocks the inhibition of KLK1 by kallistatin most likely through preventing KLK1 from docking onto kallistatin due to the electrostatic repulsion between the long heparin chain and the exosite 1 of KLK1. Conversely, heparin could promote the inhibition of proteases with positively charged exosite 1 such as KLK1-70Lm (Figure 4A, lanes 6 and 7), or thrombin by kallistatin with its P1 residue mutated to Arg as shown previously [12].

4. Discussion

Serpins inhibit their target proteases mainly through a two-step process (Figure 5A). The reactive center loop of the serpin is firstly docked into the substrate binding pocket of the protease forming a Michaelis complex which is reversible. The second step, which is irreversible, involves cleavage of the reactive loop and subsequent dramatic serpin conformational changes leading to the formation of a covalently linked serpin-protease complex and inactivation of the protease. The specificity of serpins is primarily determined by the P1 and immediately adjacent residues. However, serpins have also adopted the use of cofactors such as heparin, vitronectin, and protein Z etc., to further refine their overall specificity and activity mainly through optimization of the Michaelis complex formation [9,34]. Heparin binds to helix D of antithrombin, heparin cofactor II, PAI-1 or PN1, and promotes the inhibition of target proteases either through an allosteric mechanism as seen in FXa inhibition by antithrombin where heparin induces an optimal conformation of antithrombin [22], or a structurally well-defined bridging mechanism as seen in the heparin medicated inhibition of thrombin by antithrombin where heparin links the serpin and thrombin simultaneously [34]. Interestingly, it has been shown that heparin binding on kallistatin and PCI would block their inhibition of KLK1, but promote their inhibition of other serine proteases such as APC and thrombin [12,52]. The heparin binding site on PCI has been elucidated structurally and heparin promotes the inhibition of thrombin or APC through the bridging mechanism where heparin binds hH of PCI and exosite 2 of thrombin or exosite 1 of APC [35]. However, it remains unclear how heparin would block the inhibition of KLK1 by these two serpins.

Here we solved crystal structures of the reactive loop cleaved kallistatin and its complex with heparin and revealed that the heparin binding site of kallistatin is located around a four-residue insertion ($R^{306}KRN^{309}$) between hH and s2C. As the heparin pentasaccharide was soaked into the crystal of kallistatin and some surface residues of kallistain are involved in crystal packing, the heparin binding orientation on kallistatin in solution is likely to be different and there could even be alternative ways for heparin to bind the same serpin as shown previously with PCI [35]. Mutagenesis study showed that the heparin binding site involved key residues such as R259, R300, R308, and R394 of kallistatin, which mirrored a similar heparin binding surface on PCI. This indicated that heparin bound on the similar areas of these two serpins could block the inhibition of KLK1 through a similar molecular mechanism. We tested the role of the heparin binding residues of kallistatin in KLK1 inhibition. There was only a minor decrease in association rate (≈ 2-fold) between kallistatin mutants (rKAL-312/313D) and KLK1(Table 2). KLK1 inhibition by this mutant could still be blocked at higher concentrations of heparin (data not shown). Similarly, shortening the long kallikrein loop of KLK1 did not affect the blocking function of heparin either (Figure 4A). This indicated that the blocking effect of heparin on KLK1 inhibition by kallistatin was not due to steric hindrance of the exosite interactions between KLK1 and kallistatin. This finding is in line with previous studies on PCI-KLK1 interactions which excluded the direct involvement of basic amino acid residues present in the heparin biding site of PCI on the KLK1-PCI interaction [52].

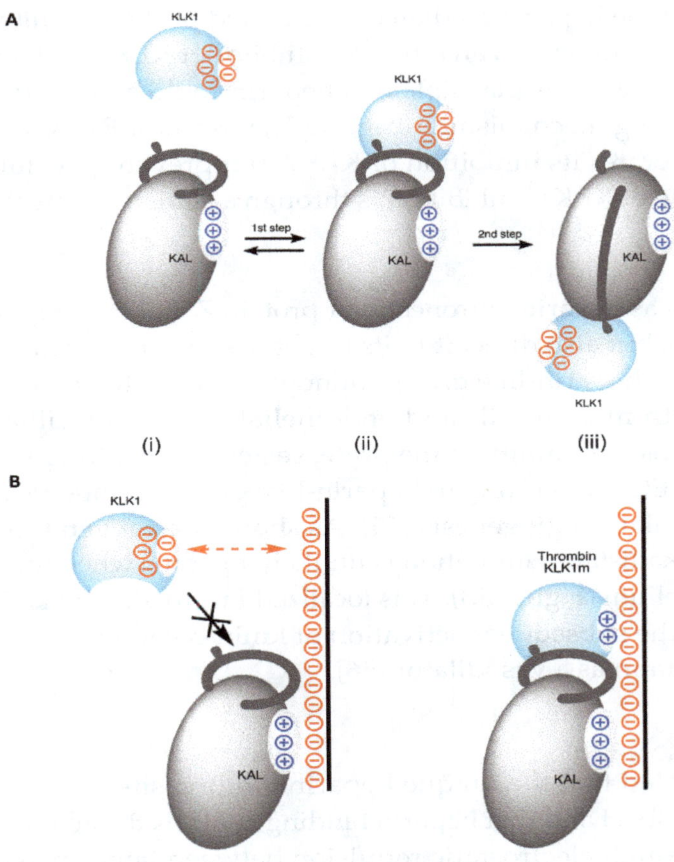

Figure 5. Heparin blocks the inhibition of KLK1 through electrostatic repulsion. (**A**) Kallistatin inhibits KLK1 through the classical two-step serpin inhibition mechanism. Kallistatin (i) in solution or in circulation can form an initial encounter or Michaelis complex with KLK1 (ii). In general, this step is reversible and often subject to modulations by cofactors as seen with many serpins. Subsequently the reactive center loop of kallistatin is cleaved by KLK1 and kallistatin undergoes profound conformational changes leading to an SDS-stable KAL-KLK1 complex linked through an ester bond (iii). This second step of the reaction is irreversible. (**B**) The specificity or activity of kallistatin is regulated by heparin through affecting its Michaelis complex formation. KLK1 is prevented from docking onto kallistatin when kallistatin is bound on heparin or heparinoids in endothelium due to electrostatic repulsion between KLK1 and the negatively charged heparin-like molecules. In contrast, heparin promotes the Michaelis complex formation between kallistatin and proteases such as KLK1 mutant (KLK1m) and thrombin with exosite 1 through the typical bridging mechanism as seen with heparin mediated antithrombin-thrombin interactions. This leads to an accelerated protease inhibition by the serpin.

The method or manner by which heparin blocks the inhibition of KLK1 by kallistatin became apparent during molecular modelling of the Michaelis complex of kallistatin with KLK1. The surface electrostatic calculation revealed that KLK1 has a molecular surface with a high negative electrostatic potential. When KLK1 forms a Michaelis complex with kallistatin, in which the reactive center loop of kallistatin is inserted in the active site pocket of KLK1, the heparin binding surface of kallistatin with positive electrostatic potential is spatially very close to KLK1. If heparin were bound on kallistatin before the formation of the Michaelis complex, most plausibly, it would prevent KLK1 from docking onto kallistatin due to electrostatic repulsion between negatively charged heparin saccharides and KLK1 (Figure 5B). It is highly likely that heparin blocks the inhibition of KLK1 by PCI through the similar mechanism. This blockade is largely due to the unique heparin binding sites around hH on kallistatin and PCI, which are very close to where proteases would dock, and the unusual surface property of KLK1 amongst serine proteases. Our subsequent charge-reversal mutagenesis study on the exosite 1 of KLK1 further established that heparin could promote the inhibition of KLK1-70Lm by kallistatin (Figure 4E), reminiscent of the heparin mediated accelerated protease-inhibition by other serpins [34] (Figure S1C). Notably kallistatin is also an efficient inhibitor of KLK7 [10], which has many positively charged residues in its exosite 1, it is plausible that heparin could accelerate the inhibition of KLK7 by kallistatin through a bridging mechanism. Intriguingly, vaspin/SERPINA12 inhibits both KLK7 and KLK14, but heparin accelerates its inhibition of KLK7, but prevents the inhibition of KLK14 [53,54]. It is unclear if this blockade of KLK14 inhibition is through a similar electrostatic expulsion mechanism shown here.

Serpin cofactors, such as heparin, vitronectin or protein Z, not only regulate the inhibitory activity or specificity of the serpin, but also direct it to its target tissues to perform its functions in a localized environment. For example, heparin-like glycosaminoglycans located on extracellular matrix and the surface of vascular smooth muscle cells and endothelial cells will facilitate protease inhibition by bringing the serpin into close proximity to the protease generation. Interestingly, kallistatin has been shown to compete with VEGF in binding to heparin-like glycosaminoglycans in extracellular matrix and to consequently modulate angiogenesis [55]. As shown here, even though KLK1 is the putative in vivo target protease of kallistatin, inhibition is unlikely to occur when the kallistatin is bound to the heparinoids of the endothelium (Figure 5B). This localized inactivation of kallistatin will facilitate kinin generation by KLK1 and the subsequent activation of kinin-receptor on the cell surface—in keeping with the function of kallistatin as a vasodilator [56].

5. Conclusions

Our study here revealed that the unique heparin binding site of kallistatin is located around a protruded 3^{10} helix near helix H and that heparin binding controls the activity of kallistatin by blocking its inhibition of KLK1 through electrostatic repulsion between heparin and the negatively charged surface of KLK1.

Author Contributions: L.M., J.W., Z.S., Z.W. performed the experiments. Y.Z., R.W.C. and A.Z. supervised experiments and aided in interpreting data. Y.S. provided reagents for the study. A.Z. designed the study and wrote the manuscript with input from all authors. All authors have read and agreed to the published version of the manuscript.

Acknowledgments: We thank the staff of BL17U beamlines at Shanghai Synchrotron Radiation Facility for assistance with data collection.

References

1. Chao, J.; Li, P.; Chao, L. Kallistatin suppresses cancer development by multi-factorial actions. *Crit. Rev. Oncol. Hematol.* **2017**, *113*, 71–78. [CrossRef] [PubMed]
2. Chao, J.; Chai, K.X.; Chen, L.M.; Xiong, W.; Chao, S.; Woodleymiller, C.; Wang, L.X.; Lu, H.S.; Chao, L. Tissue kallikrein-binding protein is a serpin. I. Purification, characterization, and distribution in normotensive and spontaneously hypertensive rats. *J. Biol. Chem.* **1990**, *265*, 16394–16401. [PubMed]
3. Chai, K.X.; Chen, L.M.; Chao, J.; Chao, L. Kallistatin: A novel human serine proteinase inhibitor. Molecular cloning, tissue distribution, and expression in Escherichia coli. *J. Biol. Chem.* **1993**, *268*, 24498–24505. [PubMed]
4. Chao, J.; Li, P.; Chao, L. Kallistatin: Double-edged role in angiogenesis, apoptosis and oxidative stress. *Biol. Chem.* **2017**, *398*, 1309–1317. [CrossRef] [PubMed]

5. Huber, R.; Carrell, R.W. Implications of the three-dimensional structure of alpha 1-antitrypsin for structure and function of serpins. *Biochemistry* **1989**, *28*, 8951–8966. [CrossRef]
6. Silverman, G.A.; Bird, P.I.; Carrell, R.W.; Church, F.C.; Coughlin, P.B.; Gettins, P.G.; Irving, J.A.; Lomas, D.A.; Luke, C.J.; Moyer, R.W.; et al. The serpins are an expanding superfamily of structurally similar but functionally diverse proteins. Evolution, mechanism of inhibition, novel functions, and a revised nomenclature. *J. Biol. Chem.* **2001**, *276*, 33293–33296. [CrossRef]
7. Huntington, J.A.; Read, R.J.; Carrell, R.W. Structure of a serpin-protease complex shows inhibition by deformation. *Nature* **2000**, *407*, 923. [CrossRef]
8. Schechter, I.; Berger, A. On the size of active sites in proteases I. Papain. *Biochem. Biophys. Res. Commun.* **1967**, *27*, 157–162. [CrossRef]
9. Gettins, P.G.W. Serpin Structure, Mechanism, and Function. *Chem. Rev.* **2003**, *34*, 4751–4804. [CrossRef]
10. Luo, L.Y.; Jiang, W. Inhibition profiles of human tissue kallikreins by serine protease inhibitors. *Biol. Chem.* **2006**, *387*, 813–816. [CrossRef]
11. Gettins, P.G.; Olson, S.T. Exosite determinants of serpin specificity. *J. Biol. Chem.* **2009**, *284*, 20441–20445. [CrossRef] [PubMed]
12. Chen, V.C.; Chao, L.; Chao, J. Roles of the P1, P2, and P3 residues in determining inhibitory specificity of kallistatin toward human tissue kallikrein. *J. Biol. Chem.* **2000**, *275*, 38457–38466. [CrossRef] [PubMed]
13. Chen, V.C.; Chao, L.; Chao, J. Reactive-site specificity of human kallistatin toward tissue kallikrein probed by site-directed mutagenesis. *Biochim. Biophys. Acta* **2000**, *1479*, 237–246. [CrossRef]
14. Raspi, G. Kallikrein and kallikrein-like proteinases: Purification and determination by chromatographic and electrophoretic methods. *J. Chromatogr. B Biomed. Appl.* **1996**, *684*, 265–287. [CrossRef]
15. Diamandis, E.P.; Yousef, G.M.; Luo, L.Y.; Magklara, A.; Obiezu, C.V. The new human kallikrein gene family: Implications in carcinogenesis. *Trends Endocrin. Metab. Tem.* **2000**, *11*, 54–60. [CrossRef]
16. Yousef, G.M.; Diamandis, E.P. Human tissue kallikreins: A new enzymatic cascade pathway? *Biol. Chem.* **2002**, *383*, 1045. [CrossRef]
17. Akiyama, K.; Nakamura, T.; Iwanaga, S.; Hara, M. The chymotrypsin-like activity of human prostate-specific antigen, gamma-seminoprotein. *FEBS Lett.* **1987**, *225*, 168. [CrossRef]
18. Alexander-Curtis, M.; Pauls, R.; Chao, J.; Volpi, J.J.; Bath, P.M.; Verdoorn, T.A. Human tissue kallikrein in the treatment of acute ischemic stroke. *Ther. Adv. Neurol. Disord.* **2019**, *12*, 1756286418821918. [CrossRef]
19. Johnson, D.J.; Li, W.; Adams, T.E.; Huntington, J.A. Antithrombin–S195A factor Xa-heparin structure reveals the allosteric mechanism of antithrombin activation. *EMBO J.* **2006**, *25*, 2029–2037. [CrossRef]
20. Storoni, L.C.; McCoy, A.J.; Read, R.J. Likelihood-enhanced fast rotation functions. *Acta Crystallogr. D Biol. Crystallogr.* **2004**, *60*, 432–438. [CrossRef]
21. Dementiev, A.; Petitou, M.; Herbert, J.M.; Gettins, P.G. The ternary complex of antithrombin-anhydrothrombin -heparin reveals the basis of inhibitor specificity. *Nat. Struct. Mol. Biol.* **2004**, *11*, 863. [CrossRef]
22. Jin, L.; Abrahams, J.P.; Skinner, R.; Petitou, M.; Pike, R.N.; Carrell, R.W. The anticoagulant activation of antithrombin by heparin. *Proc. Natl. Acad. Sci. USA* **1997**, *94*, 14683–14688. [CrossRef] [PubMed]
23. Ersdalbadju, E.; Lu, A.; Zuo, Y.; Picard, V.; Bock, S.C. Identification of the antithrombin III heparin binding site. *J. Biol. Chem.* **1997**, *272*, 19393. [CrossRef] [PubMed]
24. Baglin, T.P.; Carrell, R.W.; Church, F.C.; Esmon, C.T.; Huntington, J.A. Crystal Structures of Native and Thrombin-Complexed Heparin Cofactor II Reveal a Multistep Allosteric Mechanism. *Proc. Natl. Acad. Sci. USA* **2002**, *99*, 11079–11084. [CrossRef]
25. Tollefsen, D.M. Heparin cofactor II. *Oxyg. Transport. Tissue XXXIII* **1997**, *425*, 35–44.
26. Ragg, H.; Ulshöfer, T.; Gerewitz, J. Glycosaminoglycan-mediated leuserpin-2/thrombin interaction. Structure-function relationships. *J. Biol. Chem.* **1990**, *265*, 22386. [PubMed]
27. Li, W.; Huntington, J.A. Crystal structures of protease nexin-1 in complex with heparin and thrombin suggest a 2-step recognition mechanism. *Blood* **2012**, *120*, 459–467. [CrossRef]
28. Stone, S.R.; Brown-Luedi, M.L.; Rovelli, G.; Guidolin, A.; Mcglynn, E.; Monard, D. Localization of the heparin-binding site of glia-derived nexin/protease nexin-1 by site-directed mutagenesis. *Biochemistry* **1994**, *33*, 7731. [CrossRef]
29. Keijer, J.; Linders, M.; Wegman, J.J.; Ehrlich, H.J.; Mertens, K.; Pannekoek, H. On the target specificity of plasminogen activator inhibitor 1: The role of heparin, vitronectin, and the reactive site. *Blood* **1991**, *78*, 1254–1261. [CrossRef]

30. Yang, L.; Ding, Q.; Huang, X.; Olson, S.T.; Rezaie, A.R. Characterization of the heparin-binding site of the protein z-dependent protease inhibitor. *Biochemistry* **2012**, *51*, 4078–4085. [CrossRef]
31. Huang, X.; Rezaie, A.R.; Broze, G.J.; Olson, S.T. Heparin Is a Major Activator of the Anticoagulant Serpin, Protein Z-dependent Protease Inhibitor. *J. Biol. Chem.* **2011**, *286*, 8740–8751. [CrossRef] [PubMed]
32. Wei, H.; Cai, H.; Wu, J.; Wei, Z.; Zhang, F.; Huang, X.; Ma, L.; Feng, L.; Zhang, R.; Wang, Y.; et al. Heparin Binds Lamprey Angiotensinogen and Promotes Thrombin Inhibition through a Template Mechanism. *J. Biol. Chem.* **2016**, *291*, 24900–24911. [CrossRef] [PubMed]
33. Rein, C.M.; Desai, U.R.; Church, F.C. Serpin-glycosaminoglycan interactions. *Methods Enzymol.* **2011**, *501*, 105. [PubMed]
34. Huntington, J.A. Thrombin inhibition by the serpins. *J. Thromb Haemost* **2013**, *11* (Suppl. 1), 254–264. [CrossRef] [PubMed]
35. Li, W.; Huntington, J.A. The heparin binding site of protein C inhibitor is protease-dependent. *J. Biol. Chem.* **2008**, *283*, 36039–36045. [CrossRef]
36. Li, W.; Adams, T.E.; Nangalia, J.; Esmon, C.T.; Huntington, J.A. Molecular basis of thrombin recognition by protein C inhibitor revealed by the 1.6-Å structure of the heparin-bridged complex. *Proc. Natl. Acad. Sci. USA* **2008**, *105*, 4661. [CrossRef]
37. Chen, V.C.; Chao, L.; Pimenta, D.C.; Bledsoe, G.; Juliano, L.; Chao, J. Identification of a major heparin-binding site in kallistatin. *J. Biol. Chem.* **2001**, *276*, 1276–1284. [CrossRef]
38. Lin, F.; Zhou, A.; Wei, Z. Crystallization and crystallographic studies of kallistatin. *Acta Crystallogr. F Struct. Biol. Commun.* **2015**, *71*, 1135–1138. [CrossRef]
39. Zakabunin, A.I.; Mishukova, O.V.; Khrapov, E.A.; Sergievichev, D.S.; Boyarskikh, U.A.; Sverdlov, E.D.; Filipenko, M.L. Cloning and expression of the gene of the human chymotrypsin-like kallikrein-7 protease in Escherichia coli and isolation of the recombinant protein. *Mol. Gen. Microbiol. Virol.* **2007**, *22*, 64–67. [CrossRef]
40. Takayama, T.K.; McMullen, B.A.; Nelson, P.S.; Matsumura, M.; Fujikawa, K. Characterization of hK4 (Prostase), a Prostate-Specific Serine Protease:? Activation of the Precursor of Prostate Specific Antigen (pro-PSA) and Single-Chain Urokinase-Type Plasminogen Activator and Degradation of Prostatic Acid Phosphatase\\r. *Biochemistry* **2001**, *40*, 15341–15348. [CrossRef]
41. Battye, T.G.G.; Luke, K.; Owen, J.; Powell, H.R.; Leslie, A.G.W. iMOSFLM: A new graphical interface for diffraction-image processing withMOSFLM. *Acta Crystallogr.* **2011**, *67*, 271–281. [CrossRef] [PubMed]
42. Evans, P.R. An introduction to data reduction: Space-group determination, scaling and intensity statistics. *Acta Crystallogr.* **2011**, *67*, 282–292. [CrossRef]
43. Winn, M.D.; Ballard, C.C.; Cowtan, K.D.; Dodson, E.J.; Emsley, P.; Evans, P.R.; Keegan, R.M.; Krissinel, E.B.; Leslie, A.G.W.; Mccoy, A. Overview of the CCP4 suite and current developments. *Acta Crystallogr.* **2011**, *67*, 235–242.
44. McCoy, A.J.; Grosse-Kunstleve, R.W.; Storoni, L.C.; Read, R.J. Likelihood-enhanced fast translation functions. *Acta Crystallogr. D Biol. Crystallogr.* **2005**, *61*, 458–464. [CrossRef] [PubMed]
45. Emsley, P.; Cowtan, K. Coot: Model-building tools for molecular graphics. *Acta Crystallogr. D Biol. Crystallogr.* **2004**, *60*, 2126–2132. [CrossRef]
46. Adams, P.D.; Afonine, P.V.; Bunkoczi, G.; Chen, V.B.; Davis, I.W.; Echols, N.; Headd, J.J.; Hung, L.W.; Kapral, G.J.; Grosse-Kunstleve, R.W.; et al. PHENIX: A comprehensive Python-based system for macromolecular structure solution. *Acta Crystallogr. D Biol. Crystallogr.* **2010**, *66*, 213–221. [CrossRef]
47. Ritchie, A.W.; Webb, L.J. Optimizing Electrostatic Field Calculations with the Adaptive Poisson–Boltzmann Solver to Predict Electric Fields at Protein–Protein Interfaces II: Explicit Near-Probe and Hydrogen-Bonding Water Molecules. *J. Phys. Chem. B* **2014**, *118*, 7692–7702. [CrossRef]
48. Zhou, G.X.; Chao, L.; Chao, J. Kallistatin: A novel human tissue kallikrein inhibitor. Purification, characterization, and reactive center sequence. *J. Biol. Chem.* **1992**, *267*, 25873–25880.
49. Kozakov, D.; Hall, D.R.; Xia, B.; Porter, K.A.; Padhorny, D.; Yueh, C.; Beglov, D.; Vajda, S. The ClusPro web server for protein-protein docking. *Nat. Protoc.* **2017**, *12*, 255–278. [CrossRef]
50. Ellisdon, A.M.; Zhang, Q.; Henstridge, M.A.; Johnson, T.K.; Warr, C.G.; Law, R.H.; Whisstock, J.C. High resolution structure of cleaved Serpin 42 Da from Drosophila melanogaster. *BMC Struct. Biol.* **2014**, *14*, 14. [CrossRef]
51. Zhou, A.; Wei, Z.; Read, R.J.; Carrell, R.W. Structural mechanism for the carriage and release of thyroxine in the blood. *Proc. Natl. Acad. Sci. USA* **2006**, *103*, 13321–13326. [CrossRef] [PubMed]

52. Ecke, S.; Geiger, M.; Binder, B.R. Heparin binding of protein-C inhibitor–analysis of the effect of heparin on the interaction of protein-C inhibitor with tissue kallikrein. *Eur. J. Biochem.* **1997**, *248*, 475–480. [CrossRef] [PubMed]
53. Ulbricht, D.; Tindall, C.A.; Oertwig, K.; Hanke, S.; Sträter, N.; Heiker, J.T. Kallikrein-related peptidase 14 is the second KLK protease targeted by the serpin vaspin. *Biol. Chem.* **2018**, *399*, 1079–1084. [CrossRef]
54. Ulbricht, D.; Oertwig, K.; Arnsburg, K.; Saalbach, A.; Pippel, J.; Sträter, N.; Heiker, J.T. Basic Residues of beta-Sheet A Contribute to Heparin Binding and Activation of Vaspin (Serpin A12). *J. Biol. Chem.* **2017**. [CrossRef] [PubMed]
55. Miao, R.Q.; Agata, J.; Chao, L.; Chao, J. Kallistatin is a new inhibitor of angiogenesis and tumor growth. *Blood* **2002**, *100*, 3245–3252. [CrossRef]
56. Chao, J.; Stallone, J.N.; Liang, Y.M.; Chen, L.M.; Wang, D.Z.; Chao, L. Kallistatin is a potent new. vasodilator. *J. Clin. Invest.* **1997**, *100*, 11–17. [CrossRef] [PubMed]

3

The Challenge of Modulating Heparan Sulfate Turnover by Multitarget Heparin Derivatives

Noemi Veraldi [1], Nawel Zouggari [2] and Ariane de Agostini [3,*]

1 Division of Clinical Pathology, Department of Diagnostics, Geneva University Hospitals, 1211 Geneva 14, Switzerland; noemi.veraldi@gmail.com
2 Department of Biochemistry, Faculty of Science and Department of Pathology and Immunology, School of Medicine, University of Geneva, 1211 Geneva 14, Switzerland; nawel.zouggari@unige.ch
3 Department of Pathology and Immunology, School of Medicine, University of Geneva and Division of Clinical Pathology, Department of Diagnostics, Geneva University Hospitals, 1211 Geneva 14, Switzerland
* Correspondence: ariane.deagostini@unige.ch.

Academic Editors: Giangiacomo Torri, Jawed Fareed and Job Harenberg

Abstract: This review comes as a part of the special issue "Emerging frontiers in GAGs and mimetics". Our interest is in the manipulation of heparan sulfate (HS) turnover by employing HS mimetics/heparin derivatives that exert pleiotropic effects and are interesting for interfering at multiple levels with pathways in which HS is implicated. Due to the important role of heparanase in HS post-biosynthetic modification and catabolism, we focus on the possibility to target heparanase, at both extracellular and intracellular levels, a strategy that can be applied to many conditions, from inflammation to cancer and neurodegeneration.

Keywords: heparan sulfate; heparin derivatives; neurodegenerative disorders; heparanase; cancer; mucopolysaccharidosis

1. Introduction

1.1. HS Turnover and the Role of Heparanase

Heparan sulfate (HS) is an anionic polysaccharide belonging to the glycosaminoglycan family that assembles as disaccharide building blocks of glucuronic acid (GlcA) linked α1-4 to N-acetyl-glucosamine (GlcNAc) and undergoes extensive modification through the action of at least four families of sulfotransferases and one epimerase. The sulfation of HS is carefully regulated in the ER-Golgi pathway where the first modification is introduced by N-deacetylase/N-sulfotransferase (NDST) enzymes and plays a key role in determining the subsequent modifications, dictating the position of the sulfated domains. Epimerization of some GlcA residues into iduronic acid (IdoA) can occur and it is followed by 2-O-sulfation of some iduronic acid residues, catalyzed by heparan sulfate 2-O-sulfotransferase (HS2ST), which can also act on some GlcA units. Next, on selected glucosamine residues sulfate groups are introduced by HS6ST1-3 transferases in the 6-O position and, finally, the relatively rare 3-O-sulfation is catalyzed by HS3ST1-6 [1]. Not only the length, but also the pattern of sulfation of HS is specific to the tissue and the moment of expression, and may be dynamically remodeled. For instance, high levels of 3-O-sulfated glucosamine were found in HS from follicular fluid, where nearly 50% of total HS is endowed with anticoagulant activity [2] and participates in the anticoagulant state of preovulatory follicular fluid. HS chains are usually attached to a core protein to form proteoglycans (HSPGs) that can be expressed on the cell membrane (syndecans and glypicans), or released in the extracellular matrix (ECM) where they constitute major structural molecules (agrin, perlecan, and type XVIII collagen) or be present in secretory vesicles [3].

HS is expressed on the cell surfaces of all mammalian cells where HSPGs participate in a variety of cellular processes and their functions depend on both HS and the protein core; for example, they serve as endocytic receptors and storage for macromolecules, such as lipid, growth factors, and morphogens [3,4], as modulators of cell mobility [5], and can participate in transportation of solutes between vessels and ECM (for review, see [6]). Also, heparan sulfate accounts for 60–90% of the total amount of the glycocalyx synthesized by endothelial cells [7] and whose anticoagulant and overall charge are very important for the repulsion of negatively charged molecules, including albumin, leukocytes, red blood cells, and platelets. Thus, the network of interactions of HS regulates fundamental biochemical and developmental processes and has been called the "HS-interactome" [8]. The last step of HS biosynthesis which is 6-O-desulfation by endosulfatases (SULF1 and SULF2), takes place on the cell surface and results in release of growth factors and cytokines immobilized on HSPGs and regulation of the effects of signal transduction [9,10]. In fact, the removal of sulfate groups from HS causes the release of HSPG-sequestered ligands that can act back on the cells and, indeed, overexpression of SULFs has been reported in a wide range of human tumors [11,12].

HSPGs expressed on the cell surface can be subjected to limited proteolysis and release in the medium or can be internalized by endocytosis and degraded by a multi-step process terminating in the lysosomes. The best characterized degradation pathway is that of ovarian granulosa cells in which two pathways have been described [13]. HSPGs anchored to the membrane by glycosylphosphatidylinositol (GPI) are quickly transported to lysosomes after endocytosis. Instead, HSPGs with transmembrane protein domains are first treated in prelysosomal compartments for removal of the protein core and partial degradation of HS chains. Secondly, HS chains are completely degraded in lysosomes. Differently, HSPGs in cultured rat hepatocytes have been shown to be long recycled back to the plasma membrane or to be associated with intracellular compartments before being degraded in lysosomes with no preliminary processing in early endosomes [14]. At the moment it is not clear if differences in HSPGs endocytosis reported in literature could be justified by the cellular context and the type of extracellular ligand.

The only known mammalian endoglycosidase able to cleave HS is heparanase (HPSE), which is secreted as a latent 65-kDa enzyme, which rapidly binds to HSPGs and the complex is then internalized by endocytosis [15]. Heparanase uptake is a prerequisite for the delivery to lysosomes where it is activated by cathepsin L and cuts HS at a limited number of sites, specifically the β-(1,4) glycosidic linkage between GlcA and GlcNS, producing fragments that are 10–20 saccharide units in length and still able to interact with protein ligands [16,17]. Also, a second HPSE protein named heparanase-2, without enzymatic activity, has been discovered and can compete for the substrate thus inhibiting HPSE activity but, its role in healthy tissues is broadly unknown [18]. Upon heparanase action, another nine exo-enzymes are responsible for the rapid and complete degradation of HS fragments: five sulfatases, three glycosidases, and an integral membrane enzyme required for the transfer of acetyl groups [19]. The process is influenced by the structure of the to-be-degraded HS: in CHO mutant cells, HS bearing reduced 2-O-sulfation was less cleaved by intracellular heparanase thus allowing recycling of unprocessed proteoglycans. In fact, higher amounts of extracellular HS chains were detected and accounted for the missing intermediate and small fragments observed inside the cells [20]. It has also been shown that heparanase drives fusion of lysosomes with autophagosomes thus controlling the basal levels of autophagy and contributing to maintain homeostasis [21] (Figure 1). Although numerous studies have accumulated regarding HS turnover especially in the last years, there is still debate on certain aspects which remain unclear. For example, the exact location and moment of activation of heparanase, whether in late endosomes or lysosomes, is still not precisely defined, together with the mechanism of HSPGs trafficking. We can speculate that a certain number of possibilities are available rather than a single linear mechanism, all converging to a final aim which is the reaction of the cell to different types of stimuli.

Synthesis and degradation of HS are both complex pathways involving a variety of different enzymes, spatially and temporarily tuned to produce heterogeneous chains with different sulfation degree but tissue-specific expression of ligand-binding sequences. The overall pattern of HS modification appears relatively constant within a specific cell type or organ; therefore, the control of HS biosynthesis must be strictly regulated [22]. Not unexpectedly, altered levels of HSPGs or altered expression of genes coding for HS biosynthetic enzymes have been associated with the development of many diseases [23–29].

Today, all genes responsible for HS biosynthesis have been cloned and identified, which helps investigate the possible association of these genes with several pathologies. Also, mouse models in which different genes important for HS biosynthesis have been knocked out have helped understanding that genetic ablation of biosynthetic enzymes does not strictly correlate with a predicted phenotype in vivo [30,31], probably due to the existence of compensation mechanisms and to functional redundancy between gene family members involved in HSPG biosynthesis and redundancy in HS sequence–activity relationships. For example, ablation of the gene EXT1 in mice, which codes for a polymerase involved in the elongation of HS chains, resulted in loss of HS, disruption of gastrulation, and embryonic lethality before E8.5 [32]. In other cases, the outcome of a gene knockout may be complex as several enzymes occur in isoforms [22]. Mice that lack 3-O-sulfotransferase-1 (3-OST-1) do not show a procoagulant phenotype, although the 3-O-sulfate group is essential for the interaction of vascular HS with antithrombin [26]. Nevertheless, the other existing 3-OST isoforms have distinct substrate preferences, and may therefore regulate different biologic properties of HS [33,34]; therefore, the final phenotype is not explained by their compensatory activity. Actually, all experimental data accumulated cannot be summarized by a simple scheme.

1.2. The Use of HS Mimetics

Due to the pleiotropic effects that HS can exert and to the fact that HSPGs are ubiquitous, the idea of interfering with HS turnover can either be seen as the intriguing possibility to obtain multiple effects or the limiting fear that non-specificity would impact undesired pathways. According to most of the observations reported to date, only certain interactions rely on specific oligosaccharide sequences [35,36], whereas many others rely on a certain type of sulfation or negative charge density [37,38]. Nevertheless, the interest in HS-protein interactions is continuously growing also thanks to advance in analytical techniques and chemical synthesis of oligosaccharides with precise structures which bring light on the structural requirements for HS activity [39,40].

It is well known that heparin, which can be considered a highly sulfated version of heparan sulfate, has been used clinically for more than half a century as anticoagulant drug and has been shown to possess a number of beneficial effects in other diseases than thrombosis [41]. Prolonged administration of heparin can cause adverse effects, mostly related to bleeding [42], but also an immunological reaction, heparin-induced thrombocytopenia [43–45]. Other side effects are clinically irrelevant, despite the possible interactions that can be established following heparin diffusion into tissues, suggesting that they may be absorbed by the network of proteins with which heparin and heparan sulfate interact. These considerations support investigation on the use of heparin as a starting material to generate derivatives or HS mimetics as therapeutic agents to interfere with pathways in which HS is involved as a means of intervening in biochemical processes for medical purposes.

A plethora of different compounds both of GAG and not-GAG nature have been synthesized, the potential use of which has been comprehensively and recently reviewed [46–48]. A body of evidence indicates that the altered expression or activity of heparanase determines a profound impact on tumor behavior; indeed, heparin analogs able to inhibit heparanase have been developed to primarily target cancer and some proved very active and have been tested in clinical trials [49].

This review will focus on the possibility to control HS turnover by acting upon heparanase, at both extracellular and intracellular levels, a strategy that can be applied to many conditions, from inflammation to cancer and neurodegeneration. Many papers on HPSE have been written, and it is not our purpose to review exhaustively the biological literature on heparanase and the use of heparin derivatives, which has been undertaken successfully elsewhere [46,47,49].

Heparanase has a role intracellularly where it is involved in the catabolism of HS but it is also present extracellularly. On one hand, heparanase is overexpressed in many tumors and the active form of the enzyme is released extracellularly, therefore, explaining the rational of employing HPSE inhibitors to block tumor progression. On the other hand, in different conditions such as mucopolysaccharidosis, and, in particular, Sanfilippo syndrome, which is a neurodegenerative lysosomal storage disease, the use of HPSE inhibitors may impact HPSE action and influence the global distribution of HSPGs.

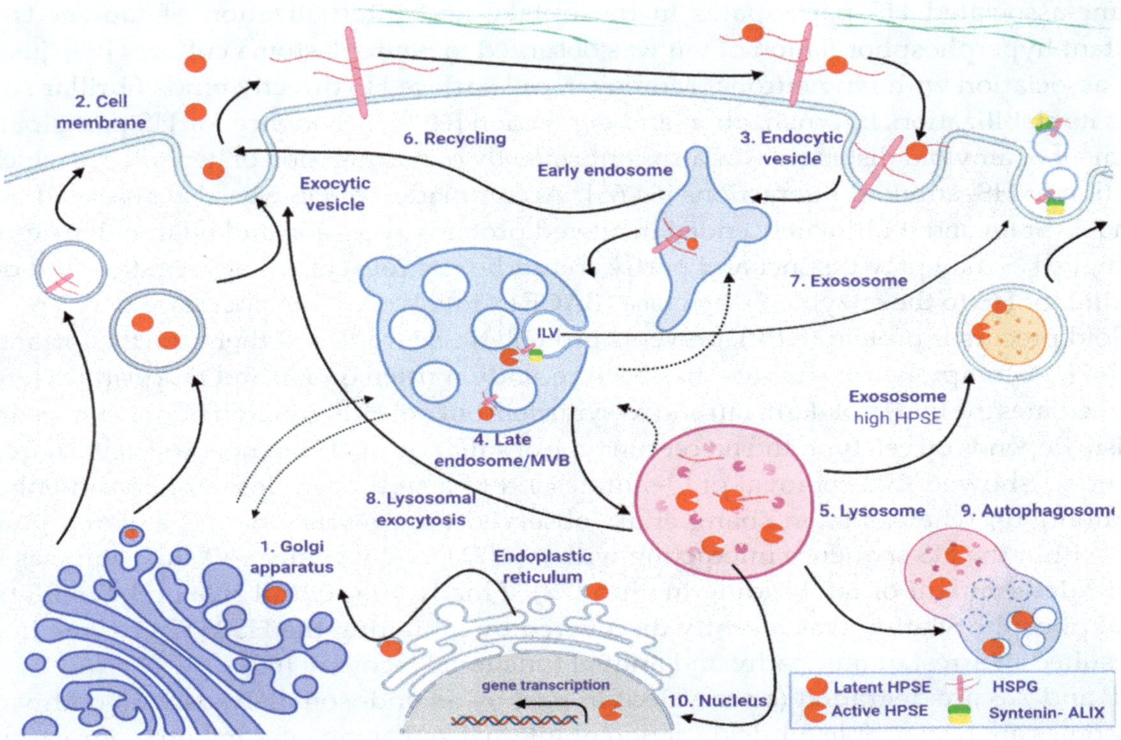

Figure 1. Schematic model of heparan sulfate proteoglycans and heparanase trafficking. (1) In the Golgi apparatus HS chains are polymerized and preHPSE is processed to produce proHPSE by the elimination of the N-terminal signal peptide. (2) The newly biosynthesized HSPGs are then shifted to the cell membrane where they can interact with the proHPSE and (3) the complex is rapidly internalized by endocytosis and then (4) accumulated in the late endosome. (5) Upon fusion of the late endosome with lysosome, proHPSE is activated and cleaves HS chains that are completely degraded by lysosomal hydrolases. (6) HPSE and HSPGs can be recycled to the cell surface from endosomes. It appears that active HPSE pursues other paths in the cells. (7) Trimming of HS from syndecans by active HPSE present in late endosomes leads to formation of the syndecan-syntenin-ALIX complex [50]. Intraluminal vesicles (ILV) are then formed by the invagination of endosomal membranes, resulting in the formation of multivesicular bodies (MVBs). MVBs release ILVs as exosomes upon fusion with the cell membrane and deliver their cargo to recipient cells. In the presence of high levels of HPSE, the enzyme can be found on the surface of exosomes and modulates tumor microenvironment. (8) Lysosomal exocytosis has been observed in malignant cells. (9) HPSE also regulates autophagy by driving fusion of lysosomes with autophagosomes which degrade macromolecules into monomeric units. (10) Perinuclear lysosomal HPSE can also translocate into the nucleus and regulate gene transcription and cell differentiation.

2. HS in Neurodegenerative Disorders

2.1. Different Involvement of HS in Neurodegenerative Disorders

Convergent phenotypes have been observed among the major pathologies affecting the brain. Neurodegenerative diseases are characterized by progressive accumulation of specific protein aggregates in the brain, e.g., amyloid-β (Aβ) in Alzheimer's disease (AD), α-synuclein in Parkinson's disease (PD) [51], and proteins with expanded polyglutamine (polyQ) in Huntington's disease (HD) [52].

According to the concept of "seeding", soluble proteins with nonnative conformations could assemble to form long unbranched structures called amyloid fibrils, able to trigger further incorporation of monomers into the fibrils. Regardless of the nature of the amyloid protein, HS has been found in all extracellular amyloid deposits [53,54], and HSPGs have been shown to be present at all stages of the degeneration process: neuron, intracellular and extracellular neurofibrillary tangles (NFTs). These fibrillary aggregates are formed by hyperphosphorylated forms of the microtubule-associated protein tau and have been detected in many neurodegenerative disorders, including AD [53,55–59]. Membrane-associated HS participates in the uptake and internalization of tau seeds [54], and concomitant hyperphosphorylation of tau was observed in neuroblastoma cultures [60], justifying the possible association with tau neurons. Moreover, cell surface HS directly binds fibrillar Aβ [61] and mediates its stabilization, internalization and deposition [62,63]. Evidence for HS participation in the development of amyloid disorders was also confirmed by overexpression of heparanase which resulted in inhibition of HS–amyloid interactions [64,65]. Accumulation of HS was also observed in neuronal nuclei in AD brain and it ultimately ended in altered protein expression and neuronal dysfunction [66]. Interestingly, HS may play distinct and partly contradictory roles in Aβ aggregation and deposit. In fact, binding of HS to the enzyme β-secretase (BACE1), involved in the liberation of Aβ peptide from the amyloid precursor protein (APP), prevents proteolytic cleavage and therefore the formation of Aβ peptide [67]. A comprehensive review has been recently written on HS and tauopathies [68].

HS mediates the fibril uptake of tau and α-synuclein but not Hungtington fibrils, suggesting that the mechanism depends on cell type and on certain type of sulfation of HS but not on specific sequences [69]. Castillo et al. showed that removal of O-sulfates led to a significant loss of heparin-enhanced Aβ fibrillization [70], whereas later Zhang et al. observed the presence of 6-O-sulfated glucosamine residues within the HS sequence interacting with Aβ [71], and recently 6-O sulfation was identified as a major determinant of tau binding in vitro [72]. Finally, the central role of 3-O-sulfation in tau abnormal phosphorylation was recently discovered by inhibiting the HS3ST2 enzyme in zebrafish, which resulted in arrest of tauopathy and animal functional recovery [60].

APP and Aβ are degraded (or recycled) in part by an endosomal–lysosomal pathway [73–75], and lysosomes are responsible for degradation of internalized aggregates in both neurons and in glial cells [76]. Efficient clearance of extracellular protein aggregates would prevent their transfer between cells, whereas compromised lysosomal efficiency may impair the degradation of many molecules normally processed within these organelles. Indeed, deficiency of lysosomal hydrolases is associated with the development of many human diseases, referred to as lysosomal storage disorders, which are often characterized by neurodegeneration [77]. Particularly, shortage or lack of specific lysosomal GAG-degrading enzymes impairs the autophagosome–lysosome fusion and leads to accumulation of GAGs; these diseases are called mucopolysaccharidoses (MPS) and many subtypes have been identified depending on the type of GAG and the specific enzyme affected. MPS III, called also Sanfilippo syndrome, is caused by deficiency of the lysosomal enzyme N-sulfoglucosamine sulfohydrolase (SGSH), resulting in incomplete degradation of HS and dramatic effects on the central nervous system with devastating consequences. Undegraded HS can affect cell functions not only due to its storage into lysosomes, but also when present outside the cell; probably, failure to degrade GAGs in MPS results in secretion and deposition in the ECM, as dysregulation of the ECM has been identified in several case reports [78,79]. Increased levels of protein markers associated with AD and PD have been detected in the brains of MPSIII mice: deposition of hyperphosphorylated tau and tau kinase, lysozyme, amyloid-β and amyloid precursor protein are all evident [80]. Moreover, α-synuclein aggregation and accumulation with neurons were observed both in MPSIII patients [81,82] and in MPSIIIA mice [83,84].

2.2. The Use of HS Derivatives in Neurodegenerative Disorders

Therapeutic approaches that target the central nervous system (CNS) are challenging due to the presence of the blood–brain barrier (BBB), which in healthy brain impedes most compounds from transiting from the blood to the brain. BBB permeability is influenced by molecular weight, charge, lipid solubility, surface activity, and relative size of the molecule [85]. If active compounds are small enough or lipid soluble they can pass the BBB by passive diffusion, alternatively they may be actively uptaken by receptors, transporters or carriers expressed by the cells of the BBB (endothelial cells, pericytes, astrocytes and neurons). The components of the BBB continuously adapt in response to various physiological changes in the brain and the integrity of the BBB is compromised in many pathological conditions including PD, AD, and MPS [81,86,87]. As a consequence, cytokines and immune cells could enter the CNS, activate glial cells, and cause alterations in the extracellular environment with consequent inflammation and damage [88,89].

A body of evidence supports targeting of HS-protein interactions in tauopathies as a therapeutic strategy. As already mentioned, studies on amyloidosis showed that overexpression of heparanase resulted in disruption of the HS–amyloid interactions, suggesting a potential strategy to interfere with the formation of fibrils. Indeed, administration of exogenous GAGs could competitively inhibit the harmful processes mediated by endogenous GAGs [90] and, in fact, heparin disaccharides were shown in vitro to pass the BBB and to efficiently decrease Aβ deposition [91], whereas chemically synthesized heparin-like oligosaccharides up to decasaccharides proved able to reduce the uptake of tau oligomers limiting their infectivity [92]. Neuroparin, a mixture of oligosaccharides with average MW of 2.1 kDa obtained by gamma irradiation of heparin, crosses the blood–brain barrier and was reported to attenuate the abnormal tau immunoreactivity in rat hippocampus and to have neuroprotective effects in several animal models of AD [93,94]. These compounds were small enough to cross the BBB and indeed an important consideration for therapeutic purposes is the extent of bioavailability of the administered GAG in the CNS. Nevertheless, in inflammatory conditions and highly damaged tissues, it is probable that increased permeability of the BBB would allow the entrance of compounds that would normally be rejected.

2.3. *The Possible Use of HS Derivatives in MPS III*

In MPS III disease, neurodegeneration is a consequence of HS accumulation in lysosomes [95]. To date, no treatments have shown promise in modifying the progression of this exceptionally rare, but ultimately lethal, disease. A review has been recently published summarizing treatment approaches for the brain in MPS [96]; therefore, only a brief summary on possible therapies will be treated in this paragraph, with a final focus on the use of heparin derivatives.

The promising Enzyme Replacement Therapy (ERT), which works for MPS I, MPS II, MPS IVA, and MPS VI, is more difficult in MPS III, where it should cross the blood–brain barrier. The approach is based on systemic delivery of recombinant lysosomal hydrolases which are internalized through mannose-6-phosphate receptors [97–99]. Intravenously delivered enzyme has been shown not to cross the BBB in an adequate amount to prevent progression of neurological manifestations [100]. Gene therapy as a treatment for MPS can potentially provide a stable and continuous source of enzyme in combination with immunosuppression to prevent an immune response against the vector. Indeed, intracerebral injection of the vector AAVrh10-hMPS3A in four children with MPS IIIA and of the vector ABO-102 in six MPS IIIA patients showed good tolerability and evidence of decreased neurocognitive decline [101]. Fusion of the recombinant enzyme to a monoclonal antibody against the human insulin receptor has been shown by Boado and coworkers to facilitate the uptake in the brain by exploiting the transport mechanisms already present in the BBB [102,103]. Another strategy called substrate reduction therapy (SRT), aims to inhibit the early stage of the lysosomal degradation pathway, reducing GAGs synthesis [104]; however, results of a 6-month clinical trial with miglustat—an imminosugar used in the treatment of type I Gaucher disease—showed no improvement of cognition or behavior in MPS III patients [105]. Another approach under investigation is chaperone therapy, with the aim of partially restore the missing enzymatic activity. In fact, 10% activity is considered sufficient to prevent lysosomal GAG storage in MPS patients [106]. Lastly, also hematopoietic stem cells transplantation (HSCT) which consist in delivery of donor stem cells producing the deficient lysosomal enzyme, has been extensively studied over the past decades with variable results [107].

HS in MPS patients is not only accumulated in lysosomes, but seems to be redistributed to different cellular and extracellular localizations [108,109]. De Pasquale et al. recently published an innovative approach called substrate-masking technology based on sequestering of extracellular excess HS (and/or DS) with consequent restoring of the natural equilibrium. Treatment of primary fibroblasts from MPS IIIA- and MPS IIIB-patients with the protein NK1 resulted in decreased GAGs accumulation and restoration of FGF2 signaling [110].

As already suggested [111], targeting HPSE in lysosomes may be an interesting way to affect autophagy either by employing HPSE inhibitors, whose ability to cross the BBB is nevertheless still unclear, or by decreasing the lysosomal content of HPSE. For example, treatment with the inhibitor PG545 was shown to decrease autophagy and promote accumulation of HPSE extracellularly while reducing its level in the lysosomes [112]. Our strategy is to employ HPSE inhibitors as a mean to affect HS turnover, based on the idea that uncleaved HS chains may fuel recycling of HSPGs and lead to a lower amount of HS degraded in lysosomes. We have tested several HPSE inhibitors on primary fibroblast from KO MPS-IIIA and spontaneously mutated MPS-IIIA mouse models [113]. Indeed, treatment with these compounds could affect HS turnover, leading to decreased HSPGs production.

3. HS in Cancer

3.1. Expression of HSPGs in Tumorigenesis

Heparan sulfate and HSPGs are expressed on all eukaryotic cells, including cancerous cells and stromal cells surrounding the tumor and play an important role in tumor–stroma cross-talk, and thus in cancer development, transformation, growth, and metastasis. Therefore, alteration of the normal expression levels of HSPGs has often been described in tumors. Several HSPGs have been shown to be upregulated in many cancers [114]; for example, increasing expression level of Agrin in hepatocellular carcinoma [115] and of glypican-1 in pancreas carcinoma was detected and associated with poor prognosis [116]. Levels of glypican-1 and syndecan-2 are also increased in colorectal cancer [117]. Syndecan-1 has been demonstrated to regulate $\alpha v\beta 3$ and $\alpha v\beta 5$ integrin activation during angiogenesis and tumorigenesis on mammary carcinoma cells [118], whereas shedding of syndecan-2 has an antiangiogenic effect on the endothelium [119]. Moreover, breast cancer was found to upregulate glypican-1 [120] and syndecan-4 [121] and to downregulate glypican-3 [122], whereas low expression of glypican-3 promotes tumor proliferation and metastasis [123]. Contrarily, glypican-3 was found to be overexpressed in approximately 70% to 80% of hepatocellular carcinomas [124] and high glypican-5 expression levels in non-small cell lung cancer were associated with poor differentiation, vascular invasion, regional lymph node metastasis, and a higher TNM stage (TNM classification of malignant tumors) [125]. In addition, glypican-2 is upregulated in neuroblastoma and associated with poor overall survival [117].

In general, remodeling of HSPGs through enzymatic modification of HS chains is associated with malignant transformation of cells and can potentially serve as molecular biomarker to aid in the diagnosis and prognosis of cancer [114,126]. Also, alteration of glycosylation affects cellular adhesion and is associated with oncogenic transformation and metastasis [114]. Indeed, altered HSPGs glycosylation has been described in lung and brain cancer [127].

3.2. Tumor–Stroma Cross-talk

Tumor stroma is composed of the ECM including proteoglycans, fibronectin, collagen, cytokines, and growth factors. As the tumor evolves, the stroma undergoes tissue remodeling under the action of enzymes able to modify the glycosidic chains of the ECM, i.e., glycosyltransferases, sulfotransferases, sulfatases, and heparanase [128]. The presence and amount of these GAG-related enzymes help to identify high-risk patients and to develop personalized therapeutics [129]. Indeed, Barkeer and collaborators demonstrated that elevated O-glycosyltransferases GALNT3 and B3GNT3 expression regulates cancer stem cell markers in pancreatic cancer and their knockdown leads to decreased clonogenicity and migratory capacity [130]. Increased heparanase expression is also often described to promote an aggressive tumor behavior via multiple mechanisms [71,83]. It has been demonstrated that tumors are more aggressive when developed in transgenic mice overexpressing heparanase (Hpa-Tg and MMTV-heparanase), whereas smaller tumors develop in Hpa-KO mice [95,120].

HPSE functions inside the cell to promote autophagy and tumor growth by driving fusion of lysosomes with autophagosomes thus controlling the basal levels of autophagy [111]. Heparanase is an important player not only in maintaining homeostasis, as a postsynthetic modification enzyme for HS structure but also for its non-enzymatic and HS-independent effects which may contribute to tumor aggressiveness [131,132]. Therefore, heparanase orchestrates cellular responses in both normal and pathologic conditions. HSPGs bind to numerous bioactive molecules, i.e., growth factors, cytokines, chemokines, enzymes, which are stored in the ECM and can be released upon cleavage by extracellular heparanase. This strategy is adopted by tumor cells to ensure rapid tissue response as a fast-acting mechanism independent from *de novo* protein synthesis that meets their needs to promote tumor growth, angiogenesis, peripheral immune tolerance and formation of a metastatic niche. Briefly, tumor cells can change the nature of the microenvironment and vice versa the microenvironment can affect how a tumor grows and spreads [133].

Heparanase promotes signal transduction, including Akt, STAT, Src, Erk, HGF-, IGF- and EGF-receptor signaling [131]. Moreover, HPSE regulates the transcription of many other factors spanning from proangiogenic (i.e., VEGF-A, VEGF-C, COX-2, and MMP-9), to pro-thrombotic (i.e., tissue factor), proinflammatory (i.e., TNFα, IL-1, and IL-6), profibrotic (i.e., TGFβ), mitogenic (i.e., HGF), and osteolyic (RANKL) [133–135]. In summary, more and more functions of HPSE are being discovered, thus confirming its importance also in normal cell processes and the need of controlling its action and expression. The presence of heparanase was reported in Langerhans cells [136], where its function still has to be elucidated, and in astrocytes in mice after ischemia, where it can participate in the repair process [137]. Interestingly, increased expression of heparanase was found in placentas with preeclampsia [138,139], where it would enhance the increase of VEGF release and it would influence the invasion of trophoblast, similarly to the invasion of cancer cells [140].

While heparanase upregulation by tumor cells is well documented, not enough attention has been given to the protumorigenic function of heparanase expressed by non-tumor cells residing in the tumor microenvironment. In fact, heparanase released from platelets, neutrophils and mast cells upon degranulation participates in ECM degradation, facilitating diapedesis and extravasation of inflammatory cells [141–145]. HPSE release can therefore be a strategy used by metastatic tumor cells to invade blood and lymphatic vessels. Moreover, HPSE was discovered to mediate TLR activation at the cell membrane, followed by Erk/p38/JNK activation therefore regulating cytokine expression by macrophages, their activation and function in tumorigenesis and cross-talk with the tumor microenvironment [146].

Tumor cells are able to influence the responses of surrounding healthy cells as demonstrated by experiments in which healthy lymphocytes were co-cultured with sera from breast cancer patients or media from MCF-7 cells. Increased expression of HPSE and secretion of exosomes was indeed observed, thus revealing the importance of cross-talk [147,148]. Exosomes serve as mediators for intercellular communication through the delivery of proteins, factors and HS chains, important for signaling processes. Heparanase overexpression dramatically increases exosome secretion in human cancer cells of myeloma, lymphoblastoid, and breast cancer [149].

It has been recently discovered that chemotherapy upregulates heparanase expression in myeloma surviving cells and induces secretion of chemoexosomes with heparanase loaded on surface [150]. These tumor chemoexosomes can remodel extracellular matrix by degrading ECM heparan sulfate and/or by transferring their heparanase cargo to cells where HS degradation will induce signal activation [150], resulting in enhanced secretion of an important myeloma growth factor, TNF-α, by macrophages. Additionally, heparanase stimulates the expression of MMP-9 via ERK signaling, promoting shedding of syndecan-1 proteoglycan (CD138) from the myeloma cell surface [150]. Shed syndecan-1 ectodomain was shown to capture VEGF and form a complex that activates integrin and VEGF receptors on adjacent endothelial cells thereby stimulating tumor angiogenesis [151].

3.3. Heparanase Targeting by Heparin and Its Derivatives in Cancer Therapy

As venous thromboembolism is a well-known cause of death in patients with cancer [152], heparin has been frequently used in the treatment of cancer-associated thromboembolism. Accordingly, accumulation of clinical evidence shows that cancer patients treated with unfractionated and low-molecular weight heparin (LMWH) survive longer than patients treated with other anticoagulants, especially patients in the early stage of the disease [153–157]. Heparin has been showned to possess anticancer, antiangiogenic, and antimetastatic activity [158,159], including inhibition of heparanase, blocking of P- and L-selectin-mediated cell adhesion, and inhibition of angiogenesis, but its anticoagulant activity and the possible side effects as bleeding and heparin-induced thrombocytopenia limit long-term treatment. As already mentioned, heparin derivatives or HS mimetics have been synthesized with reduced or absent anticoagulant activity but maintaining their binding selectivity potential towards a vast array of HS-binding proteins, many of which with pivotal roles in cancer growth and progression [46].

Nowadays the interest of researchers in oncology is not only limited to tumor cells but especially on tumor microenvironment. Information gathered on the two topics is so vast that they appear as two different specialized areas of research that are, on the contrary, profoundly interconnected. The separation into the following sections is based on experimental observations either directed on the tumor itself or on the components of the tumor microenvironment.

3.3.1. Targeting the Tumor

Numerous clinical association studies have consistently demonstrated that upregulation of heparanase expression correlates with increased tumor size, tumor angiogenesis, enhanced metastasis, and poor prognosis [160,161]. In contrast, knockdown of heparanase or treatments of tumor-bearing mice with heparanase-inhibiting compounds markedly attenuate tumor progression [162–164], further underscoring the potential of anti-heparanase therapy for multiple types of cancer.

Extensive research was done on targeting HS-degrading activity of heparanase [49,128,165,166]. The heparanase inhibitory effects of non-anticoagulant heparin have been described by Bar-Ner et al., suggesting that heparanase inhibition was dependent on polysaccharide size, degree and pattern of sulfation, and N-substitution of hexosamines [167].

Some supersulfated low-molecular weight heparins (ssLMWH) have been synthesized with low anticoagulant activity despite the high degree of sulfation and were shown to reduce synovial sarcoma growth and metastases in vitro and in vivo by interfering with the activity of heparanase, growth factor/receptor axes and proinflammatory molecules (e.g., leucocyte elastase and cathepsin G) [168]. Another compound, SSLMW-19, a key factor in the regulation of iron metabolism, and also involved in carcinogenesis and metastasis, was shown to rapidly and strongly inhibit the expression of hepcidin in vitro and in vivo [169].

Glycol-splitting of unsubstituted uronic acids obtained by periodate oxidation and borohydride reduction has been applied to a variety of heparin derivatives and increased the flexibility of the molecules for a better interaction and inhibition of heparanase or growth factors. M402 (Necuparanib) is a glycol-split LMWH with reduced anticoagulant activity [170] that was found to reduce tumor burden in vivo in KPFMC pancreatic cancer mice model at a dose of 40 mg/kg/day and reduce AsPC-1 pancreatic cancer cell line proliferation and invasion in vitro in a 3D-culture model [171]. Boothello et al. synthesized a non-saccharide compound, G2.2, which is structurally homogeneous and easy to obtain by chemical synthesis, as a mimetic of an HS hexasaccharide active on cancer stem cells. This HS mimetic reduced in a dose-dependent manner the growth of colon subcutaneous xenografts in mice and delayed the growth when added to oxaliplatin and 5-fluorouracil, which are the most frequently used chemotherapy treatment for colon cancer [172]. Also, polysaccharides from different sources are potentially able to interfere with tumorigenesis. For example, an oversulfated heparin-like polysaccharide from marine origin was recently evaluated for its ability to reduce cancer cell characteristics on human endometrioid cancer cell line in vitro. This compound effectively reduces the ability of tumor cells to initiate migration by inducing 51.6% of slowdown and induces 87% of inhibition of tumor cell invasion on Transwell compared to non-treated cells (unpublished data). It also inhibits endometrial tumor cell proliferation and is well tolerated at concentrations of 100, 75, 50, and 25μg/mL (unpublished data). A sulfated oligosaccharide mimetic of heparan sulfate, PI-88, was used to inhibit HS effector functions and heparanase activity. PI-88 reduced tumor volume by 66–70% in RIP1-Tag2 mice model of pancreatic islet cell carcinogenesis [173]. Joyce and collaborators also noticed decreased tumor cell proliferation, increased apoptosis and impaired angiogenesis associated with reduction of VEGF-A and its receptor VEGF-R2 on the tumor endothelium [173].

3.3.2. Targeting the Tumor Microenvironment

Impact of heparanase on tumor progression is related to its function in mediating tumor-host cross-talk, priming the tumor microenvironment to better support tumor seeding and growth [174]. Targeting of heparanase in the tumor microenvironment is a promising strategy to restrain tumor growth and dissemination. Indeed, a study showed the effect of heparanase-neutralizing antibodies to attenuate the growth of lymphoma cells that do not express heparanase, implying that targeting microenvironment may be sufficient [175].

Heparin derivatives and HS mimetics can also affect invasion and metastatic tumor behavior by counteracting HSPGs functions.. Yoshitomi et al. observed reduced tumor growth dissemination on several murine metastatic models by employing a glycol-split weak anticoagulant heparin [176].

Another strategy to contain metastatic progression could be targeting the angiogenic pathway. A low-molecular-weight glycol-split heparin (ST2184), generated by nitrous acid depolymerization of an undersulfated glycol-split heparin derivative (ST1514), was shown to act as VEGF antagonist by exploiting binding to VEGF165 while preventing receptor engagement [177]. This molecule inhibited neovascularization in the chick embryo chorioallantoic membrane, metastatic dissemination to the lung in the B16-BL6 mouse model of melanoma and significantly reduced angiogenesis of human MeVo melanoma xenografts [46,177]. Naggi and coworkers developed a 100% N-acetylated and 25% glycol split heparin, known as SST0001 (Roneparstat) [178], which is a potent heparanase inhibitor that is also able to suppress angiogenesis and to downregulate HGF, VEGF, and the expression of ECM-remodeling proteins (Matrix metalloproteinase 9, pentraxin, and urokinase-type plasminogen activator) [179]. Also, in combination with dexamethasone it was able to inhibit myeloma tumor growth in vivo through dual targeting of the tumor and its microenvironment via the heparanase/syndecan-1 axis [180].

We previously mentioned that M402 heparin mimetic effectively targeted pancreatic tumor cells. Interestingly, MacDonald et al. observed that M402 also targeted the stromal compartment. On a co-culture of pancreatic tumor cells and stellate cells that mimics epithelial–stromal interactions, treatment of M402 significantly decreased the invasive behavior in a dose-dependent manner, whereas in vivo it extended survival and reduced metastasis by reducing the protein levels of matrix metalloprotease 1 and by increasing the tissue inhibitor of metalloproteinase 3 (TIMP3) [171]. Karoli et al. demonstrated that carbohydrate-based HS-mimicking compounds, PI-88 and analogues, inhibit heparanase and compete with growth factors (FGF-1, FGF-2, and VEGF) for binding to HS, and therefore impact anti-angiogenic and anti-metastatic activity [48,181]. Another octasaccharide-based heparin mimetic synthesized by Dollé and coworkers was characterized in vitro for its binding affinities and towards VEGF-A, FGF-2, PDGF-β, and SDF1-α using the BIAcore technology and for the potential inhibition in an heparanase activity assay [182]. This novel molecule could thus potentially inhibit angiogenesis by interfering with components of the extracellular matrix. Lim and collaborators developed saccharide-free polyproline-based GAG mimetics (PGMs) that recapitulate key GAG structural features, notably the sized repeating units, periodicity, and helicity. GAG activities were also maintained, indeed PGMs effectively inhibited chondroitin sulfate-E binding to P-selectin which is implicated in metastasis, thrombosis and inflammation and successfully attenuate hematogenous metastasis in vivo in mice model as effectively as heparin and tinzaparin without any adverse effects on mice model, suggesting its safe use in vivo [183].

3.4. Clinical Considerations

Over the last 30 years of active research, there has been an explosion of information about the molecular biology of cancer. The challenge remains to translate this information into advances in patient care to convert new molecular information into drug therapy. According to all these studies, high levels of heparanase could be used as predictive and prognostic molecular marker for cancer. In a study published in 2016, high level of HPSE in the melanoma metastases predicted poor prognosis in patients stage IVc [184]. However, HPSE expression in the primary tumor does not always reflect metastatic output. This is the case in breast cancer patients, where the primary lesion stained positive for heparanase in some cases while the metastasis stained negative, and vice versa [185]. In addition, we observed high HPSE expression in all primary lesions from endometrioid cancer grade 1 patients despite different patterns and degree of invasions.

A number of preclinical and clinical studies have suggested that heparin and LMWH treatment in addition to conventional treatment significantly improves overall survival in cancer patients with advanced stage cancer but increasing the risk for bleeding complications [186,187]. Regarding the use of heparanase inhibitors to block tumor progression and their weak anticoagulant activity, Muparfostat PI-88 was the first heparanase inhibitor tested in early stage clinical trials in cancer patients in 2011. PI-88 was administered both alone and together with docetaxel to cancer patients in two Phase 1 studies validating their tolerance and safety for the patients [135,136]. PI-88 was also the first to enter clinical trials reaching phase III, where it was administered as an adjuvant therapy for hepatitis virus related hepatocellular carcinoma (HV-HCC) after its surgical resection. PI-88 prolonged the disease-free survival in the microvascular invasion subgroup (40% of the trial population) and exhibited anti-inflammatory properties [137]. Liao et al. demonstrated that heparanase was upregulated in both postsurgical plasma of HCC patients and in orthotopic mouse model induced after hepatectomy [137]. Upregulation of HPSE enhanced the sensitivity of HCC cells to PI-88 and thus the inhibitory effect of PI-88 on cell proliferation and migration. Likewise, Ramani et al. also showed that heparanase is upregulated in response to chemotherapy in myeloma patients and the surviving cells acquire drug resistance due to heparanase-mediated ERK signaling [138].

SST0001 heparin mimetic effectively inhibited myeloma growth in vivo, even when confronted with an aggressively growing tumor within human bone [180]. An open-label, multicenter, phase I, first-in-human study was designed to assess the safety and tolerability profile of Roneparstat in patients with relapsed/refractory multiple myeloma, and was well tolerated by patients exposed to the drug at dose levels of 200 and 400 mg/day without any clinically relevant toxicities [188]. Consequently, Roneparstat was found to be highly effective and overcome initial chemoresistance when used in combination with chemotherapeutic agents against established and aggressive myeloma tumors growing within bone or to treat brain metastatic breast cancer [189,190].

Analysis of plasma samples of patients with metastatic pancreatic cancer enrolled in a phase I/II study show that treatment with necuparanib in addition to the standard of care significantly increased TIMP3 plasma protein levels confirming the in vivo and in vitro studies on pancreatic cancer models [171].

PG545 has been selected over the PG500 series of heparan sulfate mimetics for the ability to inhibit both angiogenesis and heparanase activity and was selected as the lead clinical candidate for oncology [191]. Eight years after, PG545 was then evaluated on a Phase I study in patients with advanced solid malignancies that had relapsed or was refractory to standard therapy, and showed a disease control up to 24 weeks in 38% of evaluable subjects with increases in innate immune cell activation, plasma IFNγ, TNFα, IP-10, and MCP-1 [192].

These heparin mimetics that inhibit heparanase enzymatic activity are being evaluated in numerous clinical trials for various types of cancer, and appear to be well tolerated and also beneficial in combination with conventional anticancer drugs, thus providing a strong rationale for applying anti-heparanase therapy. Another strategy uses heparanase-neutralizing monoclonal antibodies to target the interaction of heparanase with HS and has been tested in pre-clinical studies for various types of cancer, including myeloma, pancreatic carcinoma, and hepatocellular carcinoma [175]. These heparanase-neutralizing mAbs profoundly attenuated myeloma and lymphoma tumor growth and dissemination of tumor xenografts produced by human lymphoma cells in preclinical models [175].

Although clinical trials focus on cancer patients, the same heparanase inhibitors are likely to be applied in other applications as chronic inflammation, sepsis, autoimmune diabetes, diabetic nephropathy, bone osteolysis, pancreatitis, viral infection, acute kidney injury, thrombosis, and atherosclerosis, as well as various rare diseases like mucopolysaccharidosis. Additional opportunities for development of anti-heparanase therapeutics include monoclonal antibodies and the use of the recently published crystal structure of heparanase for identification of small inhibitory molecules [81].

4. Conclusions

We gathered existing data around the idea of interfering with HS turnover by affecting heparanase and, indeed, the literature does support this working hypothesis. It is hoped that the review will promote discussion regarding the concrete possibility to therapeutically use HS mimetics/heparin derivatives which are able to act on existing pathways and to modulate them. We are confident that new discoveries will help clarify the aspects of HS turnover which are still foggy.

Author Contributions: Conceptualization, writing—original preparation, review and editing, N.V. and N.Z.; supervision, A.d.A. All authors have read and agreed to the published version of the manuscript.

Acknowledgments: We thank Antonella Bisio and MD Jean-Christophe Tille for critical reading of the manuscript.

References

1. Esko, J.D.; Selleck, S.B. Order out of chaos: Assembly of ligand binding sites in heparan sulfate. *Annu. Rev. Biochem.* **2002**, *71*, 435–471. [CrossRef] [PubMed]
2. de Agostini, A.I.; Dong, J.C.; de Vantery Arrighi, C.; Ramus, M.A.; Dentand-Quadri, I.; Thalmann, S.; Ventura, P.; Ibecheole, V.; Monge, F.; Fischer, A.M.; et al. Human follicular fluid heparan sulfate contains abundant 3-o-sulfated chains with anticoagulant activity. *J. Biol. Chem.* **2008**, *283*, 28115–28124. [CrossRef] [PubMed]
3. Sarrazin, S.; Lamanna, W.C.; Esko, J.D. Heparan sulfate proteoglycans. *Cold Spring Harb. Perspect. Biol.* **2011**, *3*, a004952. [CrossRef] [PubMed]
4. Christianson, H.C.; Belting, M. Heparan sulfate proteoglycan as a cell-surface endocytosis receptor. *Matrix Biol.* **2014**, *35*, 51–55. [CrossRef]
5. Asplund, A.; Ostergren-Lunden, G.; Camejo, G.; Stillemark-Billton, P.; Bondjers, G. Hypoxia increases macrophage motility, possibly by decreasing the heparan sulfate proteoglycan biosynthesis. *J. Leukoc. Biol.* **2009**, *86*, 381–388. [CrossRef]
6. Bishop, J.R.; Schuksz, M.; Esko, J.D. Heparan sulphate proteoglycans fine-tune mammalian physiology. *Nature* **2007**, *446*, 1030–1037. [CrossRef]
7. Reitsma, S.; Slaaf, D.W.; Vink, H.; van Zandvoort, M.A.; Oude Egbrink, M.G. The endothelial glycocalyx: Composition, functions, and visualization. *Pflugers Arch.* **2007**, *454*, 345–359. [CrossRef]
8. Ori, A.; Free, P.; Courty, J.; Wilkinson, M.C.; Fernig, D.G. Identification of heparin-binding sites in proteins by selective labeling. *Mol. Cell. Proteom.* **2009**, *8*, 2256–2265. [CrossRef]
9. Uchimura, K.; Morimoto-Tomita, M.; Bistrup, A.; Li, J.; Lyon, M.; Gallagher, J.; Werb, Z.; Rosen, S.D. Hsulf-2, an extracellular endoglucosamine-6-sulfatase, selectively mobilizes heparin-bound growth factors and chemokines: Effects on vegf, fgf-1, and sdf-1. *BMC Biochem.* **2006**, *7*, 2. [CrossRef]

10. Dhoot, G.K.; Gustafsson, M.K.; Ai, X.; Sun, W.; Standiford, D.M.; Emerson, C.P., Jr. Regulation of wnt signaling and embryo patterning by an extracellular sulfatase. *Science* **2001**, *293*, 1663–1666. [CrossRef]
11. Lemjabbar-Alaoui, H.; van Zante, A.; Singer, M.S.; Xue, Q.; Wang, Y.Q.; Tsay, D.; He, B.; Jablons, D.M.; Rosen, S.D. Sulf-2, a heparan sulfate endosulfatase, promotes human lung carcinogenesis. *Oncogene* **2010**, *29*, 635–646. [CrossRef] [PubMed]
12. Tatrai, P.; Egedi, K.; Somoracz, A.; van Kuppevelt, T.H.; Ten Dam, G.; Lyon, M.; Deakin, J.A.; Kiss, A.; Schaff, Z.; Kovalszky, I. Quantitative and qualitative alterations of heparan sulfate in fibrogenic liver diseases and hepatocellular cancer. *J. Histochem. Cytochem.* **2010**, *58*, 429–441. [CrossRef] [PubMed]
13. Yanagishita, M. Glycosylphosphatidylinositol-anchored and core protein-intercalated heparan sulfate proteoglycans in rat ovarian granulosa cells have distinct secretory, endocytotic, and intracellular degradative pathways. *J. Biol. Chem.* **1992**, *267*, 9505–9511. [PubMed]
14. Egeberg, M.; Kjeken, R.; Kolset, S.O.; Berg, T.; Prydz, K. Internalization and stepwise degradation of heparan sulfate proteoglycans in rat hepatocytes. *Biochim. Biophys. Acta* **2001**, *1541*, 135–149. [CrossRef]
15. Gingis-Velitski, S.; Zetser, A.; Kaplan, V.; Ben-Zaken, O.; Cohen, E.; Levy-Adam, F.; Bashenko, Y.; Flugelman, M.Y.; Vlodavsky, I.; Ilan, N. Heparanase uptake is mediated by cell membrane heparan sulfate proteoglycans. *J. Biol. Chem.* **2004**, *279*, 44084–44092. [CrossRef]
16. Zetser, A.; Levy-Adam, F.; Kaplan, V.; Gingis-Velitski, S.; Bashenko, Y.; Schubert, S.; Flugelman, M.Y.; Vlodavsky, I.; Ilan, N. Processing and activation of latent heparanase occurs in lysosomes. *J. Cell. Sci.* **2004**, *117*, 2249–2258. [CrossRef]
17. Secchi, M.F.; Masola, V.; Zaza, G.; Lupo, A.; Gambaro, G.; Onisto, M. Recent data concerning heparanase: Focus on fibrosis, inflammation and cancer. *Biomol. Concepts* **2015**, *6*, 415–421. [CrossRef]
18. Levy-Adam, F.; Feld, S.; Cohen-Kaplan, V.; Shteingauz, A.; Gross, M.; Arvatz, G.; Naroditsky, I.; Ilan, N.; Doweck, I.; Vlodavsky, I. Heparanase 2 interacts with heparan sulfate with high affinity and inhibits heparanase activity. *J. Biol. Chem.* **2010**, *285*, 28010–28019. [CrossRef]
19. Hopwood, J.J. Enzymes that Degrade Heparin and Heparan Sulfate. In *Heparin, Chemical and Biological Properties, Clinical Applications*; Lane, D.A., Lindahl, U., Eds.; CRC Press Inc.: Boca Raton, FL, USA, 1989; pp. 191–228.
20. Bai, X.; Bame, K.J.; Habuchi, H.; Kimata, K.; Esko, J.D. Turnover of heparan sulfate depends on 2-o-sulfation of uronic acids. *J. Biol. Chem.* **1997**, *272*, 23172–23179. [CrossRef]
21. Shteingauz, A.; Boyango, I.; Naroditsky, I.; Hammond, E.; Gruber, M.; Doweck, I.; Ilan, N.; Vlodavsky, I. Heparanase enhances tumor growth and chemoresistance by promoting autophagy. *Cancer Res.* **2015**, *75*, 3946–3957. [CrossRef]
22. Esko, J.D.; Lindahl, U. Molecular diversity of heparan sulfate. *J. Clin. Investig.* **2001**, *108*, 169–173. [CrossRef] [PubMed]
23. Gotte, M.; Joussen, A.M.; Klein, C.; Andre, P.; Wagner, D.D.; Hinkes, M.T.; Kirchhof, B.; Adamis, A.P.; Bernfield, M. Role of syndecan-1 in leukocyte-endothelial interactions in the ocular vasculature. *Invest Ophthalmol. Vis. Sci.* **2002**, *43*, 1135–1141. [PubMed]
24. Xu, J.; Park, P.W.; Kheradmand, F.; Corry, D.B. Endogenous attenuation of allergic lung inflammation by syndecan-1. *J. Immunol.* **2005**, *174*, 5758–5765. [CrossRef] [PubMed]
25. Grobe, K.; Inatani, M.; Pallerla, S.R.; Castagnola, J.; Yamaguchi, Y.; Esko, J.D. Cerebral hypoplasia and craniofacial defects in mice lacking heparan sulfate ndst1 gene function. *Development* **2005**, *132*, 3777–3786. [CrossRef]
26. HajMohammadi, S.; Enjyoji, K.; Princivalle, M.; Christi, P.; Lech, M.; Beeler, D.; Rayburn, H.; Schwartz, J.J.; Barzegar, S.; de Agostini, A.I.; et al. Normal levels of anticoagulant heparan sulfate are not essential for normal hemostasis. *J. Clin. Investig.* **2003**, *111*, 989–999. [CrossRef]
27. Westphal, V.; Murch, S.; Kim, S.; Srikrishna, G.; Winchester, B.; Day, R.; Freeze, H.H. Reduced heparan sulfate accumulation in enterocytes contributes to protein-losing enteropathy in a congenital disorder of glycosylation. *Am. J. Pathol.* **2000**, *157*, 1917–1925. [CrossRef]
28. Morita, H.; Yoshimura, A.; Inui, K.; Ideura, T.; Watanabe, H.; Wang, L.; Soininen, R.; Tryggvason, K. Heparan sulfate of perlecan is involved in glomerular filtration. *J. Am. Soc. Nephrol.* **2005**, *16*, 1703–1710. [CrossRef]
29. Arikawa-Hirasawa, E.; Watanabe, H.; Takami, H.; Hassell, J.R.; Yamada, Y. Perlecan is essential for cartilage and cephalic development. *Nat. Genet.* **1999**, *23*, 354–358. [CrossRef]

30. Bullock, S.L.; Fletcher, J.M.; Beddington, R.S.; Wilson, V.A. Renal agenesis in mice homozygous for a gene trap mutation in the gene encoding heparan sulfate 2-sulfotransferase. *Genes Dev.* **1998**, *12*, 1894–1906. [CrossRef]
31. Li, J.P.; Gong, F.; Hagner-McWhirter, A.; Forsberg, E.; Abrink, M.; Kisilevsky, R.; Zhang, X.; Lindahl, U. Targeted disruption of a murine glucuronyl c5-epimerase gene results in heparan sulfate lacking l-iduronic acid and in neonatal lethality. *J. Biol. Chem.* **2003**, *278*, 28363–28366. [CrossRef]
32. Lin, X.; Wei, G.; Shi, Z.; Dryer, L.; Esko, J.D.; Wells, D.E.; Matzuk, M.M. Disruption of gastrulation and heparan sulfate biosynthesis in ext1-deficient mice. *Dev. Biol.* **2000**, *224*, 299–311. [CrossRef] [PubMed]
33. Shworak, N.W.; Liu, J.; Petros, L.M.; Zhang, L.; Kobayashi, M.; Copeland, N.G.; Jenkins, N.A.; Rosenberg, R.D. Multiple isoforms of heparan sulfate d-glucosaminyl 3-o-sulfotransferase. Isolation, characterization, and expression of human cdnas and identification of distinct genomic loci. *J. Biol. Chem.* **1999**, *274*, 5170–5184. [CrossRef] [PubMed]
34. Shukla, D.; Liu, J.; Blaiklock, P.; Shworak, N.W.; Bai, X.; Esko, J.D.; Cohen, G.H.; Eisenberg, R.J.; Rosenberg, R.D.; Spear, P.G. A novel role for 3-o-sulfated heparan sulfate in herpes simplex virus 1 entry. *Cell* **1999**, *99*, 13–22. [CrossRef]
35. Thunberg, L.; Backstrom, G.; Lindahl, U. Further characterization of the antithrombin-binding sequence in heparin. *Carbohydr. Res.* **1982**, *100*, 393–410. [CrossRef]
36. de Paz, J.L.; Moseman, E.A.; Noti, C.; Polito, L.; von Andrian, U.H.; Seeberger, P.H. Profiling heparin-chemokine interactions using synthetic tools. *ACS Chem. Biol.* **2007**, *2*, 735–744. [CrossRef]
37. Ashikari-Hada, S.; Habuchi, H.; Kariya, Y.; Itoh, N.; Reddi, A.H.; Kimata, K. Characterization of growth factor-binding structures in heparin/heparan sulfate using an octasaccharide library. *J. Biol. Chem.* **2004**, *279*, 12346–12354. [CrossRef]
38. Lindahl, U.; Li, J.P. Interactions between heparan sulfate and proteins-design and functional implications. *Int. Rev. Cell. Mol. Biol.* **2009**, *276*, 105–159.
39. Zhang, X.; Pagadala, V.; Jester, H.M.; Lim, A.M.; Pham, T.Q.; Goulas, A.M.P.; Liu, J.; Linhardt, R.J. Chemoenzymatic synthesis of heparan sulfate and heparin oligosaccharides and nmr analysis: Paving the way to a diverse library for glycobiologists. *Chem. Sci.* **2017**, *8*, 7932–7940. [CrossRef]
40. Yates, E.A.; Rudd, T.R. Recent innovations in the structural analysis of heparin. *Int. J. Cardiol.* **2016**, *212*, S5–S9. [CrossRef]
41. Ludwig, R.J. Therapeutic use of heparin beyond anticoagulation. *Curr. Drug Discov. Technol.* **2009**, *6*, 281–289. [CrossRef]
42. Alban, S. Adverse effects of heparin. *Handb. Exp. Pharmacol.* **2012**, *207*, 211–263.
43. Warkentin, T.E.; Sheppard, J.A.; Horsewood, P.; Simpson, P.J.; Moore, J.C.; Kelton, J.G. Impact of the patient population on the risk for heparin-induced thrombocytopenia. *Blood* **2000**, *96*, 1703–1708. [CrossRef] [PubMed]
44. Andreescu, A.C.; Possidente, C.; Hsieh, M.; Cushman, M. Evaluation of a pharmacy-based surveillance program for heparin-induced thrombocytopenia. *Pharmacotherapy* **2000**, *20*, 974–980. [CrossRef] [PubMed]
45. Jang, I.K.; Hursting, M.J. When heparins promote thrombosis: Review of heparin-induced thrombocytopenia. *Circulation* **2005**, *111*, 2671–2683. [CrossRef] [PubMed]
46. Lanzi, C.; Cassinelli, G. Heparan sulfate mimetics in cancer therapy: The challenge to define structural determinants and the relevance of targets for optimal activity. *Molecules* **2018**, *23*, 2915. [CrossRef] [PubMed]
47. Mohamed, S.; Coombe, D.R. Heparin mimetics: Their therapeutic potential. *Pharmaceuticals (Basel)* **2017**, *10*, 78. [CrossRef] [PubMed]
48. Morla, S. Glycosaminoglycans and glycosaminoglycan mimetics in cancer and inflammation. *Int. J. Mol. Sci.* **2019**, *20*, 1963. [CrossRef]
49. Cassinelli, G.; Zaffaroni, N.; Lanzi, C. The heparanase/heparan sulfate proteoglycan axis: A potential new therapeutic target in sarcomas. *Cancer Lett.* **2016**, *382*, 245–254. [CrossRef]
50. Friand, V.; David, G.; Zimmermann, P. Syntenin and syndecan in the biogenesis of exosomes. *Biol. Cell.* **2015**, *107*, 331–341. [CrossRef]
51. Selkoe, D.J. Cell biology of protein misfolding: The examples of alzheimer's and parkinson's diseases. *Nat. Cell. Biol.* **2004**, *6*, 1054–1061. [CrossRef]
52. Ross, C.A.; Poirier, M.A. Protein aggregation and neurodegenerative disease. *Nat. Med.* **2004**, *10*, S10–S17. [CrossRef] [PubMed]

53. Goedert, M.; Spillantini, M.G.; Davies, S.W. Filamentous nerve cell inclusions in neurodegenerative diseases. *Curr. Opin. Neurobiol.* **1998**, *8*, 619–632. [CrossRef]
54. Holmes, B.B.; DeVos, S.L.; Kfoury, N.; Li, M.; Jacks, R.; Yanamandra, K.; Ouidja, M.O.; Brodsky, F.M.; Marasa, J.; Bagchi, D.P.; et al. Heparan sulfate proteoglycans mediate internalization and propagation of specific proteopathic seeds. *Proc. Natl. Acad. Sci. USA* **2013**, *110*, E3138–E3147. [CrossRef] [PubMed]
55. Grundke-Iqbal, I.; Iqbal, K.; Quinlan, M.; Tung, Y.C.; Zaidi, M.S.; Wisniewski, H.M. Microtubule-associated protein tau. A component of alzheimer paired helical filaments. *J. Biol. Chem.* **1986**, *261*, 6084–6089.
56. Grundke-Iqbal, I.; Iqbal, K.; Tung, Y.C.; Quinlan, M.; Wisniewski, H.M.; Binder, L.I. Abnormal phosphorylation of the microtubule-associated protein tau (tau) in alzheimer cytoskeletal pathology. *Proc. Natl. Acad. Sci. USA* **1986**, *83*, 4913–4917. [CrossRef] [PubMed]
57. Nieto, A.; Correas, I.; Montejo de Garcini, E.; Avila, J. A modified form of microtubule-associated tau protein is the main component of paired helical filaments. *Biochem. Biophys. Res. Commun.* **1988**, *154*, 660–667. [CrossRef]
58. Perez, M.; Valpuesta, J.M.; Medina, M.; Montejo de Garcini, E.; Avila, J. Polymerization of tau into filaments in the presence of heparin: The minimal sequence required for tau-tau interaction. *J. Neurochem.* **1996**, *67*, 1183–1190. [CrossRef]
59. Wood, J.G.; Mirra, S.S.; Pollock, N.J.; Binder, L.I. Neurofibrillary tangles of alzheimer disease share antigenic determinants with the axonal microtubule-associated protein tau (tau). *Proc. Natl. Acad. Sci. USA* **1986**, *83*, 4040–4043. [CrossRef]
60. Sepulveda-Diaz, J.E.; Alavi Naini, S.M.; Huynh, M.B.; Ouidja, M.O.; Yanicostas, C.; Chantepie, S.; Villares, J.; Lamari, F.; Jospin, E.; van Kuppevelt, T.H.; et al. Hs3st2 expression is critical for the abnormal phosphorylation of tau in alzheimer's disease-related tau pathology. *Brain* **2015**, *138*, 1339–1354. [CrossRef]
61. Gupta-Bansal, R.; Frederickson, R.C.; Brunden, K.R. Proteoglycan-mediated inhibition of a beta proteolysis. A potential cause of senile plaque accumulation. *J. Biol. Chem.* **1995**, *270*, 18666–18671. [CrossRef]
62. Sandwall, E.; O'Callaghan, P.; Zhang, X.; Lindahl, U.; Lannfelt, L.; Li, J.P. Heparan sulfate mediates amyloid-beta internalization and cytotoxicity. *Glycobiology* **2010**, *20*, 533–541. [CrossRef] [PubMed]
63. Ancsin, J.B. Amyloidogenesis: Historical and modern observations point to heparan sulfate proteoglycans as a major culprit. *Amyloid* **2003**, *10*, 67–79. [CrossRef] [PubMed]
64. Zcharia, E.; Metzger, S.; Chajek-Shaul, T.; Aingorn, H.; Elkin, M.; Friedmann, Y.; Weinstein, T.; Li, J.P.; Lindahl, U.; Vlodavsky, I. Transgenic expression of mammalian heparanase uncovers physiological functions of heparan sulfate in tissue morphogenesis, vascularization, and feeding behavior. *FASEB J.* **2004**, *18*, 252–263. [CrossRef] [PubMed]
65. Li, J.P.; Galvis, M.L.; Gong, F.; Zhang, X.; Zcharia, E.; Metzger, S.; Vlodavsky, I.; Kisilevsky, R.; Lindahl, U. In vivo fragmentation of heparan sulfate by heparanase overexpression renders mice resistant to amyloid protein a amyloidosis. *Proc. Natl. Acad. Sci. USA* **2005**, *102*, 6473–6477. [CrossRef]
66. Su, J.H.; Cummings, B.J.; Cotman, C.W. Localization of heparan sulfate glycosaminoglycan and proteoglycan core protein in aged brain and alzheimer's disease. *Neuroscience* **1992**, *51*, 801–813. [CrossRef]
67. Scholefield, Z.; Yates, E.A.; Wayne, G.; Amour, A.; McDowell, W.; Turnbull, J.E. Heparan sulfate regulates amyloid precursor protein processing by bace1, the alzheimer's beta-secretase. *J. Cell. Biol.* **2003**, *163*, 97–107. [CrossRef]
68. Alavi Naini, S.M.; Soussi-Yanicostas, N. Heparan sulfate as a therapeutic target in tauopathies: Insights from zebrafish. *Front. Cell. Dev. Biol.* **2018**, *6*, 163. [CrossRef]
69. Ihse, E.; Yamakado, H.; van Wijk, X.M.; Lawrence, R.; Esko, J.D.; Masliah, E. Cellular internalization of alpha-synuclein aggregates by cell surface heparan sulfate depends on aggregate conformation and cell type. *Sci. Rep.* **2017**, *7*, 9008. [CrossRef]
70. Castillo, G.M.; Lukito, W.; Wight, T.N.; Snow, A.D. The sulfate moieties of glycosaminoglycans are critical for the enhancement of beta-amyloid protein fibril formation. *J. Neurochem.* **1999**, *72*, 1681–1687. [CrossRef]
71. Zhang, G.L.; Zhang, X.; Wang, X.M.; Li, J.P. Towards understanding the roles of heparan sulfate proteoglycans in alzheimer's disease. *Biomed. Res. Int.* **2014**, *2014*, 516028. [CrossRef]
72. Zhao, J.; Huvent, I.; Lippens, G.; Eliezer, D.; Zhang, A.; Li, Q.; Tessier, P.; Linhardt, R.J.; Zhang, F.; Wang, C. Glycan determinants of heparin-tau interaction. *Biophys. J.* **2017**, *112*, 921–932. [CrossRef] [PubMed]
73. Koo, E.H.; Squazzo, S.L. Evidence that production and release of amyloid beta-protein involves the endocytic pathway. *J. Biol. Chem.* **1994**, *269*, 17386–17389. [PubMed]

74. Koo, E.H.; Squazzo, S.L.; Selkoe, D.J.; Koo, C.H. Trafficking of cell-surface amyloid beta-protein precursor. I. Secretion, endocytosis and recycling as detected by labeled monoclonal antibody. *J. Cell. Sci.* **1996**, *109*, 991–998. [PubMed]
75. Yamazaki, T.; Koo, E.H.; Selkoe, D.J. Trafficking of cell-surface amyloid beta-protein precursor. Ii. Endocytosis, recycling and lysosomal targeting detected by immunolocalization. *J. Cell. Sci.* **1996**, *109*, 999–1008.
76. Lee, H.J.; Suk, J.E.; Bae, E.J.; Lee, J.H.; Paik, S.R.; Lee, S.J. Assembly-dependent endocytosis and clearance of extracellular alpha-synuclein. *Int. J. Biochem. Cell. Biol.* **2008**, *40*, 1835–1849. [CrossRef]
77. Futerman, A.H.; van Meer, G. The cell biology of lysosomal storage disorders. *Nat. Rev. Mol. Cell. Biol.* **2004**, *5*, 554–565. [CrossRef]
78. Heppner, J.M.; Zaucke, F.; Clarke, L.A. Extracellular matrix disruption is an early event in the pathogenesis of skeletal disease in mucopolysaccharidosis i. *Mol. Genet. Metab.* **2015**, *114*, 146–155. [CrossRef]
79. Young, R.D.; Liskova, P.; Pinali, C.; Palka, B.P.; Palos, M.; Jirsova, K.; Hrdlickova, E.; Tesarova, M.; Elleder, M.; Zeman, J.; et al. Large proteoglycan complexes and disturbed collagen architecture in the corneal extracellular matrix of mucopolysaccharidosis type vii (sly syndrome). *Invest. Ophthalmol. Vis. Sci.* **2011**, *52*, 6720–6728. [CrossRef]
80. Ohmi, K.; Kudo, L.C.; Ryazantsev, S.; Zhao, H.Z.; Karsten, S.L.; Neufeld, E.F. Sanfilippo syndrome type b, a lysosomal storage disease, is also a tauopathy. *Proc. Natl. Acad. Sci. USA* **2009**, *106*, 8332–8337. [CrossRef]
81. Hamano, K.; Hayashi, M.; Shioda, K.; Fukatsu, R.; Mizutani, S. Mechanisms of neurodegeneration in mucopolysaccharidoses ii and iiib: Analysis of human brain tissue. *Acta Neuropathol.* **2008**, *115*, 547–559. [CrossRef]
82. Winder-Rhodes, S.E.; Garcia-Reitbock, P.; Ban, M.; Evans, J.R.; Jacques, T.S.; Kemppinen, A.; Foltynie, T.; Williams-Gray, C.H.; Chinnery, P.F.; Hudson, G.; et al. Genetic and pathological links between parkinson's disease and the lysosomal disorder sanfilippo syndrome. *Mov. Disord.* **2012**, *27*, 312–315. [CrossRef]
83. Beard, H.; Hassiotis, S.; Gai, W.P.; Parkinson-Lawrence, E.; Hopwood, J.J.; Hemsley, K.M. Axonal dystrophy in the brain of mice with sanfilippo syndrome. *Exp. Neurol.* **2017**, *295*, 243–255. [CrossRef] [PubMed]
84. Parker, H.; Bigger, B.W. The role of innate immunity in mucopolysaccharide diseases. *J. Neurochem.* **2019**, *148*, 639–651. [CrossRef] [PubMed]
85. Goyal, D.; Shuaib, S.; Mann, S.; Goyal, B. Rationally designed peptides and peptidomimetics as inhibitors of amyloid-beta (abeta) aggregation: Potential therapeutics of alzheimer's disease. *ACS Comb. Sci.* **2017**, *19*, 55–80. [CrossRef] [PubMed]
86. Valstar, M.J.; Marchal, J.P.; Grootenhuis, M.; Colland, V.; Wijburg, F.A. Cognitive development in patients with mucopolysaccharidosis type iii (sanfilippo syndrome). *Orphanet. J. Rare Dis.* **2011**, *6*, 43. [CrossRef] [PubMed]
87. Bartels, A.L.; Willemsen, A.T.; Kortekaas, R.; de Jong, B.M.; de Vries, R.; de Klerk, O.; van Oostrom, J.C.; Portman, A.; Leenders, K.L. Decreased blood-brain barrier p-glycoprotein function in the progression of parkinson's disease, psp and msa. *J. Neural Transm. (Vienna)* **2008**, *115*, 1001–1009. [CrossRef] [PubMed]
88. Baeten, K.M.; Akassoglou, K. Extracellular matrix and matrix receptors in blood-brain barrier formation and stroke. *Dev. Neurobiol.* **2011**, *71*, 1018–1039. [CrossRef] [PubMed]
89. Kelleher, R.J.; Soiza, R.L. Evidence of endothelial dysfunction in the development of alzheimer's disease: Is alzheimer's a vascular disorder? *Am. J. Cardiovasc. Dis.* **2013**, *3*, 197–226.
90. Wang, P.; Ding, K. Proteoglycans and glycosaminoglycans in misfolded proteins formation in alzheimer's disease. *Protein Pept. Lett.* **2014**, *21*, 1048–1056. [CrossRef]
91. Leveugle, B.; Ding, W.; Laurence, F.; Dehouck, M.P.; Scanameo, A.; Cecchelli, R.; Fillit, H. Heparin oligosaccharides that pass the blood-brain barrier inhibit beta-amyloid precursor protein secretion and heparin binding to beta-amyloid peptide. *J. Neurochem.* **1998**, *70*, 736–744. [CrossRef]
92. Wang, P.; Lo Cascio, F.; Gao, J.; Kayed, R.; Huang, X. Binding and neurotoxicity mitigation of toxic tau oligomers by synthetic heparin like oligosaccharides. *Chem. Commun. (Camb.)* **2018**, *54*, 10120–10123. [CrossRef] [PubMed]
93. Dudas, B.; Cornelli, U.; Lee, J.M.; Hejna, M.J.; Walzer, M.; Lorens, S.A.; Mervis, R.F.; Fareed, J.; Hanin, I. Oral and subcutaneous administration of the glycosaminoglycan c3 attenuates abeta(25-35)-induced abnormal tau protein immunoreactivity in rat brain. *Neurobiol. Aging* **2002**, *23*, 97–104. [CrossRef]

94. Dudas, B.; Rose, M.; Cornelli, U.; Pavlovich, A.; Hanin, I. Neuroprotective properties of glycosaminoglycans: Potential treatment for neurodegenerative disorders. *Neurodegener. Dis.* **2008**, *5*, 200–205. [CrossRef] [PubMed]
95. Dwyer, C.A.; Scudder, S.L.; Lin, Y.; Dozier, L.E.; Phan, D.; Allen, N.J.; Patrick, G.N.; Esko, J.D. Neurodevelopmental changes in excitatory synaptic structure and function in the cerebral cortex of sanfilippo syndrome iiia mice. *Sci. Rep.* **2017**, *7*, 46576. [CrossRef] [PubMed]
96. Scarpa, M.; Orchard, P.J.; Schulz, A.; Dickson, P.I.; Haskins, M.E.; Escolar, M.L.; Giugliani, R. Treatment of brain disease in the mucopolysaccharidoses. *Mol. Genet. Metab.* **2017**, *122S*, 25–34. [CrossRef] [PubMed]
97. Neufeld, E.F. Enzyme replacement therapy—A brief history. In *Fabry Disease: Perspectives from 5 Years of Fos*; Mehta, A., Beck, M., Sunder-Plassmann, G., Eds.; Oxford PharmaGenesis: Oxford, UK, 2006.
98. Kakkis, E.D. Enzyme replacement therapy for the mucopolysaccharide storage disorders. *Expert Opin. Investig. Drugs* **2002**, *11*, 675–685. [CrossRef]
99. Desnick, R.J. Enzyme replacement and enhancement therapies for lysosomal diseases. *J. Inherit. Metab. Dis.* **2004**, *27*, 385–410. [CrossRef]
100. Begley, D.J.; Pontikis, C.C.; Scarpa, M. Lysosomal storage diseases and the blood-brain barrier. *Curr. Pharm. Des.* **2008**, *14*, 1566–1580. [CrossRef]
101. Tardieu, M.; Zerah, M.; Husson, B.; de Bournonville, S.; Deiva, K.; Adamsbaum, C.; Vincent, F.; Hocquemiller, M.; Broissand, C.; Furlan, V.; et al. Intracerebral administration of adeno-associated viral vector serotype rh.10 carrying human sgsh and sumf1 cdnas in children with mucopolysaccharidosis type iiia disease: Results of a phase i/ii trial. *Hum. Gene Ther.* **2014**, *25*, 506–516. [CrossRef]
102. Boado, R.J.; Hui, E.K.; Lu, J.Z.; Pardridge, W.M. Glycemic control and chronic dosing of rhesus monkeys with a fusion protein of iduronidase and a monoclonal antibody against the human insulin receptor. *Drug Metab Dispos* **2012**, *40*, 2021–2025. [CrossRef]
103. Boado, R.J.; Lu, J.Z.; Hui, E.K.; Pardridge, W.M. Insulin receptor antibody-sulfamidase fusion protein penetrates the primate blood-brain barrier and reduces glycosoaminoglycans in sanfilippo type a cells. *Mol. Pharm.* **2014**, *11*, 2928–2934. [CrossRef] [PubMed]
104. Scarpa, M.; Bellettato, C.M.; Lampe, C.; Begley, D.J. Neuronopathic lysosomal storage disorders: Approaches to treat the central nervous system. *Best Pract. Res. Clin. Endocrinol. Metab.* **2015**, *29*, 159–171. [CrossRef] [PubMed]
105. Guffon, N.; Bin-Dorel, S.; Decullier, E.; Paillet, C.; Guitton, J.; Fouilhoux, A. Evaluation of miglustat treatment in patients with type iii mucopolysaccharidosis: A randomized, double-blind, placebo-controlled study. *J. Pediatr.* **2011**, *159*, 838–844 e831. [CrossRef] [PubMed]
106. Schueler, U.H.; Kolter, T.; Kaneski, C.R.; Zirzow, G.C.; Sandhoff, K.; Brady, R.O. Correlation between enzyme activity and substrate storage in a cell culture model system for gaucher disease. *J. Inherit. Metab. Dis.* **2004**, *27*, 649–658. [CrossRef] [PubMed]
107. Krivit, W.; Sung, J.H.; Shapiro, E.G.; Lockman, L.A. Microglia: The effector cell for reconstitution of the central nervous system following bone marrow transplantation for lysosomal and peroxisomal storage diseases. *Cell Transplant.* **1995**, *4*, 385–392. [CrossRef]
108. Pan, C.; Nelson, M.S.; Reyes, M.; Koodie, L.; Brazil, J.J.; Stephenson, E.J.; Zhao, R.C.; Peters, C.; Selleck, S.B.; Stringer, S.E.; et al. Functional abnormalities of heparan sulfate in mucopolysaccharidosis-i are associated with defective biologic activity of fgf-2 on human multipotent progenitor cells. *Blood* **2005**, *106*, 1956–1964. [CrossRef]
109. Holley, R.J.; Deligny, A.; Wei, W.; Watson, H.A.; Ninonuevo, M.R.; Dagalv, A.; Leary, J.A.; Bigger, B.W.; Kjellen, L.; Merry, C.L. Mucopolysaccharidosis type i, unique structure of accumulated heparan sulfate and increased n-sulfotransferase activity in mice lacking alpha-l-iduronidase. *J. Biol. Chem.* **2011**, *286*, 37515–37524. [CrossRef]
110. De Pasquale, V.; Sarogni, P.; Pistorio, V.; Cerulo, G.; Paladino, S.; Pavone, L.M. Targeting heparan sulfate proteoglycans as a novel therapeutic strategy for mucopolysaccharidoses. *Mol. Ther. Methods Clin. Dev.* **2018**, *10*, 8–16. [CrossRef]
111. Ilan, N.; Shteingauz, A.; Vlodavsky, I. Function from within: Autophagy induction by hpse/heparanase–new possibilities for intervention. *Autophagy* **2015**, *11*, 2387–2389. [CrossRef]
112. Weissmann, M.; Bhattacharya, U.; Feld, S.; Hammond, E.; Ilan, N.; Vlodavsky, I. The heparanase inhibitor pg545 is a potent anti-lymphoma drug: Mode of action. *Matrix Biol.* **2019**, *77*, 58–72. [CrossRef]

113. Lau, A.A.; King, B.M.; Thorsen, C.L.; Hassiotis, S.; Beard, H.; Trim, P.J.; Whyte, L.S.; Tamang, S.J.; Duplock, S.K.; Snel, M.F.; et al. A novel conditional sgsh knockout mouse model recapitulates phenotypic and neuropathic deficits of sanfilippo syndrome. *J. Inherit. Metab. Dis.* **2017**, *40*, 715–724. [CrossRef] [PubMed]
114. Hull, E.E.; Montgomery, M.R.; Leyva, K.J. Epigenetic regulation of the biosynthesis & enzymatic modification of heparan sulfate proteoglycans: Implications for tumorigenesis and cancer biomarkers. *Int. J. Mol. Sci.* **2017**, *18*, 1361.
115. Zhang, Q.J.; Wan, L.; Xu, H.F. High expression of agrin is associated with tumor progression and poor prognosis in hepatocellular carcinoma. *Math. Biosci. Eng.* **2019**, *16*, 7375–7383. [CrossRef] [PubMed]
116. Melo, S.A.; Luecke, L.B.; Kahlert, C.; Fernandez, A.F.; Gammon, S.T.; Kaye, J.; LeBleu, V.S.; Mittendorf, E.A.; Weitz, J.; Rahbari, N.; et al. Glypican-1 identifies cancer exosomes and detects early pancreatic cancer. *Nature* **2015**, *523*, 177–182. [CrossRef] [PubMed]
117. Theocharis, A.D.; Karamanos, N.K. Proteoglycans remodeling in cancer: Underlying molecular mechanisms. *Matrix Biol.* **2019**, *75–76*, 220–259. [CrossRef]
118. Beauvais, D.M.; Ell, B.J.; McWhorter, A.R.; Rapraeger, A.C. Syndecan-1 regulates alphavbeta3 and alphavbeta5 integrin activation during angiogenesis and is blocked by synstatin, a novel peptide inhibitor. *J. Exp. Med.* **2009**, *206*, 691–705. [CrossRef]
119. De Rossi, G.; Evans, A.R.; Kay, E.; Woodfin, A.; McKay, T.R.; Nourshargh, S.; Whiteford, J.R. Shed syndecan-2 inhibits angiogenesis. *J. Cell. Sci.* **2014**, *127*, 4788–4799. [CrossRef]
120. Huang, G.; Ge, G.; Izzi, V.; Greenspan, D.S. Alpha3 chains of type v collagen regulate breast tumour growth via glypican-1. *Nat. Commun.* **2017**, *8*, 14351. [CrossRef]
121. Baba, F.; Swartz, K.; van Buren, R.; Eickhoff, J.; Zhang, Y.; Wolberg, W.; Friedl, A. Syndecan-1 and syndecan-4 are overexpressed in an estrogen receptor-negative, highly proliferative breast carcinoma subtype. *Breast Cancer Res. Treat.* **2006**, *98*, 91–98. [CrossRef]
122. Xiang, Y.Y.; Ladeda, V.; Filmus, J. Glypican-3 expression is silenced in human breast cancer. *Oncogene* **2001**, *20*, 7408–7412. [CrossRef]
123. Han, S.; Ma, X.; Zhao, Y.; Zhao, H.; Batista, A.; Zhou, S.; Zhou, X.; Yang, Y.; Wang, T.; Bi, J.; et al. Identification of glypican-3 as a potential metastasis suppressor gene in gastric cancer. *Oncotarget* **2016**, *7*, 44406–44416. [CrossRef] [PubMed]
124. Moek, K.L.; Fehrmann, R.S.N.; van der Vegt, B.; de Vries, E.G.E.; de Groot, D.J.A. Glypican 3 overexpression across a broad spectrum of tumor types discovered with functional genomic mrna profiling of a large cancer database. *Am. J. Pathol.* **2018**, *188*, 1973–1981. [CrossRef] [PubMed]
125. Li, Y.; Miao, L.; Cai, H.; Ding, J.; Xiao, Y.; Yang, J.; Zhang, D. The overexpression of glypican-5 promotes cancer cell migration and is associated with shorter overall survival in non-small cell lung cancer. *Oncol. Lett.* **2013**, *6*, 1565–1572. [CrossRef] [PubMed]
126. Pinho, S.S.; Reis, C.A. Glycosylation in cancer: Mechanisms and clinical implications. *Nat. Rev. Cancer* **2015**, *15*, 540–555. [CrossRef] [PubMed]
127. Lemjabbar-Alaoui, H.; McKinney, A.; Yang, Y.W.; Tran, V.M.; Phillips, J.J. Glycosylation alterations in lung and brain cancer. *Adv. Cancer Res.* **2015**, *126*, 305–344.
128. Lanzi, C.; Zaffaroni, N.; Cassinelli, G. Targeting heparan sulfate proteoglycans and their modifying enzymes to enhance anticancer chemotherapy efficacy and overcome drug resistance. *Curr. Med. Chem.* **2017**, *24*, 2860–2886. [CrossRef]
129. Subbarayan, K.; Seliger, B. Tumor-dependent effects of proteoglycans and various glycosaminoglycan synthesizing enzymes and sulfotransferases on patients' outcome. *Curr. Cancer Drug Targets* **2019**, *19*, 210–221. [CrossRef]
130. Barkeer, S.; Chugh, S.; Karmakar, S.; Kaushik, G.; Rauth, S.; Rachagani, S.; Batra, S.K.; Ponnusamy, M.P. Novel role of o-glycosyltransferases galnt3 and b3gnt3 in the self-renewal of pancreatic cancer stem cells. *BMC Cancer* **2018**, *18*, 1157. [CrossRef]
131. Fux, L.; Ilan, N.; Sanderson, R.D.; Vlodavsky, I. Heparanase: Busy at the cell surface. *Trends Biochem. Sci.* **2009**, *34*, 511–519. [CrossRef]
132. Nadir, Y.; Brenner, B. Heparanase multiple effects in cancer. *Thromb Res.* **2014**, *133*, S90–S94. [CrossRef]
133. Vlodavsky, I.; Gross-Cohen, M.; Weissmann, M.; Ilan, N.; Sanderson, R.D. Opposing functions of heparanase-1 and heparanase-2 in cancer progression. *Trends Biochem. Sci.* **2018**, *43*, 18–31. [CrossRef] [PubMed]

134. Vlodavsky, I.; Singh, P.; Boyango, I.; Gutter-Kapon, L.; Elkin, M.; Sanderson, R.D.; Ilan, N. Heparanase: From basic research to therapeutic applications in cancer and inflammation. *Drug Resist. Updat.* **2016**, *29*, 54–75. [CrossRef] [PubMed]
135. He, Y.Q.; Sutcliffe, E.L.; Bunting, K.L.; Li, J.; Goodall, K.J.; Poon, I.K.; Hulett, M.D.; Freeman, C.; Zafar, A.; McInnes, R.L.; et al. The endoglycosidase heparanase enters the nucleus of t lymphocytes and modulates h3 methylation at actively transcribed genes via the interplay with key chromatin modifying enzymes. *Transcription* **2012**, *3*, 130–145. [CrossRef] [PubMed]
136. Dvir, R.; Vlodavsky, I.; Ilan, N.; Bitan, M.; Issacov, J.; Elhasid, R. Heparanase expression in langerhans cell histiocytosis. *Pediatr. Blood Cancer* **2014**, *61*, 1883–1885. [CrossRef]
137. Li, J.; Li, J.P.; Zhang, X.; Lu, Z.; Yu, S.P.; Wei, L. Expression of heparanase in vascular cells and astrocytes of the mouse brain after focal cerebral ischemia. *Brain Res.* **2012**, *1433*, 137–144. [CrossRef]
138. Ginath, S.; Lurie, S.; Golan, A.; Amsterdam, A.; Sandbank, J.; Sadan, O.; Kovo, M. The expression of heparanase in normal and preeclamptic placentas. *J. Matern. Fetal Neonatal Med.* **2015**, *28*, 1589–1593. [CrossRef]
139. Wang, Y.Y.; Zhou, R.; Zhou, B.; Wang, T.; Zhang, L.; Luo, D. Overexpression of heparanase is associated with preeclampsia by inhibiting invasion of trophocytes. *Int. J. Clin. Exp. Med.* **2015**, *8*, 18107–18114.
140. Sela, S.; Natanson-Yaron, S.; Zcharia, E.; Vlodavsky, I.; Yagel, S.; Keshet, E. Local retention versus systemic release of soluble vegf receptor-1 are mediated by heparin-binding and regulated by heparanase. *Circ. Res.* **2011**, *108*, 1063–1070. [CrossRef]
141. Ihrcke, N.S.; Parker, W.; Reissner, K.J.; Platt, J.L. Regulation of platelet heparanase during inflammation: Role of ph and proteinases. *J. Cell. Physiol.* **1998**, *175*, 255–267. [CrossRef]
142. Bashkin, P.; Razin, E.; Eldor, A.; Vlodavsky, I. Degranulating mast cells secrete an endoglycosidase that degrades heparan sulfate in subendothelial extracellular matrix. *Blood* **1990**, *75*, 2204–2212. [CrossRef]
143. Vlodavsky, I.; Eldor, A.; Haimovitz-Friedman, A.; Matzner, Y.; Ishai-Michaeli, R.; Lider, O.; Naparstek, Y.; Cohen, I.R.; Fuks, Z. Expression of heparanase by platelets and circulating cells of the immune system: Possible involvement in diapedesis and extravasation. *Invasion Metastasis* **1992**, *12*, 112–127. [PubMed]
144. Farrugia, B.L.; Lord, M.S.; Melrose, J.; Whitelock, J.M. The role of heparan sulfate in inflammation, and the development of biomimetics as anti-inflammatory strategies. *J. Histochem. Cytochem.* **2018**, *66*, 321–336. [CrossRef]
145. Sasaki, N.; Higashi, N.; Taka, T.; Nakajima, M.; Irimura, T. Cell surface localization of heparanase on macrophages regulates degradation of extracellular matrix heparan sulfate. *J. Immunol.* **2004**, *172*, 3830–3835. [CrossRef] [PubMed]
146. Gutter-Kapon, L.; Alishekevitz, D.; Shaked, Y.; Li, J.P.; Aronheim, A.; Ilan, N.; Vlodavsky, I. Heparanase is required for activation and function of macrophages. *Proc. Natl. Acad. Sci. USA* **2016**, *113*, E7808–E7817. [CrossRef] [PubMed]
147. Theodoro, T.R.; de Matos, L.L.; Sant Anna, A.V.; Fonseca, F.L.; Semedo, P.; Martins, L.C.; Nader, H.B.; Del Giglio, A.; da Silva Pinhal, M.A. Heparanase expression in circulating lymphocytes of breast cancer patients depends on the presence of the primary tumor and/or systemic metastasis. *Neoplasia* **2007**, *9*, 504–510. [CrossRef] [PubMed]
148. Theodoro, T.R.; Matos, L.L.; Cavalheiro, R.P.; Justo, G.Z.; Nader, H.B.; Pinhal, M.A.S. Crosstalk between tumor cells and lymphocytes modulates heparanase expression. *J. Transl. Med.* **2019**, *17*, 103. [CrossRef]
149. Thompson, C.A.; Purushothaman, A.; Ramani, V.C.; Vlodavsky, I.; Sanderson, R.D. Heparanase regulates secretion, composition, and function of tumor cell-derived exosomes. *J. Biol. Chem.* **2013**, *288*, 10093–10099. [CrossRef]
150. Bandari, S.K.; Purushothaman, A.; Ramani, V.C.; Brinkley, G.J.; Chandrashekar, D.S.; Varambally, S.; Mobley, J.A.; Zhang, Y.; Brown, E.E.; Vlodavsky, I.; et al. Chemotherapy induces secretion of exosomes loaded with heparanase that degrades extracellular matrix and impacts tumor and host cell behavior. *Matrix Biol.* **2018**, *65*, 104–118. [CrossRef]
151. Purushothaman, A.; Uyama, T.; Kobayashi, F.; Yamada, S.; Sugahara, K.; Rapraeger, A.C.; Sanderson, R.D. Heparanase-enhanced shedding of syndecan-1 by myeloma cells promotes endothelial invasion and angiogenesis. *Blood* **2010**, *115*, 2449–2457. [CrossRef]

152. Voigtlaender, M.; Langer, F. Low-molecular-weight heparin in cancer patients: Overview and indications. *Hamostaseologie* **2019**, *39*, 67–75. [CrossRef]
153. Smorenburg, S.M.; Hettiarachchi, R.J.; Vink, R.; Buller, H.R. The effects of unfractionated heparin on survival in patients with malignancy–a systematic review. *Thromb. Haemost.* **1999**, *82*, 1600–1604. [PubMed]
154. Kakkar, A.K. Thrombosis and cancer. *Hematol. J.* **2004**, *5*, S20–S23. [CrossRef] [PubMed]
155. Kuderer, N.M.; Ortel, T.L.; Francis, C.W. Impact of venous thromboembolism and anticoagulation on cancer and cancer survival. *J. Clin. Oncol.* **2009**, *27*, 4902–4911. [CrossRef] [PubMed]
156. Lyman, G.H.; Bohlke, K.; Khorana, A.A.; Kuderer, N.M.; Lee, A.Y.; Arcelus, J.I.; Balaban, E.P.; Clarke, J.M.; Flowers, C.R.; Francis, C.W.; et al. Venous thromboembolism prophylaxis and treatment in patients with cancer: American society of clinical oncology clinical practice guideline update 2014. *J. Clin. Oncol.* **2015**, *33*, 654–656. [CrossRef]
157. Garcia-Escobar, I.; Beato-Zambrano, C.; Munoz Langa, J.; Brozos Vazquez, E.; Obispo Portero, B.; Gutierrez-Abad, D.; Munoz Martin, A.J.; Cancer and Thrombosis Working Group of the Spanish Society of Medical Oncology (SEOM). Pleiotropic effects of heparins: Does anticoagulant treatment increase survival in cancer patients? *Clin. Transl. Oncol.* **2018**, *20*, 1097–1108. [CrossRef]
158. Borsig, L. Heparin as an inhibitor of cancer progression. *Prog. Mol. Biol. Transl. Sci.* **2010**, *93*, 335–349.
159. Bobek, V.; Kovarik, J. Antitumor and antimetastatic effect of warfarin and heparins. *Biomed. Pharmacother.* **2004**, *58*, 213–219. [CrossRef]
160. Ilan, N.; Elkin, M.; Vlodavsky, I. Regulation, function and clinical significance of heparanase in cancer metastasis and angiogenesis. *Int. J. Biochem. Cell. Biol.* **2006**, *38*, 2018–2039. [CrossRef]
161. Vreys, V.; David, G. Mammalian heparanase: What is the message? *J. Cell. Mol. Med.* **2007**, *11*, 427–452. [CrossRef]
162. Vlodavsky, I.; Ilan, N.; Naggi, A.; Casu, B. Heparanase: Structure, biological functions, and inhibition by heparin-derived mimetics of heparan sulfate. *Curr. Pharm. Des.* **2007**, *13*, 2057–2073. [CrossRef]
163. Hammond, E.; Khurana, A.; Shridhar, V.; Dredge, K. The role of heparanase and sulfatases in the modification of heparan sulfate proteoglycans within the tumor microenvironment and opportunities for novel cancer therapeutics. *Front. Oncol.* **2014**, *4*, 195. [CrossRef] [PubMed]
164. Vlodavsky, I.; Beckhove, P.; Lerner, I.; Pisano, C.; Meirovitz, A.; Ilan, N.; Elkin, M. Significance of heparanase in cancer and inflammation. *Cancer Microenviron.* **2012**, *5*, 115–132. [CrossRef] [PubMed]
165. Jia, L.; Ma, S. Recent advances in the discovery of heparanase inhibitors as anti-cancer agents. *Eur. J. Med. Chem.* **2016**, *121*, 209–220. [CrossRef] [PubMed]
166. Pisano, C.; Vlodavsky, I.; Ilan, N.; Zunino, F. The potential of heparanase as a therapeutic target in cancer. *Biochem. Pharmacol.* **2014**, *89*, 12–19. [CrossRef] [PubMed]
167. Bar-Ner, M.; Eldor, A.; Wasserman, L.; Matzner, Y.; Cohen, I.R.; Fuks, Z.; Vlodavsky, I. Inhibition of heparanase-mediated degradation of extracellular matrix heparan sulfate by non-anticoagulant heparin species. *Blood* **1987**, *70*, 551–557. [CrossRef] [PubMed]
168. Cassinelli, G.; Dal Bo, L.; Favini, E.; Cominetti, D.; Pozzi, S.; Tortoreto, M.; De Cesare, M.; Lecis, D.; Scanziani, E.; Minoli, L.; et al. Supersulfated low-molecular weight heparin synergizes with igf1r/ir inhibitor to suppress synovial sarcoma growth and metastases. *Cancer Lett.* **2018**, *415*, 187–197. [CrossRef]
169. Poli, M.; Asperti, M.; Ruzzenenti, P.; Mandelli, L.; Campostrini, N.; Martini, G.; Di Somma, M.; Maccarinelli, F.; Girelli, D.; Naggi, A.; et al. Oversulfated heparins with low anticoagulant activity are strong and fast inhibitors of hepcidin expression in vitro and in vivo. *Biochem. Pharmacol.* **2014**, *92*, 467–475. [CrossRef]
170. Mohan, C.D.; Hari, S.; Preetham, H.D.; Rangappa, S.; Barash, U.; Ilan, N.; Nayak, S.C.; Gupta, V.K.; Basappa, B.; Vlodavsky, I.; et al. Targeting heparanase in cancer: Inhibition by synthetic, chemically modified, and natural compounds. *iScience* **2019**, *15*, 360–390. [CrossRef]
171. MacDonald, A.; Priess, M.; Curran, J.; Guess, J.; Farutin, V.; Oosterom, I.; Chu, C.L.; Cochran, E.; Zhang, L.; Getchell, K.; et al. Necuparanib, a multitargeting heparan sulfate mimetic, targets tumor and stromal compartments in pancreatic cancer. *Mol. Cancer Ther.* **2019**, *18*, 245–256. [CrossRef]
172. Boothello, R.S.; Patel, N.J.; Sharon, C.; Abdelfadiel, E.I.; Morla, S.; Brophy, D.F.; Lippman, H.R.; Desai, U.R.; Patel, B.B. A unique nonsaccharide mimetic of heparin hexasaccharide inhibits colon cancer stem cells via p38 map kinase activation. *Mol. Cancer Ther.* **2019**, *18*, 51–61. [CrossRef]

173. Joyce, J.A.; Freeman, C.; Meyer-Morse, N.; Parish, C.R.; Hanahan, D. A functional heparan sulfate mimetic implicates both heparanase and heparan sulfate in tumor angiogenesis and invasion in a mouse model of multistage cancer. *Oncogene* **2005**, *24*, 4037–4051. [CrossRef] [PubMed]
174. Arvatz, G.; Weissmann, M.; Ilan, N.; Vlodavsky, I. Heparanase and cancer progression: New directions, new promises. *Hum. Vaccin. Immunother.* **2016**, *12*, 2253–2256. [CrossRef] [PubMed]
175. Weissmann, M.; Arvatz, G.; Horowitz, N.; Feld, S.; Naroditsky, I.; Zhang, Y.; Ng, M.; Hammond, E.; Nevo, E.; Vlodavsky, I.; et al. Heparanase-neutralizing antibodies attenuate lymphoma tumor growth and metastasis. *Proc. Natl. Acad. Sci. USA* **2016**, *113*, 704–709. [CrossRef] [PubMed]
176. Yoshitomi, Y.; Nakanishi, H.; Kusano, Y.; Munesue, S.; Oguri, K.; Tatematsu, M.; Yamashina, I.; Okayama, M. Inhibition of experimental lung metastases of lewis lung carcinoma cells by chemically modified heparin with reduced anticoagulant activity. *Cancer Lett.* **2004**, *207*, 165–174. [CrossRef]
177. Pisano, C.; Aulicino, C.; Vesci, L.; Casu, B.; Naggi, A.; Torri, G.; Ribatti, D.; Belleri, M.; Rusnati, M.; Presta, M. Undersulfated, low-molecular-weight glycol-split heparin as an antiangiogenic vegf antagonist. *Glycobiology* **2005**, *15*, 1C–6C. [CrossRef]
178. Naggi, A.; Casu, B.; Perez, M.; Torri, G.; Cassinelli, G.; Penco, S.; Pisano, C.; Giannini, G.; Ishai-Michaeli, R.; Vlodavsky, I. Modulation of the heparanase-inhibiting activity of heparin through selective desulfation, graded n-acetylation, and glycol splitting. *J. Biol. Chem.* **2005**, *280*, 12103–12113. [CrossRef]
179. Cassinelli, G.; Lanzi, C.; Tortoreto, M.; Cominetti, D.; Petrangolini, G.; Favini, E.; Zaffaroni, N.; Pisano, C.; Penco, S.; Vlodavsky, I.; et al. Antitumor efficacy of the heparanase inhibitor sst0001 alone and in combination with antiangiogenic agents in the treatment of human pediatric sarcoma models. *Biochem. Pharmacol.* **2013**, *85*, 1424–1432. [CrossRef]
180. Ritchie, J.P.; Ramani, V.C.; Ren, Y.; Naggi, A.; Torri, G.; Casu, B.; Penco, S.; Pisano, C.; Carminati, P.; Tortoreto, M.; et al. Sst0001, a chemically modified heparin, inhibits myeloma growth and angiogenesis via disruption of the heparanase/syndecan-1 axis. *Clin. Cancer Res.* **2011**, *17*, 1382–1393. [CrossRef]
181. Karoli, T.; Liu, L.; Fairweather, J.K.; Hammond, E.; Li, C.P.; Cochran, S.; Bergefall, K.; Trybala, E.; Addison, R.S.; Ferro, V. Synthesis, biological activity, and preliminary pharmacokinetic evaluation of analogues of a phosphosulfomannan angiogenesis inhibitor (pi-88). *J. Med. Chem.* **2005**, *48*, 8229–8236. [CrossRef]
182. Kuhnast, B.; El Hadri, A.; Boisgard, R.; Hinnen, F.; Richard, S.; Caravano, A.; Nancy-Portebois, V.; Petitou, M.; Tavitian, B.; Dolle, F. Synthesis, radiolabeling with fluorine-18 and preliminary in vivo evaluation of a heparan sulphate mimetic as potent angiogenesis and heparanase inhibitor for cancer applications. *Org. Biomol. Chem.* **2016**, *14*, 1915–1920. [CrossRef]
183. Lim, T.C.; Cai, S.; Huber, R.G.; Bond, P.J.; Siew Chia, P.X.; Khou, S.L.; Gao, S.; Lee, S.S.; Lee, S.G. Facile saccharide-free mimetics that recapitulate key features of glycosaminoglycan sulfation patterns. *Chem. Sci.* **2018**, *9*, 7940–7947. [CrossRef] [PubMed]
184. Vornicova, O.; Boyango, I.; Feld, S.; Naroditsky, I.; Kazarin, O.; Zohar, Y.; Tiram, Y.; Ilan, N.; Ben-Izhak, O.; Vlodavsky, I.; et al. The prognostic significance of heparanase expression in metastatic melanoma. *Oncotarget* **2016**, *7*, 74678–74685. [CrossRef] [PubMed]
185. Vornicova, O.; Naroditsky, I.; Boyango, I.; Shachar, S.S.; Mashiach, T.; Ilan, N.; Vlodavsky, I.; Bar-Sela, G. Prognostic significance of heparanase expression in primary and metastatic breast carcinoma. *Oncotarget* **2018**, *9*, 6238–6244. [CrossRef] [PubMed]
186. Lazo-Langner, A.; Goss, G.D.; Spaans, J.N.; Rodger, M.A. The effect of low-molecular-weight heparin on cancer survival. A systematic review and meta-analysis of randomized trials. *J. Thromb. Haemost.* **2007**, *5*, 729–737. [CrossRef] [PubMed]
187. Kuderer, N.M.; Khorana, A.A.; Lyman, G.H.; Francis, C.W. A meta-analysis and systematic review of the efficacy and safety of anticoagulants as cancer treatment: Impact on survival and bleeding complications. *Cancer* **2007**, *110*, 1149–1161. [CrossRef]
188. Galli, M.; Chatterjee, M.; Grasso, M.; Specchia, G.; Magen, H.; Einsele, H.; Celeghini, I.; Barbieri, P.; Paoletti, D.; Pace, S.; et al. Phase i study of the heparanase inhibitor roneparstat: An innovative approach for ultiple myeloma therapy. *Haematologica* **2018**, *103*, e469–e472. [CrossRef]
189. Vande Broek, I.; Vanderkerken, K.; Van Camp, B.; Van Riet, I. Extravasation and homing mechanisms in multiple myeloma. *Clin. Exp. Metastasis* **2008**, *25*, 325–334. [CrossRef]
190. Ramani, V.C.; Zhan, F.; He, J.; Barbieri, P.; Noseda, A.; Tricot, G.; Sanderson, R.D. Targeting heparanase overcomes chemoresistance and diminishes relapse in myeloma. *Oncotarget* **2016**, *7*, 1598–1607. [CrossRef]

191. Dredge, K.; Hammond, E.; Davis, K.; Li, C.P.; Liu, L.; Johnstone, K.; Handley, P.; Wimmer, N.; Gonda, T.J.; Gautam, A.; et al. The pg500 series: Novel heparan sulfate mimetics as potent angiogenesis and heparanase inhibitors for cancer therapy. *Invest. New Drugs* **2010**, *28*, 276–283. [CrossRef]
192. Dredge, K.; Brennan, T.V.; Hammond, E.; Lickliter, J.D.; Lin, L.; Bampton, D.; Handley, P.; Lankesheer, F.; Morrish, G.; Yang, Y.; et al. A phase i study of the novel immunomodulatory agent pg545 (pixatimod) in subjects with advanced solid tumours. *Br. J. Cancer* **2018**, *118*, 1035–1041. [CrossRef]

4

Application of Heparin Affinity Chromatography to Produce a Differential Vaccine without Eliciting Antibodies against the Nonstructural Proteins of the Serotype O Foot-and-Mouth Disease Viruses

Sun Young Park [1,2,†], Jung-Min Lee [1,†], Ah-Young Kim [1], Sang Hyun Park [1], Jae-Seok Kim [1], Hyejin Kim [1,2], Jung-Won Park [1], Jong-Hyeon Park [1], Young-Joon Ko [1,*] and Choi-Kyu Park [2,*]

1 Animal and Plant Quarantine Agency, 177 Hyeoksin-8-ro, Gimcheon-si 39660, Gyeongsangbuk-do, Korea; sun3730@korea.kr (S.Y.P.); wjdalslee@korea.kr (J.-M.L.); mochsha@korea.kr (A.-Y.K.); shpark0205@korea.kr (S.H.P.); kimjs0728@korea.kr (J.-S.K.); hyejin86@korea.kr (H.K.); parkjw6254@korea.kr (J.-W.P.); parkjhvet@korea.kr (J.-H.P.)

2 Animal Disease Intervention Center, College of Veterinary Medicine, Kyungpook National University, Daegu 41566, Gyeongsangbuk-do, Korea

* Correspondence: koyoungjoon@korea.kr (Y.-J.K.); parkck@knu.ac.kr (C.-K.P.);

† These authors contributed equally to this work.

Academic Editor: Heidi Drummer

Abstract: Although polyethylene glycol (PEG) application is the most widely used method in removing nonstructural proteins (NSPs) for foot-and-mouth disease (FMD) vaccine production, some NSPs remaining in the antigen could elicit antibodies against these proteins after repeated vaccinations in livestock. Therefore, the purpose of this study was to purify the FMD virus (FMDV) via affinity chromatography using a heparin ligand to remove most proteins, including NSPs. Chromatography showed an intact virus (146S) particle recovery of 70% or more for three different strains of serotype O FMDV (two locally isolated strains and one genetically modified strain). The experimental vaccine made with antigens eluted via heparin affinity chromatography elicited virus-neutralizing antibodies against homologous viruses but did not induce antibodies against NSPs even after five immunizations in goats; this indicated that the NSPs were effectively removed from the vaccine antigen. This method can then be used to produce a higher-quality vaccine compared with PEG application in terms of the purity of the FMD vaccine. Therefore, this result would be an important groundwork for advanced FMD vaccine manufacturing in the near future.

Keywords: foot-and-mouth disease virus; vaccine; nonstructural protein; purification; chromatography

1. Introduction

Foot-and-mouth disease (FMD) is a highly contagious vesicular disease affecting cloven-hoofed animals and often causes enormous economic loss in the livestock industry [1].

The FMD virus (FMDV), the causative agent of FMD, belongs to the *Aphthovirus* genus of the *Picornaviridae* family [2]. It has a positive-sense, single-stranded RNA genome that is translated into a polyprotein, which is further cleaved into structural proteins (SPs) and nonstructural proteins (NSPs) [3–5].

The Republic of Korea has experienced 11 FMD outbreaks since 2000 [6]. To prevent annual outbreaks, the Korean government implemented a nationwide vaccination policy after an extensive

FMD outbreak during 2010–2011. It has imported FMD vaccines annually from Argentina, the UK, and Russia and has therefore set out to develop a domestic FMD vaccine using local virus isolates [7].

Unlike other animal vaccines, a virus purification step should be included in FMD vaccine production to remove NSPs. Since NSP antibodies are only detected in animals infected with FMDV, it is considered an indicator to differentiate between FMDV naturally infected and vaccinated animals. Therefore, only high-purity FMD vaccines without NSP could allow differential diagnosis of FMD to monitor virus circulation. Although polyethylene glycol (PEG) application is the most widely used method in removing NSPs for FMD vaccine production, some NSPs left in the antigen, made using this method, could elicit NSP antibodies after repeated vaccination in animals [8,9]. In addition, we reported that NSPs could be efficiently removed by chloroform [10]. However, this method does not purify the FMDV, and many proteins derived from cells are left in the samples. Unwanted cellular protein contaminants can cause an allergic reaction in animals after multiple vaccinations [11].

In this regard, we attempted to purify the FMDV via affinity chromatography with high purity using a heparin ligand. The FMDV has been reported to be recognized by two classes of receptors, i.e., integrin and heparan sulfate. Integrin is mainly employed when FMDV infect the animals and interact with the Arg-Gly-Asp (RGD) sequence in the GH loop of the FMDV VP1 region [12,13]. However, under the conditions of adapted cell culture, FMDV obtains the ability to utilize heparan sulfate as its receptor [12]. Heparan sulfates are negatively charged disaccharide repeating polymers of iduronic acid and glucosamine [14]. They are found as the carbohydrate component of many proteins called heparan sulfate proteoglycans. The heparan sulfate receptor binding site is located 15 Å away from the RGD motif in the reduced conformation of the FMDV [14]. In the production of FMD vaccine antigens, FMDV is cultured in baby hamster kidney 21 (BHK-21) cells, thus has an affinity for heparin that is structurally similar to heparan sulfate receptor.

Therefore, the purpose of this study was to purify FMDV by heparin affinity chromatography without nonessential proteins, including NSPs, and the purity of the FMD vaccine prepared with purified FMDV was verified by evaluating NSP antibodies after repeated immunization in goats.

2. Materials and Methods

2.1. Ethic Statement

The animal experiments in this study were approved by the Institutional Animal Care and Use Committee (IACUC) and conducted in appliance with the guidelines of laboratory animal welfare and ethic of the animals in the Animal and Plant Quarantine Agency in Republic of Korea (IACUC Approval No. 2020-542, Project identification No. 2020-428).

2.2. Cells and Viruses

BHK-21 suspension cells were developed from the original adherent cell line, BHK-21 (C-13) (ATCC, Manassas, VA, USA) by the Animal and Plant Quarantine Agency and the Korea Research Institute of Bioscience & Biotechnology for use in suspension culture with serum-free media [15]. ProVero™ 1 cell culture medium (Lonza, Basel, Switzerland), a serum-free cell culture medium, was used to culture the BHK-21 suspension cells by incubation at 110 rpm in a shaking incubator at 37 °C with 5% CO_2. In this study, three different strains of serotype O FMDV were used. Two strains were domestic isolates called FMDV O/Boeun/SKR/2017 and FMDV O Jincheon/SKR/2014. The other strain was a genetically engineered virus called the FMDV Om-O-PanAsia2 recombinant strain that was made from a recombination of the backbone region of the O1 Manisa/Turkey/69 strain with the P1 region only being replaced by the O PAK/44/2008 strain [16].

2.3. Virus Propagation

The BHK-21 suspension cells started to grow at a seeding density of 3×10^5 cells/mL and reached at least 1.5×10^6 cells/mL within 72 h. The serotype O FMDV strains were inoculated into the BHK-21 suspension cells (3×10^6 cells/mL) at a multiplicity of infection of 0.001 on a shaking platform in an incubator at 37 °C with 5% CO_2. Viruses were harvested at 16 h post-infection and clarified by centrifugation at 3000× *g* for 20 min at 4 °C to remove cell debris. Binary ethylenimine (BEI; Sigma-Aldrich, St. Louis, MO, USA) was added at 3 mM to the virus culture supernatant to inactivate the FMDV, and the mixture was incubated at 100 rpm for 28 h at 26 °C. Subsequently, the BEI was neutralized by adding 1 M sodium thiosulfate (Daejung Chemicals & Metals, Siheung, Korea) at a final concentration of 2% (*v*/*v*).

2.4. Heparin Affinity Chromatography

The AKTA Pure 150 fast protein liquid chromatography system (GE Healthcare, Uppsala, Sweden) connected to a fraction collector F9-R (GE Healthcare) was used for the liquid chromatography experiments. The chromatography system was controlled using AKTA Explorer via the Unicon version 6.4 program (GE Healthcare). Prior to column purification, the inactivated FMDV supernatant was concentrated 10-fold and exchanged with a column binding buffer (20 mM Tris-HCl, 300 mM KCl, pH 7.6) for desalting using a 10-kDa cutoff Centricon Plus-70 centrifugal unit (Merck Millipore, Billerica, MA, USA). The three strains of serotype O FMDV culture supernatant was loaded onto a HiTrap HP Heparin column (7 mm × 25 mm, column volume [CV] = 1.0 mL, GE Healthcare) at a flow rate of 1.0 mL/min. Before sample loading, the column was equilibrated with binding buffer. After loading the 2 CV of the sample, 10 CV of binding buffer was flowed through the column to wash out the remaining unbound proteins. The flow-through and washing fractions containing proteins unbound to the heparin ligand were collected to determine the recovery rates of the FMDV and total protein contents. The FMDV adsorbed on the heparin ligand was gradient-eluted with a binding buffer containing 0.3–1 M KCl. The samples were traced by UV monitoring at 280 nm and collected from the peak fraction during the elution step were pooled and stored at −70 °C until use.

2.5. Total Protein Assay

The BCA protein assay kit (Thermo Fisher Scientific, Waltham, MA, USA) was used to measure the total proteins in each sample. The total protein content was measured in accordance with the manufacturer's instructions with bovine serum albumin as a standard, and the absorbance was read at 562 nm.

2.6. Quantification of FMDV Particles (146S)

The samples (virus supernatant and flow-through/elution fraction from chromatography) were treated with chloroform (Merck KGaA, Darmstadt, Germany) and benzonase nuclease (Merck KGaA) to reduce background signals induced by protein/nucleic acid-derived impurities. First, 50% (*v*/*v*) chloroform was added to the samples and mixed by inverting for 5 min, and the aqueous layer was then harvested by centrifugation at 3000× *g* for 15 min. Thereafter, these samples were treated with benzonase nuclease at a concentration of 25 units/mL and mixed at 37 °C for 1 h. After centrifugation at 10,000× *g* for 30 min, the supernatant was harvested. The pretreated samples were then layered onto 15–45% sucrose density gradients (SDG) and ultra-centrifuged again at 100,000× *g* for 4 h at 4 °C using an SW41Ti rotor. The ultra-centrifuged SDG was fractionated using a continuous density gradient fractionator (Teledyne ISCO, Lincoln, NE, USA) [17], and the absorbance of each fraction at 254 nm was consecutively recorded by the spectrophotometer component of the instrument. The area under the peak for specific fractions was measured to calculate the quantity of 146S (μg/mL) according to the formula presented in a previous study [17].

2.7. SDS-PAGE, Western Blot Analysis

The protein samples of each fraction obtained in the purification process were subjected to sodium dodecyl sulfate polyacrylamide gel electrophoresis (SDS-PAGE). The protein samples were mixed with 4× non-reducing lithium dodecyl sulfate sample buffer (Invitrogen, Carlsbad, CA, USA) and 10×

reducing agent (1M dithiothreitol; Merck KGaA). The pretreated samples were heated at 70 °C for 10 min and run on 4–12% Bis-Tris gradient gels (Invitrogen). The gel was stained by Coomassie Brilliant Blue R-250 staining solution (Biorad, Hercules, CA, USA) for 1 h with gentle agitation. The stained gel was then treated with the destaining solution (Biosesang, Sungnam, Korea) and agitated until the protein bands were visible. For Western blot analysis, the gel was transferred to a nitrocellulose membrane using the iBlot 2 gel-transfer device (Invitrogen). The membranes were blocked with 5% skimmed milk in phosphate-buffered saline with Tween-20 (PBST; 10 mM sodium phosphate, 132 mM NaCl, 2.7 mM KCl, and 0.05% Tween-20, pH 7.4). The membranes were washed and incubated with anti-FMDV 3B monoclonal antibody (4G24, supplied by the Median Diagnostics Inc. (Chuncheon, Republic of Korea) and diluted 1/2000 in PBST). After washing the membranes, they were incubated with goat anti-mouse horseradish peroxidase-conjugated secondary antibodies (Invitrogen) diluted 1/4000 in PBST. The proteins were visualized with Pierce ECL Substrate (Invitrogen) using the Azure C600 imaging system and the cSeries Capture Software (Azure Biosystem, Dublin, CA, USA).

2.8. Transmission Electron Microscopy (TEM)

The fractions eluted with a high concentration of salt from the heparin ligand were collected and concentrated to the same volume that was initially loaded onto a HiTrap HP Heparin column using a 10-kDa cutoff Centricon Plus-70 centrifugal unit (Merck Millipore). It was layered on top of sucrose density gradients and then centrifuged at 100,000× *g* for 4 h. The band between the 30% and 35% sucrose layers was collected and centrifuged at 100,000× *g* for 4 h. The resulting pellet was resuspended and dialyzed with Tris-KCl buffer (20 mM Tris-HCl, 300 mM KCl, pH 7.6) at 4 °C to eliminate residual sucrose. One drop of the purified FMDV suspension was placed on formvar-coated grids and negatively stained with 1% uranyl acetate. The morphology of purified FMDV particles were examined via TEM (Hitachi 7100; Hitachi, Tokyo, Japan).

2.9. Preparation of Vaccines

The experimental vaccines were prepared with the FMDV O/Boeun/SKR/2017 strain via: (i) PEG-precipitation; and (ii) heparin affinity chromatography. For the first group, the FMDV culture supernatant was treated with 7.5% (*w/v*) PEG 6000 (Sigma-Aldrich), stirred overnight at 4 °C, and centrifuged at 10,000× *g* for 30 min. After the supernatant was removed, the pellet was resuspended in Tris-KCl buffer (20 mM Tris-HCl, 300 mM KCl, pH 7.6) and adjusted to a concentration of 15 μg/mL. For the second group, the heparin column eluted antigens were concentrated to 15 μg/mL using a 10-kDa cutoff Centricon Plus-70 centrifugal unit (Merck Millipore). Saponin (Sigma-Aldrich) and aluminum hydroxide gel (General Chemical, Parsippany, NJ, USA) were added to these two kinds of antigens, and the ISA 206 VG adjuvant (Seppic, Paris, France) pre-warmed at 30 °C was then added in a ratio of 1:1. After the mixtures were incubated at 20 °C for 1 h in a water bath with blocked light, they were stored at 4 °C until use.

2.10. Animal Experiments

Korean black goats at the age of 8 months, which were not previously FMD-vaccinated, were tested via enzyme-linked immunosorbent assay (ELISA) to confirm negativity for SP and NSP antibodies. Twenty goats were injected intramuscularly with vaccines containing PEG-treated antigen ($n = 10$) and heparin affinity column purified antigen ($n = 10$). All goats were vaccinated five times every 4 weeks at a dose of 15 μg/2 mL and bled at an interval of 4 weeks after vaccination to obtain serum samples.

2.11. ELISA

PrioCHECK FMDV NSP and serotype O SP antibody detection kits (Prionics, Lelystad, The Netherlands) were used to measure the antibody levels elicited by the vaccines. The competition ELISAs were performed in accordance with the manufacturer's instructions. Test sera were added to antigen-coated plates and incubated for 1 h at 25 °C. After the plates were washed, horseradish peroxidase-conjugated monoclonal antibodies against the immobilized FMDV antigen (3ABC (NSP) and inactivated serotype O FMDV (SP)) were added to the plates, followed by incubation for 1 h. Finally, the plates were washed and 3,3,5,5-tetramethylbenzidine substrate solution was added. The colorimetric reaction was stopped with sulfuric acid solution after 15 min, and the optical density was measured at 450 nm. The ELISA results were expressed as percentage inhibition (PI) values. Samples with a PI value of ≥50% were considered to have a positive result and <50%, a negative result.

2.12. *Virus Neutralization Test*

The virus neutralization test for the FMDV antibody was performed using the methods described in the World Organization for Animal Health (OIE) terrestrial manual [18]. The sera were inactivated at 56 °C for 30 min before testing. Fifty microliters of two-fold serially diluted sera starting from 1/4 dilution were mixed with 50 μL of each virus containing 100 $TCID_{50}$ (50% tissue culture infective dose). After incubation at 37 °C for 1 h, 50 μL of fetal porcine kidney cells (LFBK, supplied by the Plum Island Animal Disease Center (Orient, NY, USA)) were added to each well at 10^6 cells/mL. The plates were sealed and incubated in an atmosphere of 5% CO_2 at 37 °C for 2–3 days. The cytopathic effect was observed under a microscope, and the virus-neutralizing (VN) titer was determined using the Spearman–Kärber method [19]. The VN antibody titer was converted to a $\log_{10}$ scale for graphical purposes. A titer of 1:45 (1.65 $\log_{10}$) or more of the final serum dilution in the serum/virus mixture was considered to indicate a positive result.

2.13. *Statistical Analysis*

The data were analyzed using an unpaired *t* test with the GraphPad Prism software version 5 (GraphPad Software, San Diego, CA, USA), in which a *p*-value of less than 0.05 was considered statistically significant.

3. Results

3.1. *Purification Efficacy of Chromatography Using the Heparin Ligand*

Most of the proteins were obtained in the flow-through fractions of the affinity chromatography using the heparin ligand for all three different virus strains. Small amounts of proteins were detected in the fractions corresponding to 0.5–0.8 M KCl in the gradient elution (Figure 1).

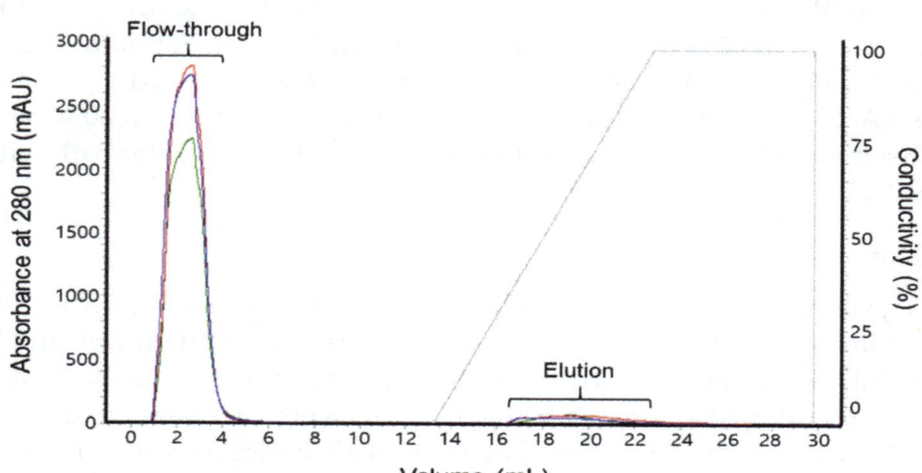

Figure 1. Chromatogram of heparin affinity chromatography. The three strains of the foot-and-mouth disease virus culture supernatant were loaded onto a HiTrap HP heparin column and traced by UV monitoring at 280 nm. The chromatogram shows the fractions obtained during the purification process. The colored lines represent each as follows: blue, O/Boeun/SKR/2017 strain; green, O/Jincheon/SKR/2014 strain; red, Om-O-PanAsia2 recombinant strain; gray, conductivity.

For FMDV O/Boeun/SKR/2017, the total amount of proteins in the flow-through and elution fractions was 61% and 6.9%, respectively (Table 1). For FMDV O/Jincheon/SKR/2014 and Om-O-PanAsia2, the amount of proteins in the flow-through fractions was 61% and 73.8%, respectively. In contrast, the amount of proteins in the elution fractions was 6.9% and 9.1%, respectively, for FMDV O/Jincheon/SKR/2014 and Om-O-PanAsia2.

Table 1. Purification efficacy by the HiTrap HP heparin column.

Strain	Step	FMDV Concentration (μg/mL)	Protein Concentration (μg/mL)	Total Protein (%)	FMDV Recovery (%)
O/Boeun/SKR/2017	Crude	27.6	5052.5	0	100
	Flow-through	ND	3084.5	61.1	-
	Elution	20.8	347.0	6.9	75.4
O/Jinchoen/SKR/2014	Crude	16.2	5211.7	0	100
	Flow-through	ND	3672.8	70.5	-
	Elution	13.2	357.1	6.9	81.5
Om-O-PanAsia2	Crude	30.0	5987.5	0	100
	Flow-through	ND	4421.2	73.8	-
	Elution	21.6	546.0	9.1	71.9

FMDV, foot-and-mouth disease virus; ND, not detected.

Meanwhile, 146S was recovered mainly in the elution fractions of the affinity chromatography, regardless of the virus strains (Table 1). The recovery rate of the virus particles for FMDV O/Boeun/SKR/2017, O/Jincheon/SKR/2014, and Om-O-PanAsia2 was 75.4%, 81.5%, and 71.9%, respectively. In contrast, no virus particles were detected in the flow-through fractions.

Sodium dodecyl sulfate–polyacrylamide gel electrophoresis (SDS-PAGE) of the chromatographic fractions revealed that there were no distinct bands corresponding to the main capsid proteins, such as VP1–VP3, in the crude samples prior to application to the column. The elution fractions only showed apparent capsid protein bands around 30 kDa, which was the same as that of the positive control (purified FMDV O/Boeun/SKR/2017 by sucrose density gradient ultracentrifugation) (Figure 2a). While the crude sample prior to chromatography showed 3AB bands around 30 kDa, no band was observed at the chromatographic elution fraction via the Western blot analysis (Figure 2b).

As shown in Figure 3, there was an intact typical FMDV particle with a diameter of 25–30 nm on electron microscopy.

3.2. Immunogenicity of the Experimental Vaccine Prepared with Heparin Affinity Column-Eluted Antigens

The experimental vaccines made with the heparin column-eluted antigens were prepared to evaluate the immunogenicity of these samples in the goats. Twenty goats were vaccinated five times at four-week intervals (Figure 4a). The vaccine was comparable to the PEG-treated vaccine in terms of the SP antibody titers. The PI values of all goats were above 50% from the first immunization and were more than 90% with the booster immunization (Figure 4b).

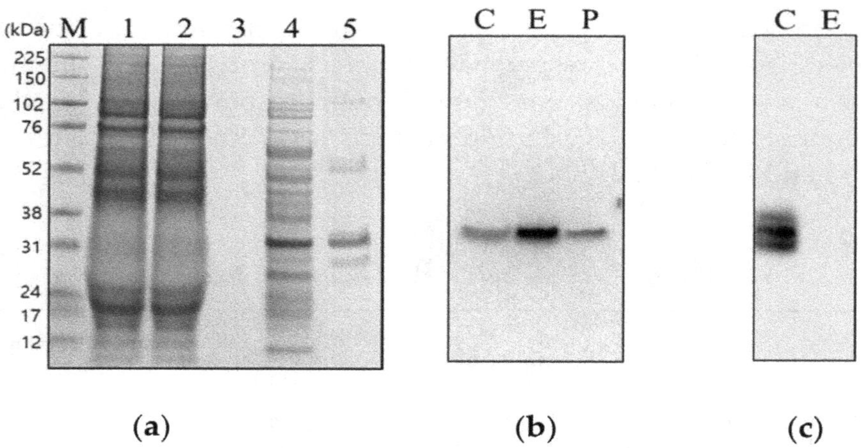

Figure 2. Identification of the purified protein after heparin affinity chromatography. The protein samples of each fraction obtained in the purification process were subjected to sodium dodecyl sulfate–polyacrylamide gel electrophoresis. (**a**) The gel was revealed by Coomassie brilliant blue staining. Lane M, molecular weight marker; Lane 1, foot-and-mouth disease virus serotype O Boeun virus culture supernatant (before column loading); Lane 2, flow-through fraction from the heparin column; Lane 3, washed fraction with the heparin column; Lane 4, eluted fraction from the heparin column (10-fold concentrated); Lane 5, Lane P, positive control (purified FMDV O/Boeun/SKR/2017 by sucrose density gradient ultracentrifugation). Western blot analysis was performed with (**b**) anti-foot-and-mouth disease virus serotype O VP1. structural protein monoclonal antibodies and (**c**) anti-foot-and-mouth disease virus 3B nonstructural protein monoclonal antibodies. Lane C, foot-and-mouth disease virus serotype O/Boeun/SKR/2017 virus supernatant; Lane E, eluted fraction from the heparin column (10-fold concentrated).

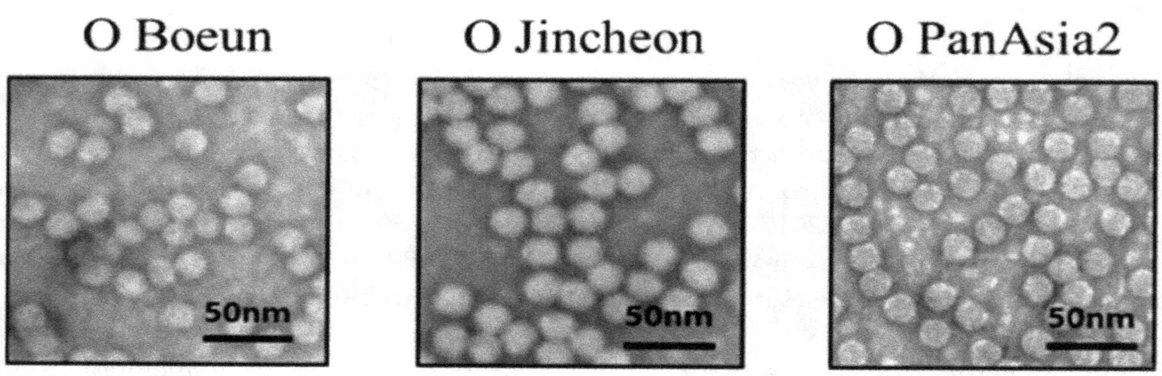

Figure 3. Morphological observation on a transmission electron microscope. The heparin affinity column purified serotype O foot-and-mouth disease viruses were negatively stained and analyzed for morphology. The bars represent 50 nm.

The VN antibody titers for the homologous virus (O/Boeun/SKR/2017) were above 1:45 (1.65 $\log_{10}$) for all goats after the first vaccination, and the subsequent titers were above 1:100 (2.00 $\log_{10}$) with the booster vaccination. The titers were the same as those of the PEG group (Figure 4c).

For the NSP antibody, the PEG group was positive for two, four, four, and five heads after the second, third, fourth, and fifth vaccinations, respectively (Figure 4d). Meanwhile, none of the goats in the heparin affinity column group showed positivity for the NSP antibody even after the fifth vaccination. In addition, the heparin affinity column group showed a mean PI value of 26.9% compared with more than 50% in the PEG group after the fifth vaccination. The heparin affinity column group had a significantly lower value ($p = 0.0226$) of mean PI value than the PEG group after the fifth vaccination.

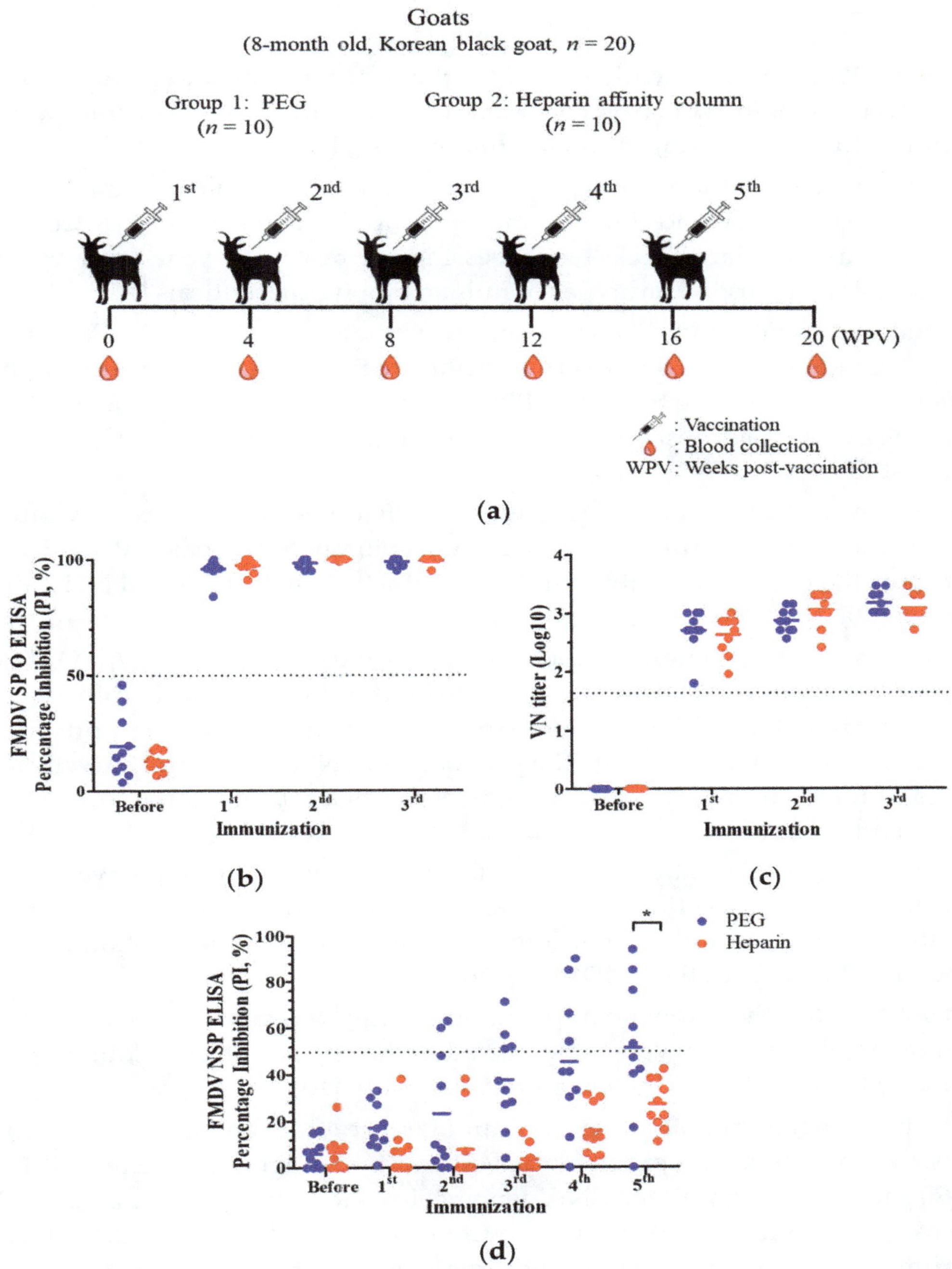

Figure 4. Antibody responses elicited by immunizations with polyethylene glycol (PEG)-treated and heparin affinity column purified serotype O foot-and-mouth disease (FMD) Boeun/SKR/2017 vaccines. (**a**) Scheme of the animal experiment. Twenty goats were vaccinated five times at a four-week interval with PEG-treated (n = 10) and heparin affinity column purified (n = 10) FMD vaccines. Blood samples were collected every four weeks after vaccination. (**b**) The antibody titers of the structural proteins were measured via enzyme-linked immunosorbent assay (ELISA). The antibody values were expressed as percentage inhibition (PI) values. A PI value of ≥50% (dotted line) was considered to indicate positivity. (**c**) The homologous virus-neutralizing (VN) antibody titers were measured using the virus neutralization test. The VN titers were expressed as a $\log_{10}$ value. A titer of $\geq 1.65 \log_{10}$ (dotted line) was considered to indicate positivity. (**d**) The antibody titers of the nonstructural proteins were measured via ELISA. The antibody values were expressed as PI values. A PI value of ≥50% (dotted line) was considered to indicate positivity. The full blue and red lines represent the mean PI values in each group. A significant difference in the mean values between the two groups in the fifth vaccination was observed. * $p < 0.05$.

4. Discussion

In general, the PEG method is widely used for the concentration and purification of the FMDV; however, some NSPs remain, which is considered a problem. Thus, several studies have been performed to purify the FMDV using chromatography [20–24].

The chromatographic method using gel columns cannot be applied to large-scale production owing to its long working time and limited amount of applicable sample [21]. Conversely, affinity columns have been used in large-scale bioprocessing for nearly 40 years and are applied in the downstream processing of various serotypes of human biopharmaceuticals [25].

Previous studies also introduced heparin affinity chromatography for FMDV purification, which showed a large deviation in the 146S recovery from 40% to 90% [23]. This proved that the application conditions differ depending on the type of FMDV strain used. Importantly, the results of evaluating vaccine purity, one of the major test factors for determining the quality of FMD vaccines, were not presented in that study.

In another study, FMD vaccine antigens were purified with a 75% recovery rate as a result of combining a gel column and a hydrophobic interaction column; however, only one FMDV strain was applied. In addition, the immunogenicity of antibody induction against SPs and NSPs after vaccination was not evaluated [20].

Therefore, in this study, the conditions for purifying various strains of serotype O FMDV developed as FMD vaccine candidates in the Korea, via heparin affinity chromatography, were established. In addition, an experimental vaccine was prepared with the heparin column purified antigen and repeatedly immunized to goats to evaluate the production of NSP antibodies as well as SP antibodies. For confirming the removal of NSPs, 3AB was detected as a representative because it is the most reliable indicator [10].

The FMDV capsid proteins that were not visible before column injection were clearly observed as major bands in the elution fraction, indicating that virus purification was effectively performed. Conversely, in the SDS-PAGE result of the eluted fraction using a heparin column reported by other researchers, the capsid protein of the FMDV was not identified.

As shown in this study, the chromatographic method used was more effective than the PEG-treated method for removing NSPs. NSPs were not detected in the heparin affinity column purified antigen but remained in the PEG-treated antigen in a previous study [10].

The FMDV is known to maintain high immunogenicity when maintained as only intact virus (146S) particles. Therefore, in the process of FMD vaccine antigen production, it is important to recover the 146S particles, including the RNA genome, instead of the capsid-dissociated VP1 subunit protein [26]. From this point of view, previous studies reported that 146S particle recovery varied significantly from 40% to 90%, whereas we observed 146S particle recovery rates over 70% for all three FMDV strains. The antigen yield in this study was much higher than that in the previous study using the same heparin column, which showed 40% recovery of the FMDV and 53% recovery of the porcine reproductive and respiratory syndrome viruses [23,27]. Even our virus strains showed different antigen recovery. It is very difficult to pinpoint the reason for the difference in the antigen recovery. It might due to the different physical characteristics of each FMDV. It remains to be found which physical feature plays the main role in the affinity.

Based on the result that the FMDV was more purified via heparin affinity chromatography than the conventional PEG treatment method, it was necessary to evaluate its immunogenicity in animals by vaccination. To this end, the FMD vaccine antigen prepared via heparin chromatography was adjusted to 15 μg per dose, as determined in a previous study [10], mixed with an adjuvant, and immunized to goats three times to evaluate the antibody levels against SPs and NSPs.

In the SP ELISA and virus neutralization test, both vaccine groups showed the same pattern of antibody levels. This indicates that there was no difference in the induction of protective antibodies against the FMDV even when antigens were further purified by chromatography in comparison with the PEG method. This was a sufficiently predictable result, as shown in a previous report [24].

Another important factor in evaluating FMD vaccines is vaccine purity. According to the OIE manual, the FMD vaccine is acceptable if fewer than two out of eight cattle are positive for NSP antibodies after being vaccinated twice [18]. In this study, goats were employed rather than cattle for the detection of NSP antibody as a vaccine purity test. This was based on the preliminary data in our institute that goats produced NSP antibodies more rapidly and sensitively than cattle in repeated vaccination experiments (data not shown). The PEG-treated vaccine yielded a positive result after the second vaccination, while the vaccine made from a sample purified via heparin affinity chromatography did not induce positivity for NSP antibodies even after the fifth vaccination. In addition, the average PI value of the PEG-treated vaccine increased over 50%, whereas that of the vaccine purified via heparin affinity chromatography remained below 50% regardless of the number of immunizations. Taken together, we demonstrated that the vaccine produced in this study is a higher-purity FMD vaccine than the conventional PEG-treated vaccine.

We reported that NSPs were removed from FMDV culture supernatant by chloroform addition [10]. The immunogenicity of FMD vaccine prepared by this chromatography and chloroform were almost the same against structural and nonstructural proteins (Figure S1). However, total protein concentration of them was different. The chloroform treated vaccine antigen still contains large amount of unwanted cellular protein contaminants compared with heparin affinity column purified vaccine antigen. That is why we established chromatography as an additional purification method. This is the same situation for other FMD vaccine manufacturers that had several methods such as PEG and chromatography in case of emergency situation of further removal of NSP and other cell-derived proteins.

5. Conclusions

This study is the first to evaluate FMD vaccine purity by repeatedly immunizing animals with a vaccine prepared via heparin affinity chromatography. This result would be an important groundwork for advanced FMD vaccine manufacturing in the near future.

Author Contributions: Conceptualization, Y.-J.K.; methodology, S.Y.P. and Y.-J.K.; software, S.Y.P.; validation, S.Y.P. and Y.-J.K.; formal analysis, S.Y.P. and J.-M.L.; investigation, S.Y.P., J.-M.L., A.-Y.K., S.H.P., J.-S.K., H.K. and J.-W.P.; resources, S.Y.P. and J.-M.L.; writing—original draft preparation, S.Y.P. and Y.-J.K.; writing—review and editing, S.Y.P., C.-K.P., J.-H.P. and Y.-J.K.; visualization, S.Y.P.; supervision, C.-K.P. and Y.-J.K.; project administration, Y.-J.K.; and funding acquisition, Y.-J.K. All authors have read and agreed to the published version of the manuscript.

References

1. Knight-Jones, T.J.D.; Rushton, J. The economic impacts of foot and mouth disease—What are they, how big are they and where do they occur? *Prev. Vet. Med.* **2013**, *112*, 161–173. [CrossRef]

2. Sharma, G.K.; Mohapatra, J.K.; Mahajan, S.; Matura, R.; Subramaniam, S.; Pattnaik, B. Comparative evaluation of non-structural protein-antibody detecting ELISAs for foot-and-mouth disease sero-surveillance under intensive vaccination. *J. Virol. Methods* **2014**, *207*, 22–28. [CrossRef]

3. Grubman, M.J.; Baxt, B. Foot-and-mouth disease. *Clin. Microbiol. Rev.* **2004**, *17*, 465–493. [CrossRef] [PubMed]

4. Rueckert, R.R.; Wimmer, E. Systematic nomenclature of picornavirus proteins. *J. Virol.* **1984**, *50*, 957. [CrossRef] [PubMed]

5. Liu, Z.; Shao, J.; Zhao, F.; Zhou, G.; Gao, S.; Liu, W.; Lv, J.; Li, X.; Li, Y.; Chang, H.J.C.; et al. Chemiluminescence immunoassay for the detection of antibodies against the 2C and 3ABC nonstructural proteins induced by infecting pigs with foot-and-mouth disease virus. *Clin. Vaccine Immunol.* **2017**, *24*, e00153-17. [CrossRef] [PubMed]

6. Kim, A.-Y.; Tark, D.; Kim, H.; Kim, J.-S.; Lee, J.-M.; Kwon, M.; Bae, S.; Kim, B.; Ko, Y.-J. Determination of optimal age for single vaccination of growing pigs with foot-and-mouth disease bivalent vaccine in South Korea. *J. Vet. Med Sci.* **2017**, *79*, 1822–1825. [CrossRef] [PubMed]
7. Kim, H.; Kim, A.-Y.; Kim, J.-S.; Lee, J.-M.; Kwon, M.; Bae, S.; Kim, B.; Park, J.-W.; Park, C.-K.; Ko, Y.-J. Determination of the optimal method for the concentration and purification of 146S particles for foot-and-mouth disease vaccine production. *J. Virol. Methods* **2019**, *269*, 26–29. [CrossRef] [PubMed]
8. Jamal, S.M.; Belsham, G.J. Foot-and-mouth disease: Past, present and future. *Vet. Res.* **2013**, *44*, 116. [CrossRef]
9. Robinson, L.; Knight-Jones, T.; Charleston, B.; Rodriguez, L.; Gay, C.; Sumption, K.; Vosloo, W. Global Foot-and-Mouth Disease Research Update and Gap Analysis: 3-Vaccines. *Transbound. Emerg. Dis.* **2016**, *63*, 30–41. [CrossRef]
10. Park, S.Y.; Lee, J.-M.; Kim, A.-Y.; Park, S.H.; Lee, S.-I.; Kim, H.; Kim, J.-S.; Park, J.-H.; Ko, Y.-J.; Park, C.-K. Efficient Removal of Non-Structural Protein Using Chloroform for Foot-and-Mouth Disease Vaccine Production. *Vaccines* **2020**, *8*, e483. [CrossRef]
11. Rodriguez, L.L.; Grubman, M.J. Foot and mouth disease virus vaccines. *Vaccine* **2009**, *27*, D90–D94. [CrossRef] [PubMed]
12. Wang, G.; Wang, Y.; Shang, Y.; Zhang, Z.; Liu, X.J.V.j. How foot-and-mouth disease virus receptor mediates foot-and-mouth disease virus infection. *Virol. J.* **2015**, *12*, 9. [CrossRef] [PubMed]
13. Ruoslahti, E. RGD and other recognition sequences for integrins. *Annu. Rev. Cell Dev. Biol.* **1996**, *12*, 697–715. [CrossRef] [PubMed]
14. Fry, E.; Stuart, D.; Rowlands, D. The structure of foot-and-mouth disease virus. *Curr. Top. Microbiol. Immunol* **2005**, *288*, 71–101.
15. Lee, E.G.; Park, S.Y.; Tark, D.S.; Lee, H.S.; Ko, Y.J.; Kim, Y.G.; Park, S.Y.; Kim, C.S.; Ryu, K.H.; Lee, M.H. Novel BHK-21 Cell Line Available for Suspension Culture in Serum-Free Medium and Method for Foot-and-mouth Disease Vaccine Production Using the Same. KR101812223B1, 2017. Available online: https://patents.google.com/patent/KR101812223B1/en (accessed on 7 December 2020).
16. Lee, S.-Y.; Lee, Y.-J.; Kim, R.-H.; Park, J.-N.; Park, M.-E.; Ko, M.-K.; Choi, J.-H.; Chu, J.-Q.; Lee, K.-N.; Kim, S.-M.; et al. Rapid engineering of foot-and-mouth disease vaccine and challenge viruses. *J. Virol.* **2017**, *91*, e00155-17. [CrossRef] [PubMed]
17. Doel, T.; Fletton, B.; Staple, R. Further developments in the quantification of small RNA viruses by U.V. photometry of sucrose density gradients. *Dev. Biol. Stand.* **1981**, *50*, 209–219.
18. International Committee, Biological Standards Commission, International Office of Epizootics. *Manual of Diagnostic Tests and Vaccines for Terrestrial Animals: Mammals, Birds, and Bees*; Renouf Publishing Co. Ltd.: Ottawa, ON, Canada, 2018; Available online: https://www.oie.int/fileadmin/Home/eng/Health_standards/tahm/3.01.08_FMD.pdf (accessed on 5 October 2020).
19. Kärber, G. Beitrag zur kollektiven behandlung pharmakologischer reihenversuche. *Arch. Exp. Pathol. Phamakologie* **1931**, *162*, 480–483. [CrossRef]
20. Li, H.; Yang, Y.; Zhang, Y.; Zhang, S.; Zhao, Q.; Zhu, Y.; Zou, X.; Yu, M.; Ma, G.; Su, Z. A hydrophobic interaction chromatography strategy for purification of inactivated foot-and-mouth disease virus. *Protein Expr. Purifircation* **2015**, *113*, 23–29. [CrossRef]
21. Spitteler, M.A.; Fernández, I.; Schabes, E.; Krimer, A.; Régulier, E.G.; Guinzburg, M.; Smitsaart, E.; Levy, M.S. Foot and mouth disease (FMD) virus: Quantification of whole virus particles during the vaccine manufacturing process by size exclusion chromatography. *Vaccine* **2011**, *29*, 7182–7187. [CrossRef]
22. Cañizo, A.A.N.; Mazza, M.; Bellinzoni, R.; Cascone, O. Foot and mouth disease virus concentration and purification by affinity chromatography. *Appl. Biochem. Biotechnol.* **1997**, *61*, 399–409. [CrossRef]
23. Du, P.; Sun, S.; Dong, J.; Zhi, X.; Chang, Y.; Teng, Z.; Guo, H.; Liu, Z. Purification of foot-and-mouth disease virus by heparin as ligand for certain strains. *J. Chromatogr. B* **2017**, *1049*, 16–23. [CrossRef]
24. Cheng, H.; Chen, J.; Cai, Z.; Du, L.; Hou, J.; Qiao, X.; Zheng, Q. Development of GEM-PA-nanotrap for purification of foot-and-mouth disease virus. *Vaccine* **2019**, *37*, 3205–3213. [CrossRef] [PubMed]
25. Łącki, K.M.; Riske, F.J. Affinity Chromatography: An Enabling Technology for Large-Scale Bioprocessing. *Biotechnol. J.* **2020**, *15*, e1800397. [CrossRef] [PubMed]

26. Doel, T.R.; Chong, W.K. Comparative immunogenicity of 146S, 75S and 12S particles of foot-and-mouth disease virus. *Arch. Virol.* **1982**, *73*, 185–191. [CrossRef] [PubMed]
27. Hu, J.; Ni, Y.; Dryman, B.A.; Meng, X.Y.; Zhang, C. Purification of porcine reproductive and respiratory syndrome virus from cell culture using ultrafiltration and heparin affinity chromatography. *J. Chromatogr. A* **2010**, *1217*, 3489–3493. [CrossRef] [PubMed]

5

Characterization of Danaparoid Complex Extractive Drug by an Orthogonal Analytical Approach

Cristina Gardini [1], Elena Urso [2], Marco Guerrini [2], René van Herpen [3], Pauline de Wit [3] and Annamaria Naggi [2,*]

[1] Centro Alta Tecnologia Istituto di Ricerche Chimiche e Biochimiche G. Ronzoni S.r.l., via G. Colombo 81, 20133 Milan, Italy; gardini@cat-ronzoni.it

[2] Istituto di Ricerche Chimiche e Biochimiche G. Ronzoni S.r.l., via G. Colombo 81, 20133 Milan, Italy; urso@ronzoni.it (E.U.); guerrini@ronzoni.it (M.G.)

[3] Aspen Oss B.V., Kloosterstraat 6, 5349 AB Oss, The Netherlands; rvanherpen@nl.aspenpharma.com (R.v.H.); pdewit@nl.aspenpharma.com (P.d.W.)

* Correspondence: naggi@ronzoni.it

Abstract: Danaparoid sodium salt, is the active component of ORGARAN, an anticoagulant and antithrombotic drug constituted of three glycosaminoglycans (GAGs) obtained from porcine intestinal mucosa extracts. Heparan sulfate is the major component, dermatan sulfate and chondroitin sulfate being the minor ones. Currently dermatan sulfate and chondroitin sulfate are quantified by UV detection of their unsaturated disaccharides obtained by enzymatic depolymerization. Due to the complexity of danaparoid biopolymers and the presence of shared components, an orthogonal approach has been applied using more advanced tools and methods. To integrate the analytical profile, 2D heteronuclear single quantum coherence (HSQC) NMR spectroscopy was applied and found effective to identify and quantify GAG component signals as well as those of some process signatures of danaparoid active pharmaceutical ingredient (API) batches. Analyses of components of both API samples and size separated fractions proceeded through the determination and distribution of the molecular weight (Mw) by high performance size exclusion chromatographic triple detector array (HP-SEC-TDA), chain mapping by LC/MS, and mono- (^{1}H and ^{13}C) and bi-dimensional (HSQC) NMR spectroscopy. Finally, large scale chromatographic isolation and depolymerization of each GAG followed by LC/MS and 2D-NMR analysis, allowed the sequences to be defined and components to be evaluated of each GAG including oxidized residues of hexosamines and uronic acids at the reducing ends.

Keywords: danaparoid sodium; low molecular weight glycosaminoglycans; orthogonal multi-analytical methods; sequence and compositional investigations; component quantitative analysis

---

1. Introduction

Danaparoid sodium, constituted by a mixture of Low Molecular Weight (LMW) heparan sulfate (HS), dermatan sulfate (DS), and chondroitin sulfate (CS), extracted from porcine intestinal mucosa, is the active component of ORGARAN an anticoagulant and antithrombotic drug approved for prophylaxis of post-operative deep-vein thrombosis. Its beneficial effect upon factor IIa (thrombin) is shown by the anti-factor Xa/IIa ratio more than that of heparin [1–3].

A weight/weight (*w*/*w*) percentage maximum of 8.5% of CS and in the range of 8.0% up to 16.0% for DS, have been specified and quantified by an enzymatic method reported in the danaparoid monograph of the EC-Pharmacopoeia [4]. The chondroitinase selective depolymerization of galactosaminoglycans to UV detectable unsaturated disaccharides was originally developed to quantify

CS and DS present in API heparin batches. Alternative more feasible NMR quantifications have been developed for the components of danaparoid API batches [5] and for heparin composition [6].

The linear polymers HS, CS, and DS are the most abundant mucopolysaccharides in the body and ubiquitous components of connective tissue and cartilages. As other extracted and purified glycosaminoglycans (GAGs), they show high size, mean molecular weight (Mw) 50 kDa and heterogeneous chains [7] too great to be fully characterized as they are. Therefore, they must be partially/fully depolymerized by enzymatic or chemical methods. Lyase enzymes generally cleave hexosamine–uronic acid bonds and the final products of their exhaustive digestion are disaccharides bearing at the non-reducing end (NRE) a 4,5-unsaturated (Δ) uronic acid. Nitrous acid is also used to cleave hexosamine N-sulfated bonds at pH 1.5 and free hexosamine at pH 4.0 [8] leading to an anhydromannose at the reducing end (RE) of the depolymerized fragments. CS-A and CS-C, bearing a common repeating unit of D-glucuronic acid β-3-D-*N*-acetylgalactosamine β-4 (GlcA β-3-GalNAc β4) differ in sulfation degree of the 4-O and 6-O positions of GalNAc. DS, also known as CS-B, is a variant bearing a number of GlcA units epimerized to L-iduronic acid (L-IdoA), some of them 2-O sulfated (IdoA2S). HS, expressed on cell surface and basement membranes is a linear, highly heterogeneous, acidic GAG, in nature mainly bound to core proteins in proteoglycans. Depending on the core protein, cell types and cellular environment, the HS polysaccharides show an average chain size ranging from 5 up to 50 KDa and a polydispersity of 1.05–1.6 [7]. In the Golgi apparatus of most mammalian cells the HS precursor, constituted by the alternating (1–4) linked β-D-glucuronic acid α-N-Acetyl D-glucosamine (GlcA-GlcNAc) is synthesized. In the following complex biosynthetic steps some GlcA units are epimerized to IdoA and partially 2-O-sulfated (IdoA2S) while some GlcNAc are N-deacetylated, N-sulfated as well as 3-O and/or 6-O-sulfated leading to a plethora of diverse HS chains. Porcine intestinal mucosa is a source of HS usually in a mixture with CS and DS, remaining after the extraction of heparin [9].

To define compositional and structural characteristic of API samples an orthogonal analytical approach, already adopted for detecting potential contaminants in API heparin batches, was applied for this study [10,11].

At first, danaparoid API was characterized using NMR spectroscopy, mass spectrometry, and molecular weight determination. This allowed a general picture to be obtained of the API in which HS was observed to be the most abundant component in danaparoid. With the aim of also investigating the galactosaminoglycan component, a study was carried out. The structural information here obtained was fundamental for the subsequent part, where two paths were followed to go deeper into the characterization work: (1) fractionation of danaparoid by size and (2) isolation of the two GAG families, which are HS and CS/DS. Both groups of fractions were fully characterized as the parent sample, benefitting from the complementary information coming from the applied analytical methods.

2. Results

2.1. Danaparoid API Samples

Seven danaparoid API batches and their related size separated fractions were submitted for a full characterization by nuclear magnetic resonance experiments, mass spectrometry, and molecular weight determination.

A study in depth of digested products obtained by chondroitinase ABC (ChABC) digestion treatment (Section 2.2) and the pilot study on size exclusion chromatography (SEC) fractions, described in the first part of Section 2.3.3, were conducted only on one sample.

2.1.1. Determination of Molecular Weight Parameters

Analysis of molecular weight distribution was performed on seven API samples of danaparoid using high performance size-exclusion chromatography (HP-SEC) on polymeric columns, combined with a triple detector array (TDA) and UV detector. Using a 0.1 M $NaNO_3$ aqueous mobile phase, comparable Gaussian profiles exemplified in Figure 1a, were obtained by refractive index, viscometer, and right-angle laser light scattering [12,13].

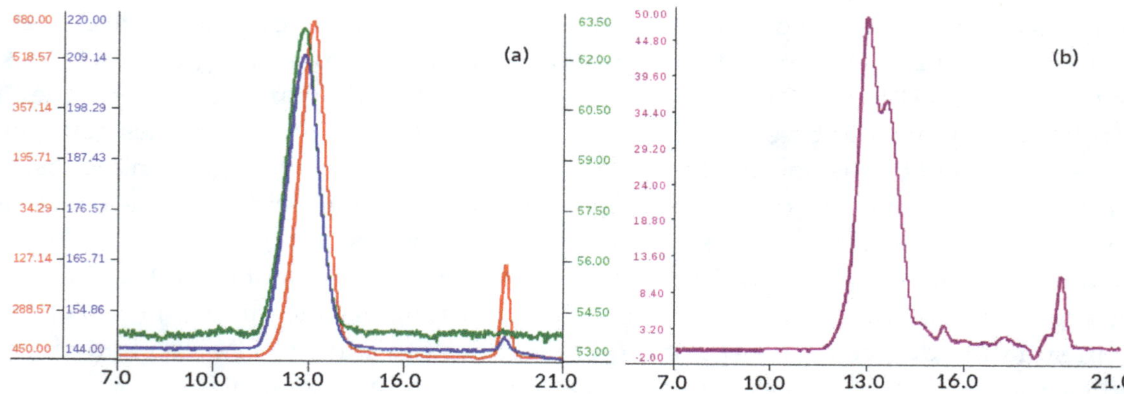

Figure 1. Size-exclusion chromatography profile of a danaparoid sample (CAT272): (**a**) red—refractive index (mV), blue—viscometer (mV) and green—right-angle laser light scattering (mV) detectors; (**b**) UV (mV) detector.

The software processed data of number average molecular weight (Mn), weight average Mw, and polydispersity (Pd) of analyzed samples were calculated as the mean of two runs. The values of Mn, Mw, and Pd ranging between 3300–3400 Da, 4200–4600 Da, and 1.27–1.36 respectively, indicate for the danaparoid analyzed samples small variation, near to the experimental error (5%).

The non-Gaussian profiles, obtained by UV detection at 260 nm (the eluent suppressed the lower λ signals) (Figure 1b) suggest an inhomogeneous distribution of different components of the complex GAG mixture. This could be ascribed to galactosaminoglycans that are present in high concentration in the higher Mw chains eluted which contain higher molar concentration of UV absorbing N-acetyl groups in comparison to the HS chains of lower Mw and N-acetyl content.

2.1.2. Determination of Sulfate to Carboxylate Ratio

The sulfate-carboxylate ratio, expressing the average disaccharide charge density, was determined in duplicate for all samples by a conductimetric titration method previously reported [14].

The resulting mean ratio of each sample, comprised in the narrow interval 1.19–1.32, indicated a substantial sample equivalence for the sulfation degree, considering the intrinsic variability of the extracted natural GAG components of API danaparoid.

Over the last forty years, the mean ratio values of several analyzed GAG samples, determined in our laboratories with the same method, were found in the range of 1.0–1.2 for CS and DS, 1.0–1.8 for HS and 2.1–2.8 for API porcine mucosal heparin.

2.1.3. Compositional Analysis by 1D and 2D NMR Spectroscopy

Both ^{1}H and ^{13}C one-dimensional NMR spectra of the samples have similar profiles, in Figures 2 and 3 a proton and a carbon spectra are displayed as examples.

In the proton spectra, the most evident difference is detected in the region of N-acetyl signals at 2.0–2.1 ppm which is correlated to the variable content of galactosaminoglycan components among samples [10,11,15]. Signals of N-acetyl galactosamine of CS are observed at 2.02 ppm, while that of DS is at 2.08 ppm. On the other hand, GlcNAc signals of HS are detected at 2.04 and 2.06 ppm, while those of oxidized N-acetyl hexosamine (ANAc-ox) are at 2.1 ppm (Figure 2b) [16–18]. A comparison between acetyl regions of different samples is reported in Figure S1.

^{13}C-NMR spectral analysis allowed signals to be attributed to each danaparoid component (Figure 3) confirmed by HSQC NMR spectra (Figure 4) and comparison with the corresponding literature data [15].

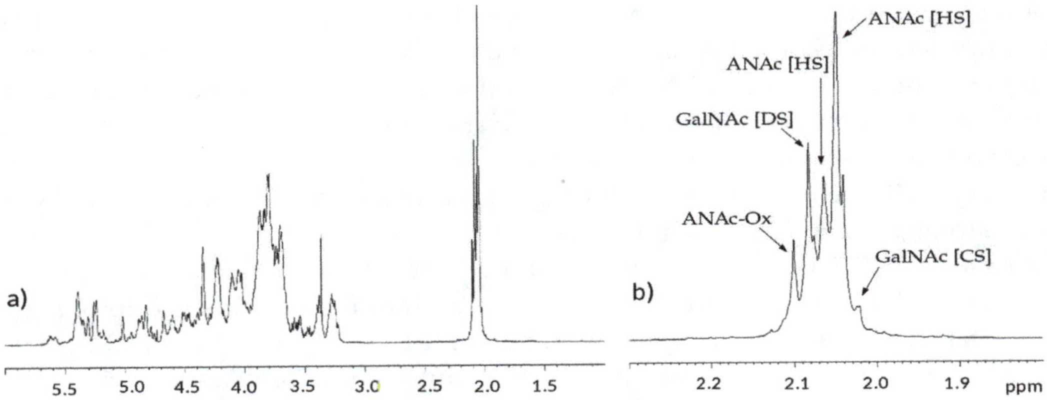

Figure 2. Example of ^{1}H-NMR spectrum of a danaparoid sample (CAT272): (**a**) whole spectrum; (**b**) expansion of the acetyl region.

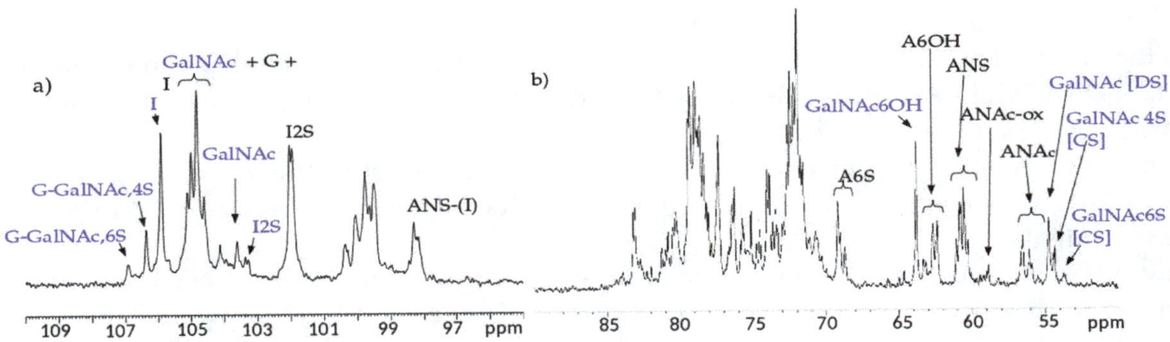

Figure 3. Example of ^{13}C-NMR spectrum of a danaparoid sample (CAT272): (**a**) anomeric region; (**b**) ring carbon region. Black: signals attributed to heparan sulfate (HS); Blue signals attributed to chondroitin sulfate (CS) and dermatan sulfate (DS).

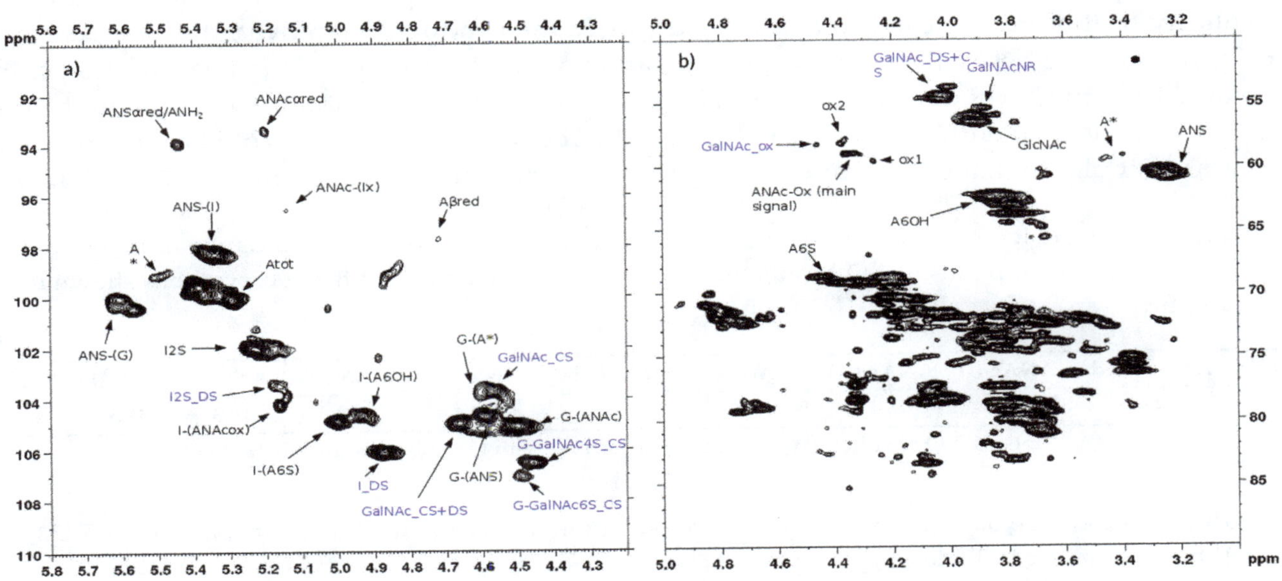

Figure 4. Example of 2D Heteronuclear Single Quantum Coherence (HSQC) NMR of a danaparoid sample (CAT272): (**a**) anomeric region; (**b**) ring region. Black: signals attributed to HS; Blue: signals attributed to DS and CS. Abbreviations in Table S1.

Heteronuclear single quantum coherence spectroscopy (HSQC) 2D NMR experiments on danaparoid samples were recorded by adapting the method recently validated for heparin samples [6].

The qualitative observation of 2D NMR spectra (Figure 4) allows the observation that the majority of peaks can be attributed to the HS component. In the ring region different signals correspond to glucosamines with various sulfation and acetylation substitution (such as ANS, A2*, ANAc, A6OH, and A6S, abbreviations in Table S1); moreover, the signals corresponding to N-acetylated galactosamines and their NRE are present and shown as GalNAc and GalNAc_NR.

In the area 4.6–4.2/57–61 ppm peaks associated to H2/C2 of N-acetyl hexosamine oxidized at the RE due to a bleaching process are observed. The assignments of this group of signals are done based on both literature [17–19] and experimental data: the cross-peak at 4.47/58.3 ppm is attributed to the oxidized N-acetylgalactosamines of CS/DS component (GalNAc-ox), whereas the signal at 4.37/58.9 ppm, shown as ANAc-ox, is assigned to oxidized reducing end (N-acetylglucosaminic acid) as described in [16,17]. The other peaks in the same area, displayed as ox1 and ox2, are associated with HS component because they are absent in the enriched CS/DS fractions described in Section 2.4. The hypothesis is that they can be associated to similar oxidized reducing ends on different oligosaccharidic sequences.

In the anomeric region, together with the HS signals, peaks related to DS and CS are displayed (I_DS, I2S_DS, G-GalNAc,4S and G-GalNAc,6S): the uronic acids of both components are useful for the characterization of the API samples.

The assignment of the peak at 5.18/104.2 ppm, previously reported [18], is confirmed as H1/C1 α-L-iduronic acid linked to oxidized N-acetylglucosamine (abbreviation I-(ANAcox)) by 2D NMR experiments.

The integration of characteristic signals of each component allows every contribution to be calculated and produces a detailed characterization of HS in a sample as shown in Tables 1 and 2.

For the analyzed samples, HS, DS, and CS the percentage ranged from 77.6–88.4%, from 9.0–16.8% and from 2.3–8.0%, respectively. The present NMR quantification was useful for the comparability of API batches. The comparability of the NMR method with the EU Pharmacopeia enzymatic method is ongoing. The NMR method should be not compared equally to the EU Pharmacopeia enzymatic method.

The composition of HS in different danaparoid batches was found very similar, supporting the validity of the process used to extract and purify the product. Moreover, the low percentage of 6-O-sulfation, agrees with the typical composition of an HS structure [20]. The sulfation degree, calculated from the NMR data, confirm the similarity of the HS composition. Values are in the range between 1.62 and 1.70 with an average value of 1.65. The IdoA/IdoA2S ratio of DS and CS-A/CS-C ratio is also similar to that of galactosaminoglycans extracted from porcine mucosa (Table 3) [21].

Table 1. Percentage of glucosamine residues of heparan sulfate (HS) of one danaparoid sample (CAT272). A* corresponds to 3-O,N-sulfated glucosamine according with the abbreviations shown in Table S1.

A *	ANAc αred	ANAc-(I)	ANAc-(G)	ANAc-ox	ANS αred	ANS βred	ANS-(G)	ANS-(I)	ANS-(I2S)	A6S
2.2	0.9	0.3	23.4	4.4	1.7	0.4	11.4	19.3	33.5	48.4

"A *" means 3-O,N-sulfated glucosamine according with the abbreviations in Table S1.

Table 2. Percentage of uronic acid residues and sulfation degree of HS of one danaparoid (CAT272). (Abbreviations are in Table S1.)

I2S	I-(A6S)	I-(A6OH)	I-(ANAcox)	G-(ANS)	G-(ANAc)	Sulfation Degree
43.5	11.2	6.7	3.2	13.3	22.1	1.63

Table 3. Sulfate distribution (percentage) of dermatan sulfate (DS) and chondroitin sulfate (CS) of one danaparoid sample (CAT272). (Abbreviations in Table S1.)

DS		CS	
I2S	**I**	**G-(GalNAc,4S)**	**G-(GalNAc,6S)**
8.7	91.3	80.0	20.0

2.1.4. Chain Mapping by HPLC/ESI MS

An optimized LC/MS method allowed fingerprints of all the samples to be recorded and compared. The ion pair reversed phase high performance liquid chromatography (IPRP-HPLC) coupled to electrospray ionization mass spectroscopic (ESI-TOF MS) detection achieved partial separation of chain components and first level structural assignment. The presence in danaparoid GAGs of epimeric hexosamines required an optimization of the method successfully applied for chain mapping of LMWHs [22,23].

Dibutylamine, the ion pair in the mobile phase, interacting with sulfate groups allowed a better peak resolution when an initial isocratic mode was followed by a linear gradient elution (Figure S2). Good repeatability in three consecutive days and inter-day precision of LC/MS chromatograms was obtained and shown in Figure S3.

Comparable profiles were obtained for all the samples showing common oligosaccharidic peaks ranging from 1200 up to 7000 Da. Complete base peak chromatogram of sample CAT272 was shown in Figure 5a: minor fluctuations were observed for some samples in the chromatogram portions at 30–40 min and at 75–85 min.

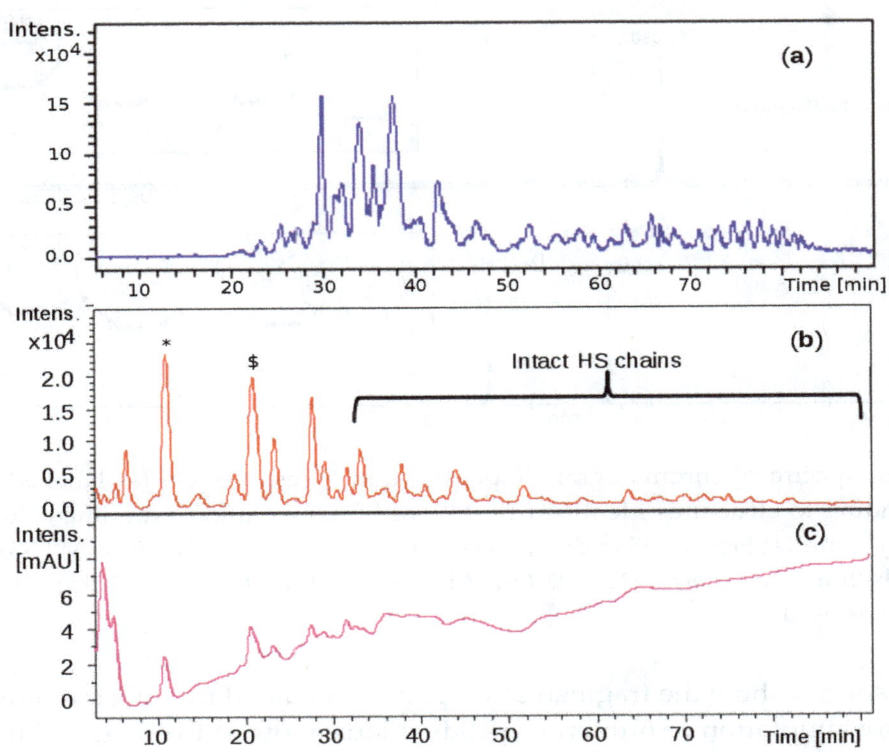

Figure 5. Liquid Chromatography-Mass Spectrometry (LC-MS) profiles: (**a**) one danaparoid sample CAT272; (**b**) ChABC danaparoid digestion product CAT469; (**c**) UV chromatogram at 232 nm of CAT469.

Only the most representative mass signals were attributed to the HS structures: several even and odd chains having 16 additional mass units than the regular oligosaccharidic sequences were identified and, supported by the previous NMR data that highlighted the presence of oxidized residues at the reducing ends, identified as 1-carboxy N-acetyl hexosamine [17,18].

2.2. Structural Study of One Danaparoid Sample

Compared to the natural porcine HS, the major component of danaparoid showed some structural modifications that could occur on galactosaminoglycan minor components of danaparoid and need to be further investigated.

One API sample was submitted to digestion with ChABC, the digest was analyzed by ^{1}H-NMR and its main signals were assigned to HS sequences. Comparing the N-acetyl region signals with those of the starting material a reduction of DS contribution (Figure S4) became evident; while at 5.9–6.0 ppm the signals of 4,5- unsaturated (Δ) uronic acids at the NRE produced by lyase were observed.

The same mixture was analyzed by LC-MS: the profile showed that the first eluted species (0 to 30 min) generated by the depolymerization of CS/DS could be detected at 232 nm for the presence of 4,5- unsaturated uronic acid due to the lyase action, followed by intact HS species detectable only by MS (Figure 5b,c).

This phase was focused on CS/DS oligosaccharides and among them two species with mass value of 934 (*m/z* 466 (z-2) RT 10′) and 1050 (*m/z* 524.0 (z-2) RT 20′) were detected (Figure 5b) and submitted to MS/MS fragmentation. Two species were identified: one as an unsaturated disulfated, di-*N*-acetyl tetrasaccharide bearing at the RE an oxidized N-acetyl galactosamine residue (ΔU4,2,2(T1)) and an unsaturated disulfated, di-*N*-acetyl pentasaccharide with a remnant (Ra) at the RE (ΔU5,2,2(Ra)) (Figure 6).

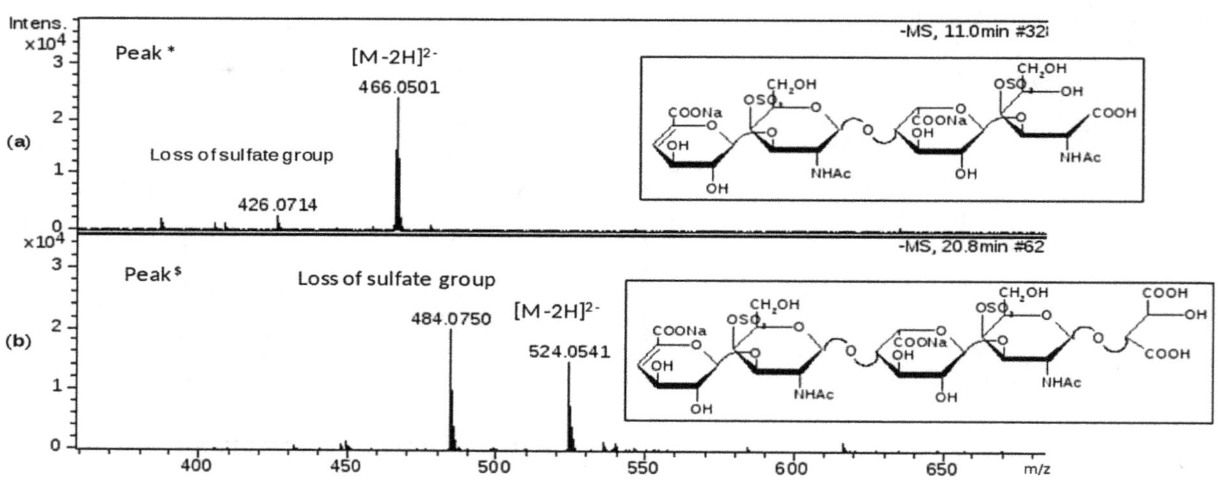

Figure 6. Mass spectra of chromatographic peaks * and $, respectively (as labelled in Figure 5b) and corresponding to structures identified by MS/MS fragmentation experiment (data shown in supplementary material Figures S5 and S6): (**a**) fragment at *m/z* 466.0501 (z-2; M 934) attributed to ΔU4,2,2(T1); (**b**) fragment at *m/z* 524.0541 (z-2; M 1050) attributed to ΔU5,2,2(Ra). The substitution pattern of DS was used.

The MS/MS spectra show the fragmentation pattern obtained by collision induced dissociation (CID) and structure annotation of numerous product ions allowed to elucidate the structure of the unknown parent ion (Figures S5 and S6). In particular, the characteristic ion product at *m/z* 316.0 (z-1) in the MS/MS spectrum of the first tetrasaccharide (M 934), revealed the oxidized galactosamine residue (ANAc,S +O labelled T1) which differs by 16 mass units from its regular form, as similarly observed for HS in Section 2.1.4. While the CID product ion at *m/z* 352.1 (z-1) generated from the second oligosaccharide (M 1050) resulted in being particularly informative for the confirmation of Ra terminal (ANAc + $C_4H_4O_5$).

Considering the whole profile, the main peaks were integrated and their assignments underlined such that the expected final product of the enzymatic cleavage ΔU2,1,1 was accompanied by the variant bearing a remnant Ra at the reducing end ΔU3,2,1(Ra). Other peaks were assigned to sequences having modified terminals T1 or Ra such as the oligosaccharides ΔU6,2,3(T1) and ΔU7,2,3(Ra), but also odd regular species such as the hexosamine A1,1,1, and trisaccharides A3,2,2 and A3,3,2 as well as the pentasaccharide ΔU5,2,2 bearing a uronic acid at the RE.

Since the digestion products detected in the mixture highlighted the presence of oligomers longer than the expected disaccharides, the conditions for an exhaustive depolymerization with ChABC were verified using a higher quantity of enzyme and repeating the reaction on the same sample, without improvement as checked by NMR. Therefore, the enzymatic efficiency was likely decreased by the presence of oxidized and remnant residues at the RE.

This study allowed the presence of unusual reducing ends on CS/DS component to be highlighted: the experimental data agreed in that T1 modification was observed on the galactosamine at the reducing end, while the terminal Ra occurred on uronic acid at the RE.

2.3. *Preparative Size Exclusion Chromatography of API Danaparoid Samples*

Seven batches of danaparoid (CAT271-277) were submitted to preparative gel filtration (SEC) on a Biogel P6 column. Comparable UV curves were detected for all the samples, an example with the indication of the collected fractions is displayed in Figure 7: the molecular weight decreases from A to N.

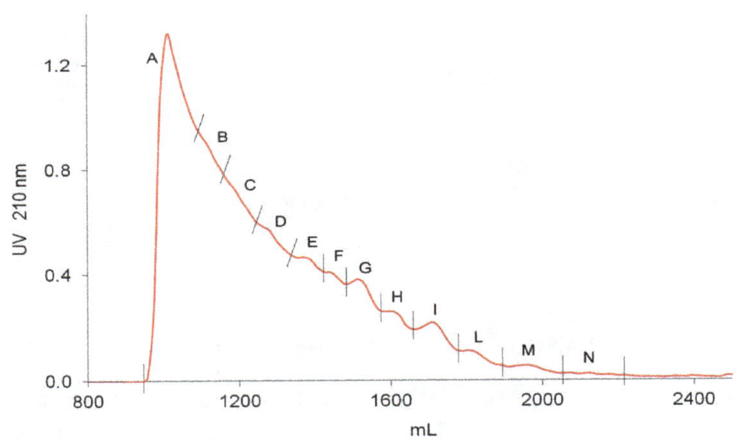

Figure 7. Preparative size exclusion chromatography (SEC) fractionation chromatographic UV 210 nm profile of a danaparoid (CAT277).

2.3.1. Determination of the Mw Distribution of SEC Fractions

The Mw distribution of fractions A, B, and C of all the seven API samples was determined and the results, reported in Table 4, showed comparable ranges of weight average Mw and polydispersity. The fraction A, constituted by the highest Mw components, was at the limit of the Biogel P6 chromatographic separation efficiency.

Table 4. Ranges of weight average molecular weight (Mw) and polydispersity (Pd) of SEC fractions of seven danaparoid Active Pharmaceutical Ingredient (API) samples.

Fractions	Mw (Da)	Pd
A	8200–8800	1.14–1.17
B	5300–5700	1.06–1.11
C	4400–4700	1.05–1.11

All SEC fractions (A–N) obtained from one danaparoid sample (CAT277) were analyzed for the determination of molecular weight parameters (Table 5): components of the subsequent fractions showed decreasing Mw and very low Pd values; the partial overlapping between adjacent fractions was displayed by their Refractive Index (RI) profiles in Figure 8.

Table 5. Weight average Mw and polydispersity (Pd) of SEC fractions of danaparoid Active Pharmaceutical Ingredient (API) sample CAT277.

Fractions	A	B	C	D	E	F	G	H	I	L	M	N
Mw (kDa)	8.2	5.4	4.4	3.9	3.3	3.0	2.8	2.5	2.3	2.1	2.1	1.9
Pd	1.17	1.06	1.06	1.04	1.05	1.06	1.05	1.05	1.05	1.04	1.04	1.01

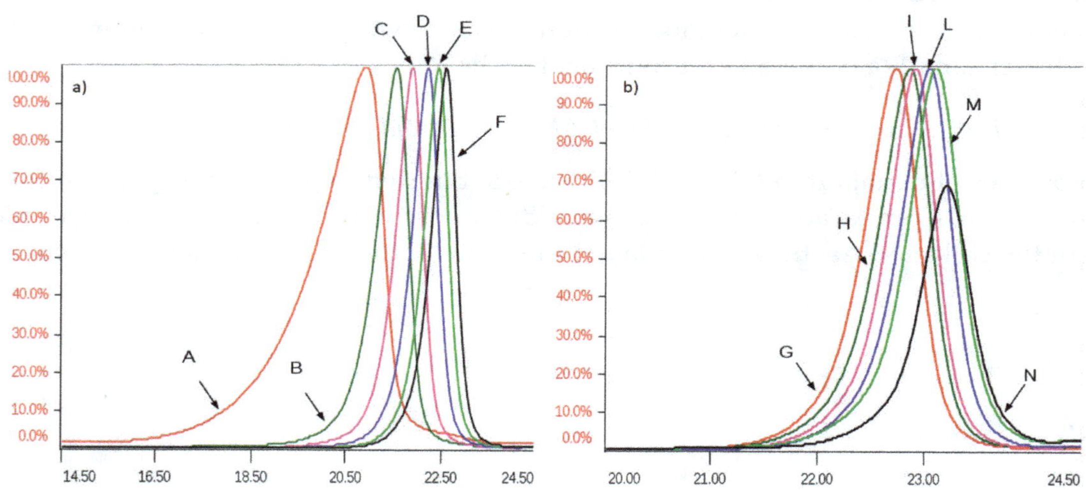

Figure 8. Overlapping of normalized Refractive Index (RI) profiles of SEC fractions of a danaparoid sample (CAT277): (**a**) fractions A–F, range volume 14–24.5 mL; (**b**) fractions G–N, range volume 20–24.5 mL.

2.3.2. 2D-NMR Spectroscopic Analysis of SEC Fractions of Danaparoid Samples

The 2D-NMR spectra of the danaparoid SEC fractions, considering some signals characteristic for each component, allowed it to be underlined how the proportion of GAG species varies over fractions.

Inspection of the H2/C2 region displays that the galactosamine (CS/DS) signals had more or equal intensity than those of glucosamine (HS) in the high Mw oligomers corresponding to fractions A and B followed by a progressive decrease in the subsequent fractions up to being absent in fractions L, M, and N.

The signal of C2/H2 of NS,3S,6S glucosamine (A2*) is present with variable intensity in almost all fractions, up to being undetected or in traces in fractions A and B.

The peaks related to oxidized RE residues at 4.6–4.2/57–61 ppm were variably present in almost all fractions.

The comparison between fractions obtained from different APIs was performed by analyzing the anomeric regions of the HSQC spectra (Figure S7), considering the peculiar disaccharides, IdoA2S-GlcN for HS, IdoA-GalNAc for DS and GlcA-GalNAc 4 and/or 6 sulfated for CS.

By visual inspection the highest content of CS and DS components was found in fraction A, the intensity of their cross-peaks being superior to those of IdoA2S of HS, then decreasing gradually in all the danaparoid samples, while the HS oligosaccharides increased upwards to become the sole components in fractions L to N. The DS components seemed to be more abundant than those of CS which disappeared early, as the signals of GlcA linked to GalN6S in comparison with those of GlcA linked to GalN4S. Variation of the CS/DS component content and distribution was qualitatively evaluated in HSQC spectra and summarized as scores in Table 6, resulting in being slightly different among the seven API danaparoid samples. This is considered normal for a natural extraction product.

Table 6. Variation of dermatan sulfate and chondroitin sulfate among SEC fractions of seven API batches by qualitative observation of peculiar HSQC anomeric signals.

		A	B	C	D	E	F	G	H	I	L	M	N
CAT271	DS	+++	+++	+++	+++	++	++	++	++	+	—	—	—
	CS	+++	+++	+++	+++	++	++	++	+	—	—	—	—
CAT272	DS	+++	+++	+++	+++	++	++	++	++	++	—	—	—
	CS	+++	+++	+++	+++	++	++	++	+	+	—	—	—
CAT273	DS	+++	+++	++	++	++	++	++	+	—	—	—	—
	CS	+++	+++	++	++	++	++	—	—	—	—	—	—
CAT274	DS	+++	+++	++	++	++	++	+	—	—	—	—	—
	CS	+++	+++	++	++	+	—	—	—	—	—	—	—
CAT275	DS	+++	+++	++	++	++	++	+	—	—	—	—	—
	CS	+++	+++	++	++	+	—	—	—	—	—	—	—
CAT276	DS	+++	+++	++	++	++	+	+	—	—	—	—	—
	CS	+++	+++	++	+	—	—	—	—	—	—	—	—
CAT277	DS	+++	+++	+++	+++	++	++	++	++	+	—	—	—
	CS	+++	+++	+++	+++	++	++	++	+	—	—	—	—

Where '—' = absent; '+' = traces; '++' = present; '+++' = more present.

2.3.3. Sequencing of Danaparoid SEC Fractions by LC/MS Analysis

A pilot study by the IPRP-HPLC/MS method was addressed to sequence the SEC fractions of a danaparoid sample (CAT277) (Figure 7) to achieve a first level structural assignment of components and identify probable modified structures on shorter chains. This explorative study was conducted by analyzing a restricted portion of each SEC fraction of the danaparoid sample, with the aim of simplifying the expected complexity of sequences and eventually identifying structure modifications. These selective analyses provided only a partial picture of the whole fractions but also the detection of minor modified sequences useful for the study.

This approach led to the identification in the fractions E to N of few HS regular sequences and a majority of HS chains bearing oxidized residues at the reducing end, likely 1-carboxylated glucosamines, shown as T1 in Figure 9 [17–19] applying the code already used for the similar modification on CS/DS (Section 2.2). Less abundant modifications were observed and displayed as T2, T3, T4 and T5 (Figure 9).

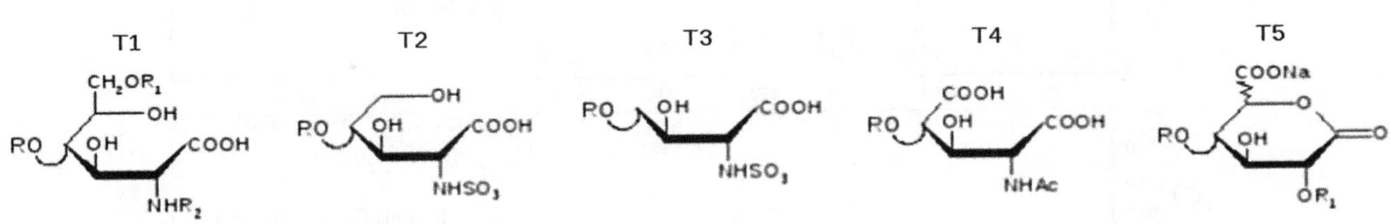

where R= GAG chain; R_1=H or SO_3; R_2=H, SO_3 or Ac

Figure 9. Structures of oxidized Reducing End (RE) residues compatible with the observed *m/z* values (the substitution pattern was in accordance with the observed species listed in Table 7).

In particular, the species exhibiting T2 and T3 end residues, detected in a minor peak of fraction N, can be explained by further oxidation of the secondary alcohol and decarboxylation steps of terminal T1 (Figure 10). Confirmation of the molecular formula is supported by a very low error (<10 ppm) between experimental and theoretical mass values.

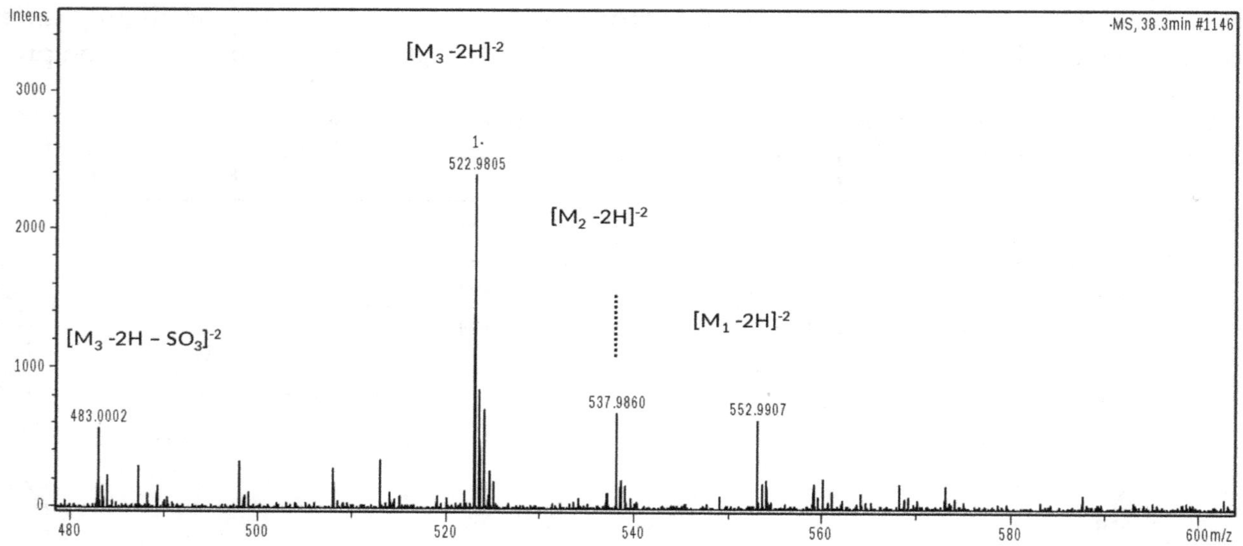

Figure 10. Mass spectrum displaying the different oxidation forms of oligosaccharide U4,5,0 from M_1 to M_3 derivative: *m/z* 552.9907 (z-2, M_1 1108) identified as U4,5,0 (T1); *m/z* 537.9860 (z-2, M_2 1078) identified as U4,5,0 (T2); *m/z* 522.9805 (z-2, M_3 1048) identified as U4,5,0 (T3).

Concerning the T4 modification, observed in fraction H, only a high resolution MS measurement allowed this oxidized residue to be discriminated from a regular structure.

The experimental mass signal at *m/z* 881.086 (z-2), shown in Figure 11, at first sight seemed to correspond to the regular hexasaccharide U6,6,3 (sum formula $C_{42}N_3O_{52}H_{65}S_6$). A more detailed mass investigation, revealing a high mass error between experimental and theoretical values (22 ppm), suggested another possible structure modification as U6,6,3(T4) corresponding to a sum formula of $C_{41}N_3O_{53}H_{61}S_6$, showing a good overlap of mass signals with a decrease of the error to 2 ppm.

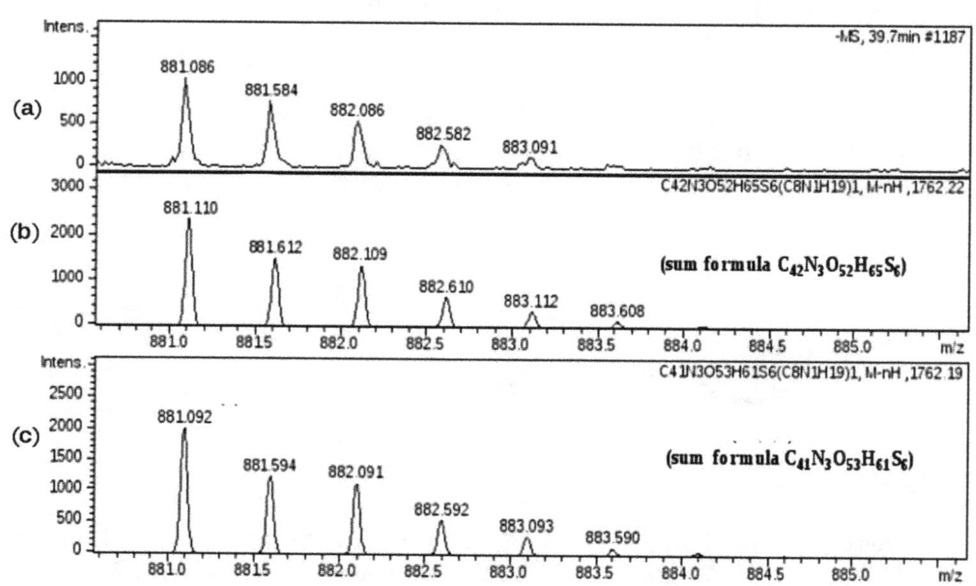

Figure 11. Mass signal at *m/z* 881.086 (z-2): (**a**) experimental *m/z* and isotopic distribution; (**b**) theoretical *m/z* and isotopic distribution corresponding to the regular structure of U6,6,3 (sum formula $C_{42}N_3O_{52}H_{65}S_6$); (**c**) theoretical *m/z* and isotopic distribution corresponding to the oxidized structure U6,6,3(T4) (sum formula $C_{41}N_3O_{53}H_{61}S_6$).

In fractions F, H, and L, some mass values differing by two Daltons (-2H) with respect to the HS regular sequences were observed. The hypothesis was that after the oxidation of carbon 1 a water loss occurred to give the lactone (T5 in Figure 9) and lacking 2 Da. The mass accuracy of both T1 and T5 modifications found in fraction F was verified also by ESI-FT MS: the error on theoretical mass was minor or equal to 1.5 ppm.

After the pilot study the same analytical method was applied to the SEC fractions isolated from seven API samples. A qualitative observation of the LC profiles of the corresponding fractions showed a good similarity mainly among fractions D to N, containing LMW chains. A higher variability was observed among the first eluted fractions (A to C), containing mainly CS/DS high Mw chains endowed with an intrinsic heterogeneity of natural extractive GAGs such as danaparoid and whose content varied among API samples. A compositional analysis was performed integrating the main peaks where the principal detected species were investigated: the structures were the same inside each fraction group, while different oligomers were observed in different fractions.

The list of main species found in SEC fractions is shown in Table 7, together with the GAG assignment and eventual additional species previously identified in the pilot study. Components are indicated by: A for hexosamines or U for uronic acids as NRE residues, followed by three numbers referring respectively to oligosaccharidic units, sulfate, and N-acetyl groups. The number of oligosaccharidic units includes both RE and/or NRE variants (T1–T5 and Ra), examples of sequences are shown in Figure 12. The assignment of the m/z value to a single GAG component was based on the knowledge of their N-acetylated, N-, O-sulfated degrees.

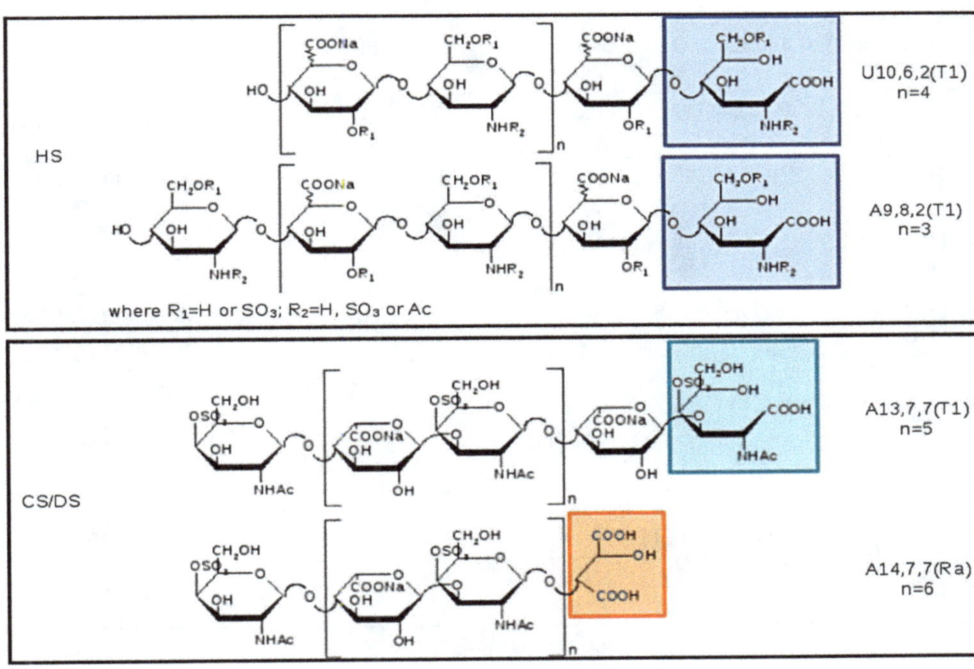

Figure 12. Example of structures detected in SEC fractions, the modified RE are highlighted in the boxes: HS sequences are displayed in the upper panel with the terminal T1 at the RE and with the uronic acid or the glucosamine at the non reducing end (NRE) in even or odd oligomers, respectively. CS/DS structures are shown in the lower panel (the substitution pattern of DS is used as example because it is more abundant than CS): two possibly reducing ends are T1 and Ra, the galactosamine is placed at the NRE.

The main components of fractions A–C were assigned to CS/DS, and those of fractions D to N to HS components. Some unassigned mass values were present, but detected in all samples.

Almost all the detected species showed a structural modification of the reducing end residue. Oxidized hexosamine T1 was present in both CS/DS and HS sequences, while the remnant Ra, of oxidized uronic acid, seems to be present only on CS/DS chains.

In principle, oxidation of reducing end residues can occur both on hexosamine and uronic acid [24]. Actually, whereas for odd sequences experimental mass data permitted the certain identification of ending residues thus confirming the presence of T1 on RE hexosamine, for even sequences terminal RE and NRE residues cannot be distinguished, and oxidized residues were not precisely assigned accordingly. Considering the literature data [17,18], in Table 7 and Figure 12 the variant T1 was attributed to the RE hexosamine of even sequences bearing a uronic acid at the NRE.

The terminal T5 (lactonized form of T2) was observed on both even and odd sequences as shown in Figure 9 and Table 7.

Table 7. Main species detected in fractions A–N of 7 API samples.

Fraction	Main Species in the Woul Fraction	GAG	Species Detect at the Top of the Fraction (Pilot Study)
A	A19,10,10(T1) to A27,14,14(T1); A20,10,10(Ra) to A26,13,13(Ra)	CS/DS	-
B	A17,9,9(T1) to A21,11,11(T1); A16,8,8(Ra) to A22,11,11(Ra)	CS/DS	-
C	A13,7,7(T1) to A15,11,8(T1); A14,7,7(Ra) to A18,9,9(Ra)	CS/DS	-
D	U10,9,3 to U10,10,3; A7,10,0(T1); A11,10,6(T1) to A11,11,6(T1); U10,10,3(T1) to U10,13,3(T1)	HS	-
E	U8,8,3(T1) to U8,10,3(T1); A11,8,2(T1) to A11,14,2(T1)	HS	U8,10,2(T1); A11,14,1(T1)
F	U10,6,2(T1) to U10,8,2(T1); U10,8,1(T1) to U10,13,1(T1)	HS	U7,8,1(T5) to U7,10,1(T5); U10,8,0(T5)
G	A9,4,2(T1) # to A9,8,2(T1); A9,8,1(T1) to A9,13,1(T1)	HS	-
H	U8,6,1(T1) to U8,10,1(T1); U6,6,3(T4) to U6,8,3(T4)	HS	A9,6,2; A9,9,1 and A9,10,1; U8,6,0(T5)
I	A7,6,1 and A7,7,1; A7,5,1(T1) to A7,10,1(T1); U6,4,1 to U6,5,1; U6,6,1(T1)	HS	A7,5,2(T1); U7,4,0(T5)
L	A7,6,1; A5,5,1; A7,5,2 # to A7,6,2; U6,5,1(T1) to U6,7,1(T1); U6,6,1(T5) #	HS	U6,3,0(T5) and U6,4,0(T5); A7,7,1; A7,8,0 to A7,9,0; A7,9,1
M	A5,4,1; U6,5,1 to U6,6,1; U6,6,0 to U6,9,0; A5,4,1(T1) to A5,7,1(T1); A5,7,0(T1)	HS	A5,8,1(T1)
N	A5,5,0 to A5,9,0; A5,5,1 and A5,6,1; A5,5,1(T1); U4,5,0(T3)	HS	U4,5,0(T1); U4,5,0(T2)

species not detected in one sample.

2.4. Isolation of GAG Components of Danaparoid and Compositional Analysis

Three danaparoid samples were chosen to perform the isolation of HS and CS/DS components, based on their different content of HS-DS-CS that range from 78.0–87.2%, from 9.8–14.0% and from 3.0–8.0%, respectively (NMR data).

The parent samples were submitted to complementary procedures to depolymerize selectively the two GAG families of danaparoid: for the isolation of HS the chondroitinase ABC was applied, while the isolation of CS/DS was performed using heparin lyase III followed by a chemical reaction using nitrous acid.

The depolymerization methods, described in Section 5, led to the isolation of three enriched fractions of HS and CS/DS. The weight recovery for the enriched HS fractions was about 78–81%, while those of CS/DS range from 15–26%.

Both components were fully characterized by NMR, molecular weight distribution, LC-MS chain mapping and only for HS fractions by LC-MS disaccharidic analysis as subsequently reported herein.

2.4.1. Molecular Weight Data

Molecular weight distribution was determined by triple detector array (TDA) for both families of samples: the enriched CS/DS fractions range from 6200 to 7100 Da, while for those enriched HS components the Mw varies from 3300 to 3500 Da and is consistent with the data of the SEC fractions. The polydispersity is lower for the HS species (1.13) than for the CS/DS ones (1.19), both are lower than the API samples.

In Figure 13 The Refractive Index (RI) profile overlay of a parent API sample and its enriched HS and CS/DS fractions displays the presence of CS/DS components in the higher Mw with respect to the API, as already observed in the NMR and MS data regarding the SEC study. On the other hand, the enriched HS fraction is observed in the mid–lower Mw range.

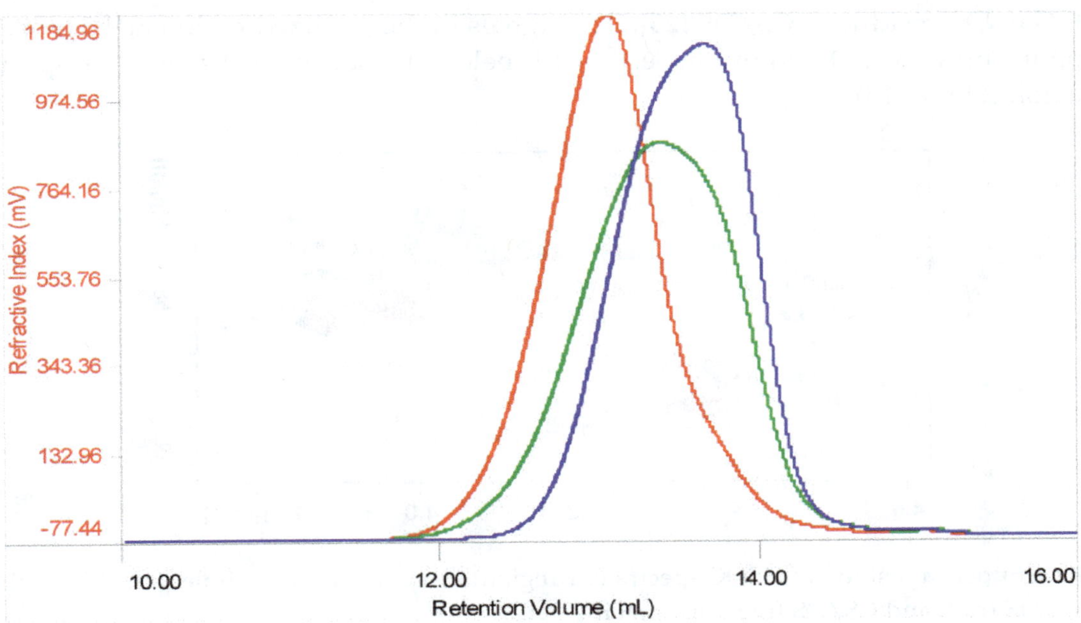

Figure 13. Refractive Index profile overlay of a danaparoid sample (CAT272 in green), its enriched CS/DS (red) and HS (blue) fractions.

2.4.2. NMR Observations

The 2D-NMR-HSQC assignments of the CS/DS component were done according to literature data [19,25,26] as shown in the spectra of one CS/DS enriched fraction (Figure 14a): the chemical shifts of 4.36/85.4 ppm and 4.19/76.8 ppm, in red, were in agreement with the positions C4′ and C5′ of remnant Ra. While the CS/DS fraction does not contain signals of HS, the spectrum of the HS fraction also shows signals typical of CS/DS oligomers, highlighted in red in Figure 14b.

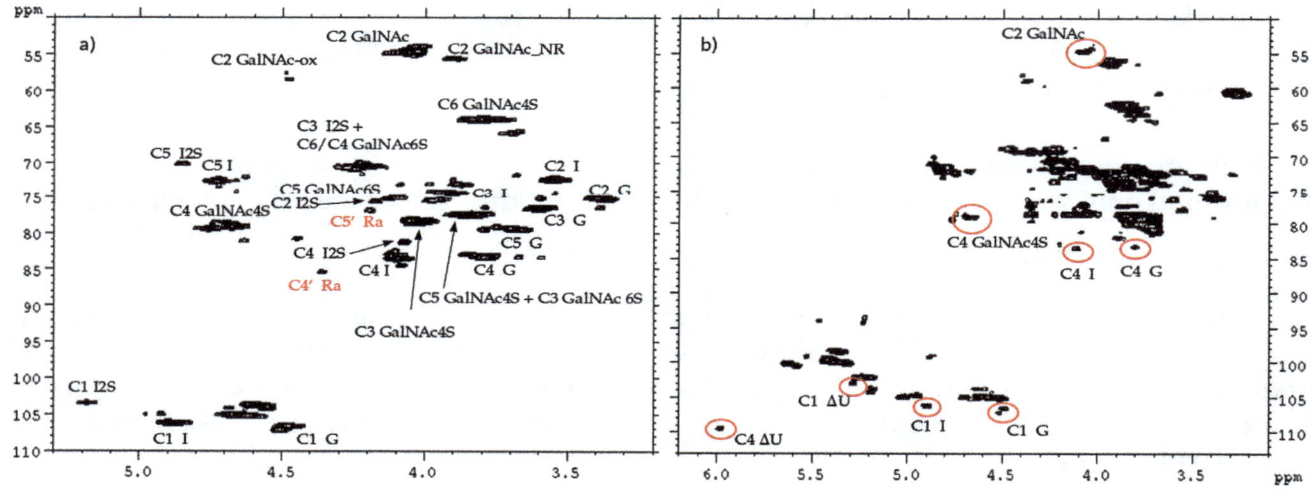

Figure 14. HSQC NMR spectra of CS/DS (**a**) and HS (**b**) fraction of danaparoid CAT272. Signals belonging to CS/DS are circled in red.

The superimposition of the HSQC spectra of HS and CS/DS fractions with that of the danaparoid starting material allows some peaks to be assigned correctly: signal at 3.90/55.5 ppm belongs to the C2 of the NRE GalNAc residue of CS/DS [25]. The signals in the oxidized region at 4.39/58.1 ppm and 4.27/59.5 ppm (shown as ox1 and ox2 in Section 2.1) belong to HS, being absent in the spectrum of the CS/DS fraction (Figure 15).

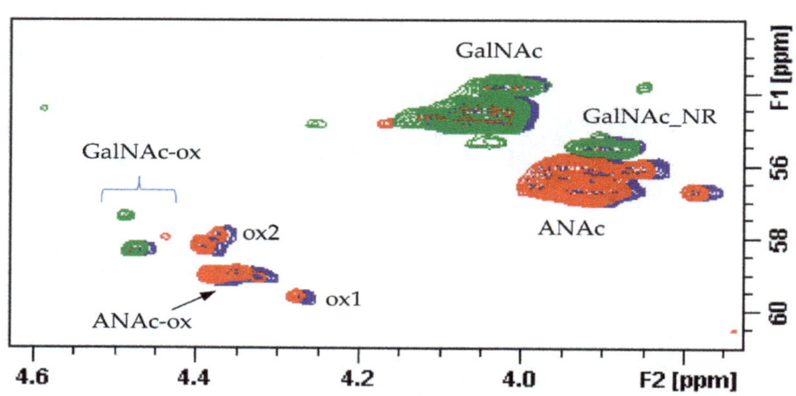

Figure 15. Superimposition of HSQC spectra (C2 region) of a danaparoid sample (CAT272 in blue), its enriched HS (red) and CS/DS fractions (green).

The composition of HS and CS/DS in the corresponding enriched fractions is very similar to that found in the parent danaparoid samples, demonstrating the robustness of the methods of separation.

The enriched CS/DS fractions, free from HS, display DS as the most abundant species ranging from 63–76%. On the contrary, the enriched HS fractions include a part of CS/DS that varies between 5% and 14%.

2.4.3. LC-MS Chain Mapping Analysis of CS/DS Fractions

The LC-MS analysis of enriched CS/DS fractions show the simplification of the region of short chains (RT 20–40 min) due to the removal of the HS component by the analytical depolymerization/purification procedure, and contemporarily the enrichment of CS/DS species in the region of long chains (RT 50–90 min).

The investigation in depth of mass spectra at the apex of each peak allows the main mass signals (Figure 16) to be assigned: CS/DS chains from A6,2,3 to A30,15,15 oligomers were identified (Table S2), almost all of them having both the oxidized variants T1 and Ra remnant due to the production process. These results are in agreement with the data obtained by SEC fractions in which the CS/DS sequences from A13,7,7 to A27,14,14 were identified. The isolation of the CS/DS component allowed their shorter oligomers previously masked by the HS component in the API danaparoid sample to be detected.

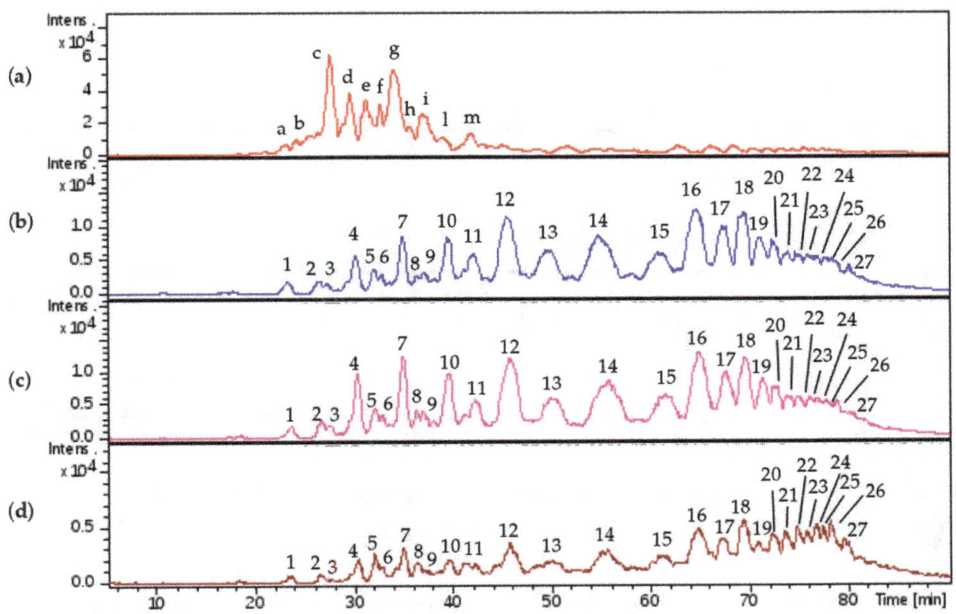

Figure 16. LC-MS profiles comparison: (**a**) danaparoid sample CAT272; (**b**) CS/DS isolated from CAT271; (**c**) CS/DS isolated from CAT272; (**d**) CS/DS isolated from CAT275.

The qualitative comparison of LC-MS profiles of the three isolated CS/DS samples underlines a good similarity between the CS/DS fractions isolated from CAT272 and CAT271, while for those isolated from CAT275 the lower molecular weight species (from 20 to 60 min) are less represented with respect to the higher Mw ones eluting from 60 to 85 min in comparison with the other two samples. This observation is in agreement with SEC data in which the variation of CS/DS content is displayed as scores in Table 6 and for CAT275 their reduction is observed in longer fractions than for CAT271 and CAT272.

2.4.4. LC-MS Chain Mapping Analysis of HS Enriched Fractions

The enriched HS fractions were also analyzed by LC-MS and compared with danaparoid (Figure 17).

The assignments were reported in accordance with the retention time, the majority of the peaks (n.7–15) were attributed to HS oligomers with the modification T1. Regular sequences of HS were observed with less intensity assigned to A5,6,0; A7,6,1; A7,5,0.

The comparison of the region from 30 to 45 min for the three isolated samples displayed slight differences in the intensity of the peaks.

The comparison of isolated HS and danaparoid (Table S3) allowed the correspondence of HS sequences in the isolated HS (peaks n.7–15) and in danaparoid (peaks from 'c' to 'm') to be observed; in the range of shorter species (peaks n.1–6 and at 29.1 min) there were pentasaccharides with 3 acetyl and hexa- and hepta-saccharides with a double bond on uronic acid, not present in the parent danaparoid that should be related to the residual presence of CS/DS fragments from the enzymatic process and not removed by purification steps (as already observed in NMR spectra).

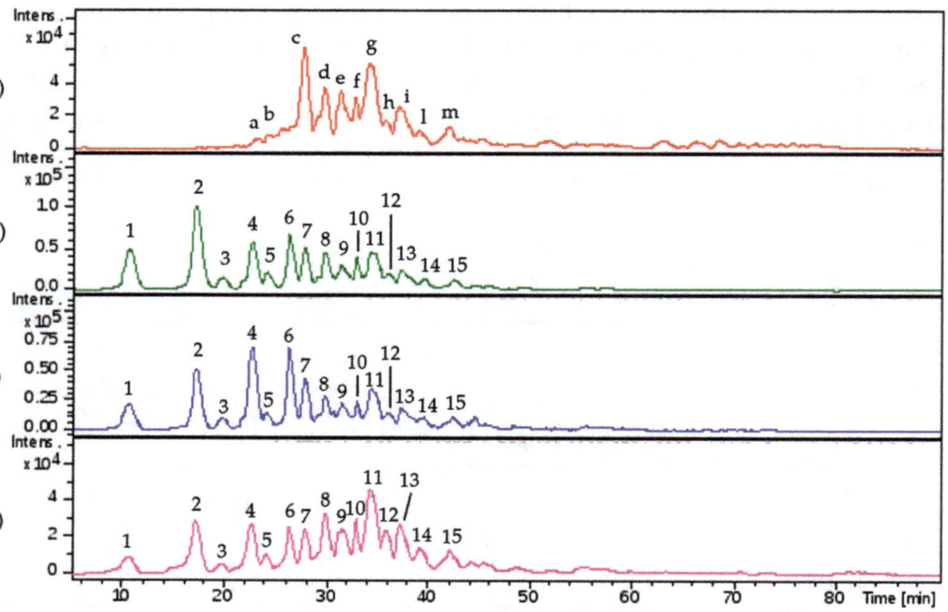

Figure 17. LC-MS profiles comparison: (**a**) danaparoid sample CAT272; (**b**) HS isolated from CAT271; (**c**) HS isolated from CAT272; (**d**) HS isolated from CAT275.

To complete the compositional analysis, the HS enriched fractions, along with a nadroparin and a heparin samples were submitted to enzymatic digestion using a mixture of heparinase I, II, III.

A qualitative inspection of the profiles highlighted a comparable oligosaccharidic composition among the digestion products of all the enriched HS fractions, some differences were observed in the nadroparin and heparin digest components (Figure 18).

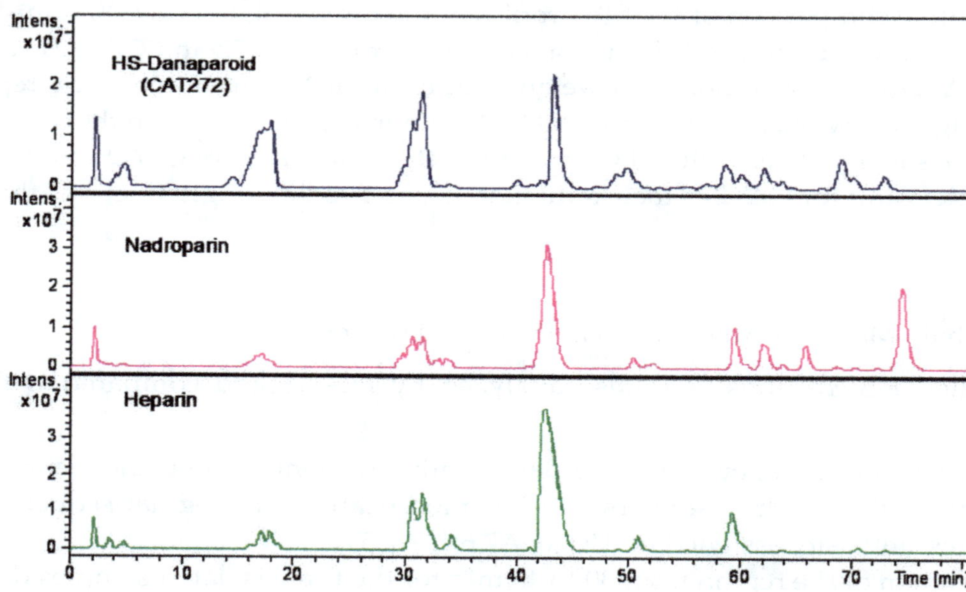

Figure 18. LC-MS profiles of HS danaparoid (CAT272), nadroparin and heparin digested by heparinases I, II, III.

The peaks identified by comparison with commercial standard disaccharides, were detected in all digested samples. As regards the species obtained from the enriched HS fractions regular unsaturated oligomers were observed together with some saturated odd and even sequences. Confirming the previously described data, some tetrasaccharides with the variant T1 at RE were present, only a very low peak corresponding to an unsaturated monosulfated, *N*-acetyl disaccharide bearing the T1 at the RE was detected supporting the hypothesis that the variants at RE inhibit the lyases.

An unsaturated tetrasaccharide with one acetyl and four sulfates was observed together with some species, Δ4,3,1, A3,4,0, and A3,5,0 that should be related to the sequence AGA*IA not cleaved by lyases [27,28].

Based on the ratio between N-acetylated and N-sulfated disaccharides, calculated by the commercial standard disaccharides peaks, the enriched HS fractions were compared with nadroparin and heparin. The data shown as percent in Table 8 allow the substantial different nature of heparin to be underlined in respect of the glucosaminoglycan component of danaparoid that has an HS structure [29,30]. This semi-quantitative analysis of N-acetylated/N-sulfated disaccharides ratio was performed on extracted ion chromatograms (EIC) of mass signals corresponding to mass values of disaccharides (the sum of ΔU-ANAc, ΔU-ANAc6S, ΔU2S-ANAc, ΔU2S-ANAc6S with respect to the sum of ΔU-ANS, ΔU-ANS6S, ΔU2S-ANS, ΔU2S-ANS6S percent).

Table 8. Ratio percentage between disaccharides N-acetylated and N-sulfated.

Sample	Ratio % N-acetylated/N-sulfated Disaccharides
HS-CAT271	41.4
HS-CAT272	39.0
HS-CAT275	39.2
nadroparin	16.8
heparin	13.2

3. Discussion

The danaparoid characterization was focused on a compositional study of intact API samples in obtaining their general picture, followed by the study of fractions differing in size and of their GAG components. Both APIs and their fractions were analyzed with complementary techniques following an orthogonal analytical approach.

The analyzed API samples resulted in similar data for every applied technique such as NMR spectra, LC-MS profiles, and HP-SEC-TDA curves; their variability was included in the natural variation typical of extractive products.

Danaparoid was a low-molecular-weight mixture of HS, CS, and DS, confirmed by experimental weight average molecular weight (Mw) ranging from 4200 to 4600 Da. The charge density determined as sulfate-to-carboxylate ratio was between 1.19 and 1.32.

By analyzing the NMR spectra, it was confirmed that the main species is an HS glucosaminoglycan, based on the sulfation/acetylation pattern. Dermatan sulfate and chondroitin sulfate were present quantitatively as secondary and tertiary components, respectively. Among the peaks relative to regular mono- or disaccharides of GAGs, some signals connected to the bleaching process were detected and attributed to oxidized gluco-/galactosamine at the reducing end (shown as T1). This modification, corresponding to the addition of one oxygen to the mass values of regular sequences, was confirmed by mass spectrometry both on HS and CS/DS. During the in-depth study on the galactosaminoglycan component, the remnant 3-O tartaric acid (Ra) at the RE was also detected.

The size fractionation was performed for all danaparoid batches and their fractions were submitted for further studies. NMR spectra were evaluated by means of the main characteristic signals of each component of danaparoid, through the variation of their anomeric peaks in every fraction and then among the starting batches: for all APIs the highest quantity of CS/DS component was found in the higher molecular weight fraction A, then decreasing down to fractions L, M, and N containing only HS. The different CS/DS content as well as their different distribution could be explained by variation in the starting natural sources. The presence of HS component in all fractions was ascertained by NMR.

The MS data of SEC fractions were evaluated qualitatively from the chromatographic profiles. These showed slight variations among batches in the range of longer chains where the major variability was expected. From the compositional point of view, the chain size decreased and sequences varied from fraction A to N, the main species found in the fraction of the same size of different API batches had an analogue composition.

In particular, investigating the main mass values, the fractions A to C showed CS/DS sequences having both T1 and Ra variants at RE; while in the subsequent fractions, structures attributed to HS were identified and characterized not only by the most abundant reducing end variant T1 but also by regular sequences and, less representative but structural interesting, variants T2, T3, T4, and T5. The majority of the HS components of all fractions were found to be odd oligosaccharides with a glucosamine (A) at the NRE; in fractions F and H only even sequences were identified; in the fractions containing shorter chains odd and even sequences were in similar abundance. Odd oligosaccharidic chains were not usually found in extractive GAG sequences even if present in low amounts in the LMWHs, enoxaparin and dalteparin [23] and highly represented in parnaparin [31] and γ-heparin [32] obtained by radical depolymerization.

The Mw range of fraction components, determined by MS is comparable with that obtained by the HP-SEC-TDA method which underlined also the closeness of contiguous fraction components, in particular for F to N included from 3000 to 1900 Da.

The isolation of components starting from three intact API samples was performed applying depolymerization procedures, using the proper enzyme and/or chemical reaction, followed by multiple purification steps. All of them were submitted for full characterization: Mw distribution, NMR, chain mapping, and only for HS fractions disaccharidic analysis by LC-MS.

The isolated CS/DS fractions were pure and the molecular weight analysis confirmed that the galactosaminoglycans were mainly present in the high molecular weight range of danaparoid, having a weight average molecular weight (Mw) from 6200 to 7100 Da. On the other hand, the HS fractions should be considered enriched HS fractions with CS/DS still being present (5–14%), their weight average Mw was found in the range from 3300 to 3500 Da, consistent with SEC fractions data.

Analyzing their NMR spectra, the fractions isolated from the three API samples showed a composition similar to that of the corresponding species present in the parent API samples, supporting the robustness of the separation procedures. Taking advantage of the purity of CS/DS fractions, some NMR signals were correctly assigned to the right component such as the C2/H2 of the NRE GalNAc residue at 3.90/55.5 ppm. In the region of oxidized residues two signals ox1 and ox2, hypothetically belonging to sequences similar to that bearing T1 variant, were attributed to HS because they were not observed in the isolated CS/DS fractions. The content of DS was evaluated by NMR in the isolated CS/DS fractions compared with that of CS and resulted ranging from 63% to 76%.

Moreover, also the LC-MS profiles of isolated CS/DS fractions were simplified by the removal of HS component, in the region of both short and long oligomers. The observed oligomeric size distribution was in good agreement with the SEC data and allowed the detection of higher oligomers (range 1271 (dp6) to 8282 Da (dp30)) bearing the variants T1 or Ra at the RE.

The study of enriched HS fractions allowed the confirmation of components already observed in danaparoid (dp5 to dp8) and the disaccharidic analysis, performed in comparison with nadroparin and heparin samples, provided compositional data in accordance with SEC data. Moreover, the evaluation of N-acetyl and N-sulfate ratio underlined that the glucosaminonoglycan component of danaparoid is heparan sulfate differing from those obtained from nadroparin and heparin samples.

4. Materials and Methods

4.1. Reagents and Starting Materials

Seven danaparoid API batches (CAT271-277), one heparin sodium USP and one Nadroparin calcium samples were provided by Aspen Oss B.V., Oss, Netherlands. Heparin lyases I (EC 4.2.2.7), II and III (EC 4.2.2.8) were purchased from Grampian Enzymes, Aberdeen, UK. Chondroitin ABC lyase from *Proteus vulgaris* (EC 4.2.2.4), ammonium acetate ($\geq$98%), sodium azide ($\geq$99.0%), sodium nitrate (≥99.0%), sodium dihydrogen phosphate monohydrate (>98%), sodium hydrogen phosphate dihydrate (≥99.0%), trimethylsilyl-3-propionic acid (TSP 98% D), dibutylamine (≥99.5%), acetic acid (glacial, 99.9%), acetonitrile (LC-MS grade), methanol (LC-MS grade), ammonium chloride (≥99.5%), sodium nitrite (>95%), sodium tetraborate (≥98%), hydrochloric acid (≥37%) were purchased from Sigma Aldrich (Milan, Italy); calcium acetate (≥97%) from BDH; sodium acetate (≥99%) and NaOH (≥99%) from Merck (Kenilworth, NJ, USA); Amberlite IR 120 H^+ and 0.1 M NaOH from Fluka Analytical (Milan, Italy).

Ethanol (96%) was purchased from Girelli Alcool (Milan, Italy); ethylenediaminetetraacetic acid (EDTA D16, 98%) from Cambridge Isotope Laboratories (Tewksbury, MA, USA) and deuterium oxide (≥99.9%) from Euriso-top (Saint-Aubin, France). Deionized water (conductivity less than 0.15 μS) was prepared with an osmosis inverse system (Culligan, Milan, Italy).

4.2. Molecular Weight Determination

Molecular weight determinations were performed using an HPLC system combined with a Viscotek mod. 305 Triple Detector Array [12,13]. The HPLC Viscotek equipment was made up by a Knauer Smartline 5100 pump, a Biotech Degasser model 2003, and an HTA autosampler model HT310L. The detector system was composed of right angle laser light scattering (90° angle geometry), refractive index and viscometer; all detectors and the separation columns were contained in an oven compartment.

Two chromatographic conditions were applied: (I) for SEC fractions (Section 2.3.1) two silica columns G3000SWXL+G4000SWXL TSK GEL (7.8 mm ID × 30 cm, Tosoh Bioscience S.r.l., Rivoli, Torino, Italy) preceded by precolumn TSK GEL SWXL GUARD (7 μm, 6.0 × 40 mm, Tosoh Bioscience) were used eluting with ammonium acetate 0.1 M, sodium azide 0.02% at 0.6 mL/min ± 10% setting up the temperature at 30 °C; (II) for API samples (Section 2.1.1) and isolated fractions CS/DS and HS (Section 2.4.1) the chromatographic elution was performed at 0.6 mL/min ± 10% with sodium nitrate 0.1 M, sodium azide 0.05% on two polymeric columns G3000PWXL+G2500PWXL TSK GEL (7.8 mm ID × 30 cm, Tosoh Bioscience) at 40 °C.

The samples were dissolved with a concentration between 8 and 12 mg/mL in the mobile phase used for the elution; 100 μL of each solution was injected. All chromatographic systems were calibrated using for (I) a pullulan (PSS, Mainz, Germany) and for (II) a polyethylene oxide (Agilent Technologies, Santa Clara, CS, USA), both are certified standards of known Mw, polydispersity and intrinsic viscosity. The data elaboration was performed with OmniSEC software, version 4.6.2 (Malvern, UK).

4.3. Sulfation Degree Determination

The sulfation degree of all samples, expressed as sulfate to carboxylate molar ratio, was determined in duplicate by conductimetric titration following the method proposed by Casu et al. [14]. A sample of ~75 mg of the acidic form of danaparoid, previously exchanged on Amberlite IR 120 H+, in 100 mL of distilled water was titrated with 0.1 M NaOH using an automatic titrator (Titrando 888, Metrohm Italiana S.r.l., Origgio, Varese, Italy) equipped with a conductivity cell (constant = 0.76 cm^{-1}).

4.4. NMR

About 250 mg of API batches were dissolved in 2.5 mL of D_2O, and analyzed by using a Bruker AV 500 MHz (125 MHz for ^{13}C) NMR spectrometer (Karlsruhe, Germany). The carbon spectra were recorded with a pulse delay of 1 s and 20 k scans.

About 35 mg of danaparoid samples were dissolved in 0.6 mL of buffer solution pH 7.1 (buffer phosphate 0.15 M, EDTA-D16 0.3 mM) in D_2O with 0.12 mM TSP; while the fractions isolated (20 or 35 mg) during the experimental activity were dissolved in 0.6 mL of D_2O. Both groups of samples were analyzed by using a Bruker Avance III HD NMR spectrometer operating at 500 MHz (^1H) equipped with TCI cryoprobe (Karlsruhe, Germany). The proton spectra were acquired with presaturation of residual HDO signal, 16 scans and 12 s of pulse delay. The Heteronuclear Single Quantum Coherence

(HSQC) spectra were recorded with the library Bruker pulse sequence hsqcetgpsisp2.2, a pulse delay of 2–5 s and 8–24 scans. The spectra elaboration was done using Bruker TopSpin software, version 3.2 (Karlsruhe, Germany).

4.5. LC-MS Analysis

LC-MS analysis of all of samples was performed using ion-pair reversed-phase separation on a Kinetex-C18 column (2.1 mm × 100 mm, ODS 2.6 μm, 100 Å, Phenomenex, Aschaffenburg, Germany) with pre-column filter (Phenomenex, Aschaffenburg, Germany) at room temperature coupled with mass spectrometer. The injected volume was 5 μL at a concentration of about 5 mg/mL.

A binary solvent system was used for a multi-step gradient elution using solvent A (dibutylamine 10 mM, acetic acid 10 mM in water) and solvent B (dibutylamine 10 mM, acetic acid 10 mM in acetonitrile) with the following schedule: (I) for SEC fractions of pilot study (first part of Section 2.3.3) at flow rate of 0.1 mL/min, 15% B for 5 min, linear gradient from 15% to 26% B in 25 min, 26% B for 20 min, linear gradient from 26% to 40% B in 35 min, fast linear gradient from 40% to 60% in 13 min, hold 60% B for 10 min, then return to 15% B in 2 min and hold for 30 min 15% B; (II) for API batches, isolated fractions of CS/DS and HS and all SEC fractions at flow rate of 0.15 mL/min, 15% B for 5 min, linear gradient from 15% to 24% B in 22 min, 24% B for 23 min, linear gradient from 24% to 40% B in 50 min, fast linear gradient from 40% to 60% B for 3 min, then 60% B for 10 min, then return to 15% B in 2 min and hold for 20 min at 15% B.

The samples were analyzed on an Ultimate 3000 HPLC-UV system (Dionex, Sunnyvale, CA, USA) coupled to an ESI-Q-TOFMS MicrOTOF-Q (Bruker Daltonics, Bremen, Germany). The mass spectrometer setting was as follows: ESI in negative ion mode (capillary voltage +3.2 kV); nitrogen, used as nebulizer and heater gas, flowed at 7 L/min, +180 °C and pressure 0.9 bar; mass range of 200–2000 m/z. Only the SEC fractions F, I–N were analyzed on an HPLC-UV system (Agilent Technologies, Santa Clara, CA, USA) coupled to an ESI FT-ICR MS Solarix (Bruker Daltonics, Bremen, Germany) using the elution schedule (II) and MS conditions were set up in negative polarity with a capillary voltage of +3.2 kV, nitrogen at the flow rate of 3.7 L/min, temperature of +180 °C and pressure of 1 bar, mass range 200–3000 m/z.

The MS^2 fragmentation experiments were performed on selected ions isolated in the quadrupole collision cell by a width of 5 Da and activated by collision-induced dissociation (CID) at the collision energy of 25 eV.

LC-MS analyses of enzymatic digested mixture (Section 2.4.4) were performed on an ESI-IT amaZon SL (Bruker Daltonics, Bremen, Germany) using solvent A (dibutylamine 10 mM, acetic acid 10 mM in water) with solvent C (dibutylamine 10 mM, acetic acid 10 mM in methanol) at flow rate of 0.1 mL/min, 10% C for 5 min, linear gradient from 10% to 35% C in 35 min, linear gradient from 35% to 50% C in 45 min, from 50% to 90% in 13 min, then hold at 90% C for 5 min, then return to 10% C in 2 min and hold for 25 min 10% C. The mass spectrometer parameters were as follows: ESI in negative ion mode with a capillary voltage of +3.8 kV, nitrogen at +200 °C, 9 L/min with a nebulizer pressure of 30 psi, mass range 200–1500 m/z.

4.6. Size-Exclusion Chromatography

The fractionation method was applied to seven API samples: about 250 mg dissolved in 2.5 mL of H_2O were loaded onto two columns in series (5.0 × 90 cm each) of Bio-Gel P6 (BIO-RAD Laboratories S.r.l., Milan, Italy), the elution was performed with 0.25 M ammonium chloride solution at a flow rate of 1.8 mL/min. Tubes of 18 mL were collected, and their absorbance at 210 nm was monitored using a variable-wavelength UV detector (Varian Cary 50scan, Agilent Technologies, Santa Clara, CA, USA). Based on the profile, twelve fractions with decreasing molecular weight were recovered (labelled from A to N).

Two desalting/purification methods were applied and described as follows: (I) one column (5.0 cm × 90 cm) filled with TSK HW40S resin (Tosoh Bioscience S.r.l., Rivoli, Torino, Italy) was eluted with 10% aqueous ethanol at the flow rate of 5 mL/min, samples elution was monitored by absorbance at 210 nm, positive fractions were pooled concentrated and lyophilized; (II) about 90–120 mg of sample were injected in a volume of 2.5 mL onto HPLC system made up by two glass columns in series (3.0 × 48 cm + 2.0 × 83 cm) filled with the resin Superdex 30 preparative grade (GE Healthcare Life Science, Milan, Italy) and a pump, a manager unit and a UV detector (KNAUER, Smartline, models 1050, 5050; and 2500, respectively) set up at 210 nm, the elution was performed with 0.25 M ammonium chloride solution at 5 mL/min, the system is managed by Clarity Chrom Preparative software, version 2.6 (Knauer, Berlin, Germany).

4.7. Depolymerization of CS/DS for the Isolation of HS Component

About 100 mg of danaparoid API sample was dissolved in phosphate sodium acetate buffer 50 mM pH 8, the enzyme Chondroitin ABC lyase was added to have a ratio enzyme/substrate equal to 7 mU/mg. The reaction was driven at 37 °C under magnetic stirring for 72 h.

At the end, to eliminate the enzyme by denaturation, the solution was heated at 95–100 °C for 5–10 min, after cooling the solution was filtered on 0.22 μm (Merck Millipore, Billerica, MA, USA), concentrated by reduced pressure and then purified by size-exclusion chromatography systems, applying TSK HW40S column, Superdex 30 and finally TSK HW40S column (Section 4.6).

4.8. Depolymerization of HS for the Isolation of CS/DS Component

About 500 mg of danaparoid API sample was dissolved in buffer 100 mM sodium acetate +10 mM calcium acetate pH 7 and incubated with the enzyme Heparinase III with a ratio of enzyme/substrate equal to 20 mU/mg, at 37 °C for 48 h under magnetic stirring. Then the solution was heated at 90–100 °C for 5–10 min for enzyme denaturation, subsequently it was cooled and filtered on 0.22 μm (Merck Millipore, Billerica, MA, USA). The solution was submitted to chemical reaction with nitrous acid twice following the procedure here described: the sample (500 mg) was dissolved in 20 mL of water, cooled to 4 °C and added to 140 mg of $NaNO_2$ dissolved in 1 mL of water. The pH was adjusted to 1.7 with HCl 4% (*w*/*v*) and the solution was stirred for 20 min. Then portions of $NaNO_2$ were added (140, 100 and 100 mg, respectively), after each addition the solution was stirred for 20 min. Subsequently, the pH was adjusted to 7 with NaOH 1 M and the solution was conditioned to room temperature. $NaBH_4$ was added as solid (400 mg) in several portions with stirring. After 2 h, the pH solution was adjusted to 4 with HCl 4% and then neutralized with NaOH 1M. The obtained product was purified by SEC systems such as TSK HW40S column, Superdex 30 and finally TSK HW40S column (Section 4.6).

4.9. Depolymerization of HS for the Isolation of CS/DS Component Exhaustive Enzymatic Digestion with Lyases I, II and III

Each isolated HS fraction was depolymerized using heparinases I, II, and III according to the USP method [33]. Each sample was solubilized in water to obtain a concentration of 20 mg/mL and 20 μL (400 μg) that were then digested in sodium/calcium acetate buffer pH 7.0 by using a mixture 1:1:1 of Heparinases I, II, and III prepared by mixing a solution 0.4 IU per mL of each one. The reaction mixture was stirred (Thermo shaker TS-100, Biosan, Riga, Latvia) at 25 °C for 48 h, then each digestion solution was boiled for two minutes at 100 °C and passed through a filter having a porosity of 0.20 μm and analyzed by LC-MS.

5. Conclusions

For the present work an orthogonal analytical approach based on complementary techniques, allowed a compositional comparison and first structural assignment of the components of different batches of danaparoid.

The in depth studies conducted on SEC fractions and on isolated CS/DS and HS components produced much structural information that completed the characterization of the starting API samples and allowed the similarity of analyzed batches to be established, ascribing slight differences to the intrinsic heterogeneity of extractive products such as danaparoid.

From the compositional point of view, both NMR and MS data confirmed the presence of different GAGs variably distributed over fractions/molecular weights, the CS/DS component represents the higher Mw species of danaparoid. LMW heparan sulfate was confirmed to be the major component of the API samples.

NMR and LC-MS analysis underlined the fact that a majority of the analyzed species showed oxidized hexosamines as T1 variant at the RE of both CS/DS and HS chains and a remnant (Ra) of an oxidized uronic acid at the reducing end of CS/DS species. Minor further oxidation products (T2, T3, T4, and T5) were present on the HS chains. Some NMR signals were correctly assigned to GAG species by studying the isolated components.

The exemplification of species through size fractionation and isolation of components allowed a good correspondence in terms of composition with the parent danaparoid samples to be observed, supporting the robustness of the separations methods and analytical tools.

Acknowledgments: The authors thank Edwin Kellenbach (Aspen Oss B.V.) and Giuseppe Cassinelli (G. Ronzoni Institute) for the critical reading of the manuscript.

Author Contributions: A.N., R.v.H. and P.d.W. conceived and designed the experiments; C.G. performed the experiments; E.U. performed and analyzed mass experiments; M.G. analyzed NMR experiments; C.G., A.N., R.v.H,. and P.d.W. analyzed the data; C.G. and A.N. wrote the paper.

References

1. Acostamadiedo, J.M.; Iyer, U.G.; Owen, J. Danaparoid sodium. *Expert Opin. Pharmacother.* **2000**, *1*, 803–814. [CrossRef] [PubMed]
2. Nurmohamed, M.T.; ten Cate, H.; ten Cate, J.W. Low molecular weight heparin(oid)s. Clinical investigations and practical recommendations. *Drugs* **1997**, *53*, 736–751. [CrossRef] [PubMed]
3. Skoutakis, V.A. Danaparoid in the prevention of thromboembolic complications. *Ann. Pharmacother.* **1997**, *31*, 876–887. [CrossRef] [PubMed]
4. Council of Europe; European Pharmacopoeia Commission. *European Pharmacopoeia*, 6th ed.; Strasbourg Council of Europe: Strasbourg, France, 2007; pp. 1644–1646.
5. Üstün, B.; Sanders, K.B.; Dani, P.; Kellenbach, E.R. Quantification of chondroitin sulfate and dermatan sulfate in danaparoid sodium by ^{1}H-NMR spectroscopy and PLS regression. *Anal. Bioanal. Chem.* **2011**, *399*, 629–634. [CrossRef] [PubMed]
6. Mauri, L.; Boccardi, G.; Torri, G.; Karfunkle, M.; Macchi, E.; Muzi, L.; Keire, D.; Guerrini, M. Qualification of HSQC methods for quantitative composition of heparin and low molecular weight heparins. *J. Pharm. Biomed. Anal.* **2016**, *136*, 92–105. [CrossRef] [PubMed]
7. Casu, B. Structure and biological activity of heparin. *Adv. Carbohydr. Chem. Biochem.* **1985**, *43*, 51–134. [PubMed]
8. Conrad, H.E. *Heparin-Binding Proteins*; Academic Press: New York, NY, USA, 1997.
9. Casu, B.; Moretti, M.; Oreste, P.; Riva, A.; Torri, G.; Vercellotti, J.R. Glycosaminoglycans from pig duodenum. *Arzneimittelforschung* **1980**, *30*, 1889–1892. [PubMed]
10. Guerrini, M.; Zhang, Z.; Shriver, Z.; Naggi, A.; Masuko, S.; Langer, R.; Casu, B.; Linhardt, R.J.; Torri, G.; Sasisekharan, R. Orthogonal analytical approaches to detect potential contaminants in heparin. *Proc. Natl. Acad. Sci. USA* **2009**, *106*, 16956–16961. [CrossRef] [PubMed]
11. Guerrini, M.; Shriver, Z.; Bisio, A.; Naggi, A.; Casu, B.; Sasisekharan, R. The tainted heparin story: An update. *Thromb. Haemost.* **2009**, *102*, 907–911. [CrossRef] [PubMed]
12. Bertini, S.; Bisio, A.; Torri, G.; Bensi, D.; Terbojevich, M. Molecular weight determination of heparin and dermatan sulfate by size exclusion chromatography with a triple detector array. *Biomacromolecules* **2005**, *6*, 168–173. [CrossRef] [PubMed]

13. Bisio, A.; Mantegazza, A.; Vecchietti, D.; Bensi, D.; Coppa, A.; Torri, G.; Bertini, S. Determination of the molecular weight of low-molecular-weight heparins by using high-pressure size exclusion chromatography on line with a triple detector array and conventional methods. *Molecules* **2015**, *20*, 5085–5098. [CrossRef] [PubMed]
14. Casu, B.; Gennaro, U. A conductimetric method for the determination of sulphate and carboxyl groups in heparin and other mucopolysaccharides. *Carbohydr. Res.* **1975**, *39*, 168–176. [CrossRef]
15. Holme, K.R.; Perlin, A.S. Nuclear magnetic resonance spectra of heparin in admixture with dermatan sulfate and other glycosaminoglycans. 2-D spectra of the chondroitin sulfates. *Carbohydr. Res.* **1989**, *186*, 301–312. [CrossRef]
16. Kellenbach, E.; Sanders, K.; Michiels, P.J.; Girard, F.C. ^{1}H-NMR signal at 2.10 ppm in the spectrum of $KMnO_4$-bleached heparin sodium: Identification of the chemical origin using an NMR-only approach. *Anal. Bioanal. Chem.* **2011**, *399*, 621–628. [CrossRef] [PubMed]
17. Becatti, D.; Roy, S.; Yu, F.; Gunay, N.S.; Capila, I.; Lech, M.; Linhardt, R.J.; Venkataraman, G. Identification of a novel structure in heparin generated by potassium permanganate oxidation. *Carbohydr. Polym.* **2010**, *82*, 699–705. [CrossRef] [PubMed]
18. Mourier, P.A.; Guichard, O.Y.; Herman, F.; Viskov, C. Heparin sodium compliance to the new proposed USP monograph: Elucidation of a minor structural modification responsible for a process dependent 2.10 ppm NMR signal. *J. Pharm. Biomed. Anal.* **2011**, *54*, 337–344. [CrossRef] [PubMed]
19. Panagos, C.; Thomson, D.; Bavington, C.D.; Uhrín, D. Structural characterisation of oligosaccharides obtained by Fenton-type radical depolymerisation of dermatan sulfate. *Carbohydr. Polym.* **2012**, *87*, 2086–2092. [CrossRef]
20. Griffin, C.C.; Linhardt, R.J.; Van Gorp, C.L.; Toida, T.; Hileman, R.E.; Schubert, R.L., II; Brown, S.E. Isolation and characterization of heparan sulfate from crude porcine intestinal mucosal peptidoglycan heparin. *Carbohydr. Res.* **1995**, *276*, 183–197. [CrossRef]
21. Huckerby, T.N.; Nieduszynski, I.A.; Giannopoulos, M.; Weeks, S.D.; Sadler, I.H.; Lauder, R.M. Characterization of oligosaccharides from the chondroitin/dermatan sulfates. ^{1}H-NMR and ^{13}C-NMR studies of reduced trisaccharides and hexasaccharides. *FEBS J.* **2005**, *272*, 6276–6286. [CrossRef] [PubMed]
22. Langeslay, D.J.; Urso, E.; Gardini, C.; Naggi, A.; Torri, G.; Larive, C.K. Reversed-phase ion-pair ultra-high-performance-liquid chromatography-mass spectrometry for fingerprinting low-molecular-weight heparins. *J. Chromatogr. A* **2013**, *1292*, 201–210. [CrossRef] [PubMed]
23. Alekseeva, A.; Casu, B.; Cassinelli, G.; Guerrini, M.; Torri, G.; Naggi, A. Structural features of glycol-split low-molecular-weight heparins and their heparin lyase generated fragments. *Anal. Bioanal. Chem.* **2014**, *406*, 249–265. [CrossRef] [PubMed]
24. Vismara, E.; Pierini, M.; Guglieri, S.; Liverani, L.; Mascellani, G.; Torri, G. Structural modification induced in heparin by a Fenton-type depolymerization process. *Semin. Thromb. Hemost.* **2007**, *33*, 466–477. [CrossRef] [PubMed]
25. Mascellani, G.; Liverani, L.; Prete, A.; Bergonzini, G.L.; Bianchini, P.; Silvestro, L.; Torri, G.; Bisio, A.; Guerrini, M.; Casu, B. Active Sites of Dermatan Sulfate for Heparin Cofactor II. Isolation of a Nonasaccharide Fragment Containing Four Disaccharide Sequences [α-L-Iduronic Acid 2-*O*-Sulfate (1, 3)-β-D-*N*-Acetylgalactosamine 4-Sulfate]. *J. Carbohydr. Chem.* **1995**, *14*, 1165–1177. [CrossRef]
26. Mucci, A.; Schenetti, L.; Volpi, N. ^{1}H and ^{13}C nuclear magnetic resonance identification and characterization of components of chondroitin sulfates of various origin. *Carbohydr. Polym.* **2000**, *41*, 37–45. [CrossRef]
27. Naggi, A.; Gardini, C.; Pedrinola, G.; Mauri, L.; Urso, E.; Alekseeva, A.; Casu, B.; Cassinelli, G.; Guerrini, M.; Iacomini, M.; et al. Structural peculiarity and antithrombin binding region profile of mucosal bovine and porcine heparins. *J. Pharm. Biomed. Anal.* **2016**, *118*, 52–63. [CrossRef] [PubMed]
28. Zhao, W.; Garron, M.L.; Yang, B.; Xiao, Z.; Esko, J.D.; Cygler, M.; Linhardt, R.J. Asparagine 405 of heparin lyase II prevents the cleavage of glycosidic linkages proximate to a 3-*O*-sulfoglucosamine residue. *FEBS Lett.* **2011**, *585*, 2461–2466. [CrossRef] [PubMed]
29. Gallagher, J.T.; Walker, A. Molecular distinctions between heparan sulphate and heparin. Analysis of sulphation patterns indicates that heparan sulphate and heparin are separate families of *N*-sulphated polysaccharides. *Biochem. J.* **1985**, *230*, 665–674. [CrossRef] [PubMed]

30. Toida, T.; Yoshida, H.; Toyoda, H.; Koshiishi, I.; Imanari, T.; Hileman, R.E.; Fromm, J.R.; Linhardt, R.J. Structural differences and the presence of unsubstituted amino groups in heparan sulphates from different tissues and species. *Biochem. J.* **1997**, *322*, 499–506. [CrossRef] [PubMed]
31. Vismara, E.; Pierini, M.; Mascellani, G.; Liverani, L.; Lima, M.; Guerrini, M.; Torri, G. Low-molecular-weight heparin from Cu^{2+} and Fe^{2+} Fenton type depolymerisation processes. *Thromb. Haemost.* **2010**, *103*, 613–622. [CrossRef] [PubMed]
32. Bisio, A.; De Ambrosi, L.; Gonella, S.; Guerrini, M.; Guglieri, S.; Maggia, G.; Torri, G. Preserving the original heparin structure of a novel low molecular weight heparin by γ-irradiation. *Arzneimittelforschung* **2001**, *51*, 806–813. [CrossRef] [PubMed]
33. U.S. Pharmacopeia–National Formulary (USP–NF). *Test for 1,6-anhydro Derivative for Enoxaparin Sodium*; U.S. Pharmacopeial Convention: Rockville, MD, USA, 2009; pp. 1–7.

6

Combining NMR Spectroscopy and Chemometrics to Monitor Structural Features of Crude Heparin

Lucio Mauri [1], Maria Marinozzi [1], Giulia Mazzini [1], Richard E. Kolinski [2], Michael Karfunkle [2], David A. Keire [2] and Marco Guerrini [1,*]

1 Institute for Chemical and Biochemical Research G. Ronzoni, via G. Colombo 81, 20133 Milan, Italy; mauri@ronzoni.it (L.M.); maria.marinozzi90@gmail.com (M.M.); giulia.mazzini@gmail.com (G.M.)

2 Division of Pharmaceutical Analysis, Office of Testing and Research, Center for Drug Evaluation and Research, U.S. Food and Drug Administration, 645 S. Newstead Ave., St. Louis, MO 63110, USA; Richard.kolinski@fda.hhs.gov (R.E.K.); michael.karfunkle@fda.hhs.gov (M.K.); David.Keire@fda.hhs.gov (D.A.K.)

* Correspondence: guerrini@ronzoni.it

Abstract: Because of the complexity and global nature of the heparin supply chain, the control of heparin quality during manufacturing steps is essential to ensure the safety of the final active pharmaceutical ingredient (API). For this reason, there is a need to develop consistent analytical methods able to assess the quality of heparin early in production (i.e., as the crude heparin before it is purified to API under cGMP conditions). Although a number of analytical techniques have been applied to characterize heparin APIs, few of them have been applied for crude heparin structure and composition analyses. Here, to address this issue, NMR spectroscopy and chemometrics were applied to characterize 88 crude heparin samples. The samples were also analyzed by strong anion exchange HPLC (SAX-HPLC) as an orthogonal check of the purity levels of the crudes analyzed by NMR. The HPLC data showed that the chemometric analysis of the NMR data differentiated the samples based on their purity. These orthogonal approaches differentiated samples according their glycosaminoglycan (GAG) composition and their mono and disaccharide composition and structure for each GAG family (e.g., heparin/heparan, dermatan sulfate, and chondroitin sulfate A). Moreover, quantitative HSQC and multivariate analysis (PCA) were used to distinguish between crude heparin of different animal and tissue sources.

Keywords: heparin; crude heparin; NMR; quantitative NMR; PCA; chemometric; HSQC

1. Introduction

In spite of its 100 year history, heparin and its lower molecular weight versions remain the most used anticoagulant and antithrombotic drug [1]. Heparin is a sulfated polysaccharide composed of alternating disaccharide sequences of uronic acid (either D-glucuronic or L-iduronic acid) and glucosamine. The glucosamine residue can be *N*-acetylated or *N*-sulfated in position 2, while both uronic acid and glucosamine can be sulfated in position 2 and 6, respectively. More rarely, the glucosamine residue can be sulfated in position 3, and found in the pentasaccharide sequence GlcNS/Ac-GlcA-GlcNS,3S,6S/OH-IdoA2S-GlcNS,6S, corresponding to the heparin binding site for antithrombin (AT). The degree of sulfation and distribution within the heparin chains depends on the animal or organ source; however, the detailed monosaccharide sequence is still largely undisclosed [2].

Until the late 1980s and early 1990s, when cases of bovine spongiform encephalopathy (BSE) were reported in United Kingdom and other countries, bovine heparin products were widely used together with those extracted from porcine intestine. As a result of BSE, bovine heparin was withdrawn from both the U.S. and European markets and entirely replaced by porcine mucosa heparin, limiting bovine heparin use to South America and some Islamic countries. The removal of bovine heparin from the market increased the market demand for porcine heparin. As a result, at present more than 50% of worldwide heparin production originates from China [3]. In addition, a shortage in the heparin supply (due also to a pig disease outbreak) was presumably the reason for the heparin contamination with the semisynthetic over-sulfated chondroitin sulfate (OSCS), an inexpensive adulterant with anticoagulant activity, which occurred in late 2007 in the US and Europe [4]. This so called heparin crisis, in addition to causing many deaths and severe side effects, demonstrated the vulnerability of the global heparin supply chain. Fortunately, the subsequent introduction of new tests (e.g., NMR and HPLC tests) to the heparin monographs of several pharmacopoeias around the world increased the degree of quality control of this drug, decreasing the risk of product adulteration [3]. However, the complexity of the heparin supply chain provides other opportunities for intentional adulteration, such as contamination with foreign substances or the addition of non-porcine sources of crude heparin (i.e., bovine or ovine heparin), which might not be detected by the current monograph test methods.

Heparin is produced from tissues of food animals, and for medical use the drug has been primarily obtained from pig or beef intestine, and can be sourced from sheep as well. Typically, the pig intestine is collected and processed in slaughterhouses approved by regulatory authorities and then transported to crude heparin processing facilities. In these facilities, the intestinal mucosa is removed and the dissociated mucosa is treated with proteolytic enzymes under alkaline conditions. After multiple steps, the highly anionic glycosaminoglycans (GAGs) can be adsorbed onto an anion exchange resin, which is washed. Then, the partially purified heparin is eluted, filtered, precipitated, and vacuum dried to form a substance known as crude heparin, where the glycosaminoglycan (GAG) fraction is concentrated. Crude heparin is then further purified at the level of active pharmaceutical ingredient (API) to remove impurities such as dermatan and chondroitins, nucleic acids, residual proteins, metal ions, and unwanted counterions. In addition, the purification involves oxidation ($KMnO_4$ or H_2O_2) and alkaline treatments to remove color and inactivate endotoxins and viruses that might be present in the product [5,6].

Whereas the purification of crude heparin to heparin sodium API is always conducted under cGMP conditions, only a few manufacturers can establish traceability back to the living animals. Many companies buy crude heparins from third parties, which have collected mucosa at multiple small slaughterhouses. These multiple sites increase the risk of un-intended or intentional contamination. Although it is impossible to eliminate all possible risks, reinforcing of appropriate requirements, controls, and best practices at the level of crude heparin as a key intermediate might help ensure the quality of the final pharmaceutical grade product.

A first step to define crude heparin as an intermediate in the production process of the API requires the specification of a normal range of composition found in heparin currently on the market. Different intermediates may exist and be qualified for use in the manufacture of heparin, such as resin bound heparin (early intermediates), a brown powder containing a large amount of RNA/DNA and galactosaminoglycans (mainly dermatan sulfate (DS) and chondroitin sulfate A (CSA)), or partly purified crude heparin, a light yellow powder containing only a small amount of dermatan sulfate [7]. Although different techniques have been used to identify and quantify OSCS in crude heparin, to our knowledge, these studies did not fully characterize the average composition of crudes produced in the global marketplace [8,9].

In the present study, 88 crude heparins collected from 2010 to 2015, representing 13 different manufacturers, have been characterized by NMR spectroscopy and strong anion exchange HPLC (SAX-HPLC). Particularly, a multivariate analysis (principal component analysis (PCA)) of one-dimensional (1D) proton NMR spectra was used to differentiate the crudes on the basis of their structural features and animal/organ of origin. Moreover, the quantitative composition of crude samples was performed using an adapted version of the HSQC method recently described in [10].

2. Results

2.1. Protocol for Sample Preparation

Crude heparin samples are often not completely soluble in water. Therefore, to avoid the presence of insoluble material in the NMR tube, a protocol of sample separation by centrifugation was developed. Three parameters of the separation protocol were evaluated for their effect on the supernatant content, including: the amount of insoluble material present, crude concentration, and the method of solution equilibration (with or without stirring). Each of the eight combinations of the parameters was tested. Moreover, three separations were performed for a single parameter set to evaluate the precision of the data, giving a total of ten separations. For each separation, two parameters were measured after lyophilization of the supernatant or the pellet: the total weight loss and the amount of precipitate, both expressed as a percentage of the original weight (Table 1).

Table 1. Recovering of soluble and insoluble material obtained by two crude heparin samples. Weightings before and after the separation and lyophilization procedure are shown.

Sample	Crude (mg/mL)	Stirring	Supernatant (mg)	Precipitate (mg)	Weight loss % (%w)	Precipitate (%w)
G9709	40.4	No	35.3	1.2	9.7	3.3
G9709	40.8	No	35.4	1.0	10.8	2.7
G9709	38.9	No	33.7	1.2	10.3	3.4
G9709	39.0	Yes	34.0	1.1	10.0	3.1
G9709	79.7	No	60.4	10.0	11.7	14.2
G9709	81.4	Yes	62.4	9.4	11.8	13.1
G9710	39.0	No	33.8	2.7	6.4	7.4
G9710	39.3	Yes	33.2	2.1	10.2	5.9
G9710	79.5	No	56.8	13.8	11.2	19.5
G9710	80.5	Yes	59.3	13.0	10.2	18.0

With the exclusion of one result, the loss of water due to lyophilization was around 10%, regardless of sample concentration. While the stirring procedure during solution equilibration did not affect the yield on a percentage basis, the amount of precipitate was related to the sample concentration, showing that the precipitate still contains soluble material. To verify that the procedure does not result in the selective separation of glycosaminoglycan species, a precipitate obtained at a higher concentration (80 mg/mL) was re-suspended in 1 mL of D_2O, centrifuged, and the spectrum of the supernatant compared with that obtained after the first solubilization. While no differences in the glycosamonoglycan pattern were found, higher non-GAG signals in the re-suspended precipitate were observed (Figure S1). Based on these results, to collect enough soluble material for the NMR characterization, an aliquot of 60 mg of crude heparin was determined to be sufficient for analysis in 1.5 mL of D_2O. The average weights of the 88 crude samples are shown in Table S1.

The proton chemical shifts of heparin are affected both by the pH and concentration of the solution [11,12]. Crude heparin does not contain only heparin, but also other GAGs (heparan, dermatan, and chondroitin sulfate), as well as non-GAG material, mainly DNA and RNA, some proteinaceous material, and a variable amount of water and salts. For these reasons, the proton spectra of crude heparins in D_2O were not fully reproducible, and a shift of signals, particularly those of anomeric glucosamine and iduronic acid residues, was often observed (Figure S2). The maximum shift of both peaks observed was about 10–12 Hz (0.015–0.020 ppm), presumably due to the different concentration of GAG components in the samples, which affect the pH of the solution. These spectra cannot be easily compared, particularly when they are analysed by multivariate analysis (e.g., PCA). To remove the effect of pH variability, the samples were solubilized in 0.15 M of phosphate buffer at pH 7.1, containing 3 mM of perdeuterated EDTA. The complexation of bivalent or paramagnetic ions induced by the addition of perdeuterated EDTA provides narrower lines and improved resolution. A comparison of crude proton spectra recorded in water and the buffer solution is shown in Figure S2.

2.2. One-Dimensional (1D) Spectra Library and PCA

The proton spectra of eighty-eight crude heparin samples were registered by the NMR analysis protocol indicated in the experimental section. The spectra show very high variability of composition, both in terms of non-GAGs components (broad signals at both aromatic and aliphatic regions due to DNA/RNA and other impurities, Figure S1) and galactosaminoglycans components, mainly dermatan and chondroitin sulfate (Figure 1).

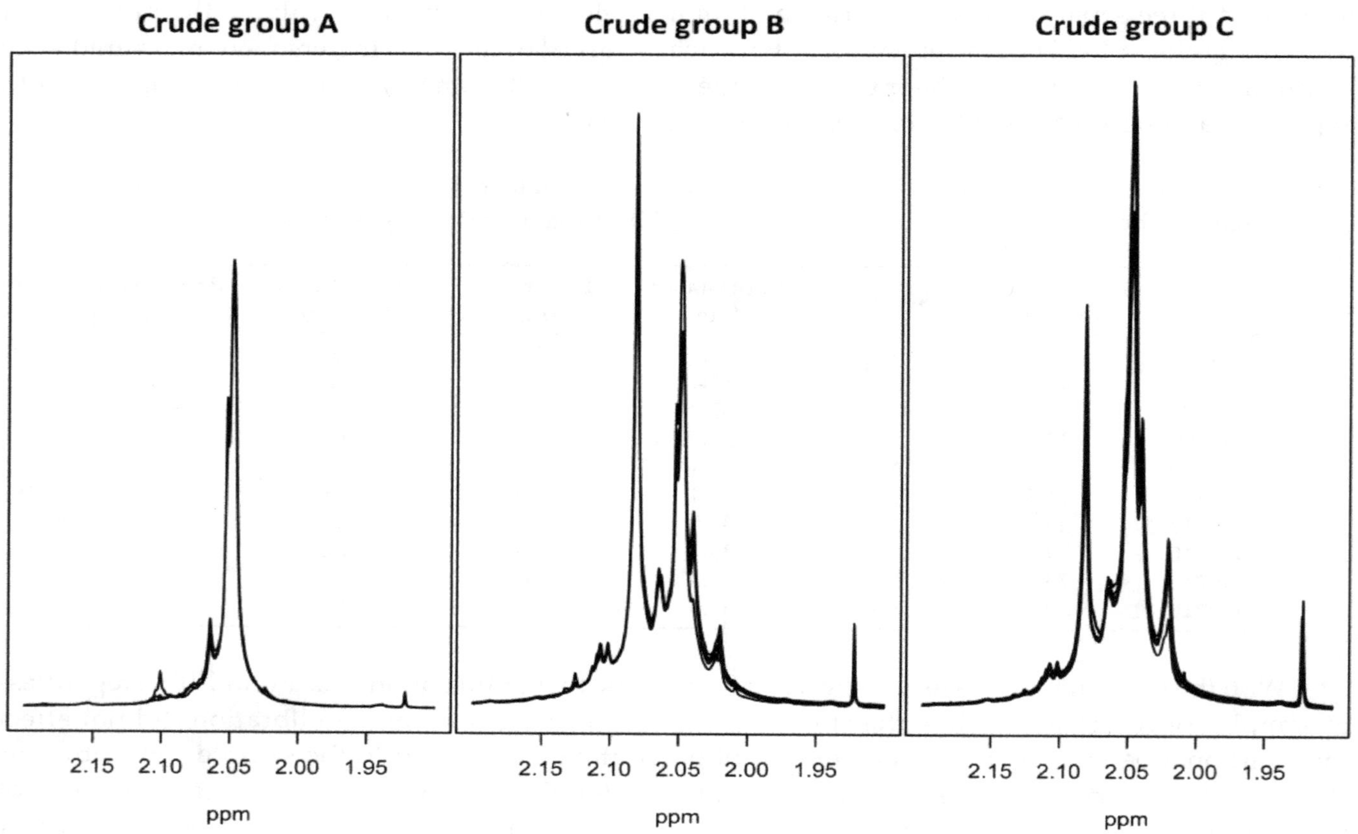

Figure 1. ^{1}H-NMR spectra. Acetyl region of proton spectra of samples of group A, group B, and group C (see Figure 2) registered at 600 MHz, showing methyl signals of Dermatan (2.08 ppm), Heparin (2.05 ppm), and Chondoritin (2.02 ppm) components.

Due to this variability and the difficulties in establishing quantitative ratios among diagnostic signals, the spectral complexity was reduced to the basic elements which best define the crucial differences between samples by employing chemometric techniques.

One of the most common tools used to explore a complex dataset is principal component analysis (PCA). Typically, this tool takes a large number of correlated variables and transforms the data into a smaller number of uncorrelated variables (principal components), while extracting the maximal amount of variation, thus making it easier to analyse the data and make predictions [13].

The score plot of the first two components, generated by the PCA of 88 ^{1}H-NMR spectra of the crude samples, is shown in Figure 2. The graph, displaying the variance accounted for by the principal components, shows that only two components are necessary to account for more than 80% of the total variance, indicating that the differences among the samples are mainly distributed along the components **1** and **2**.

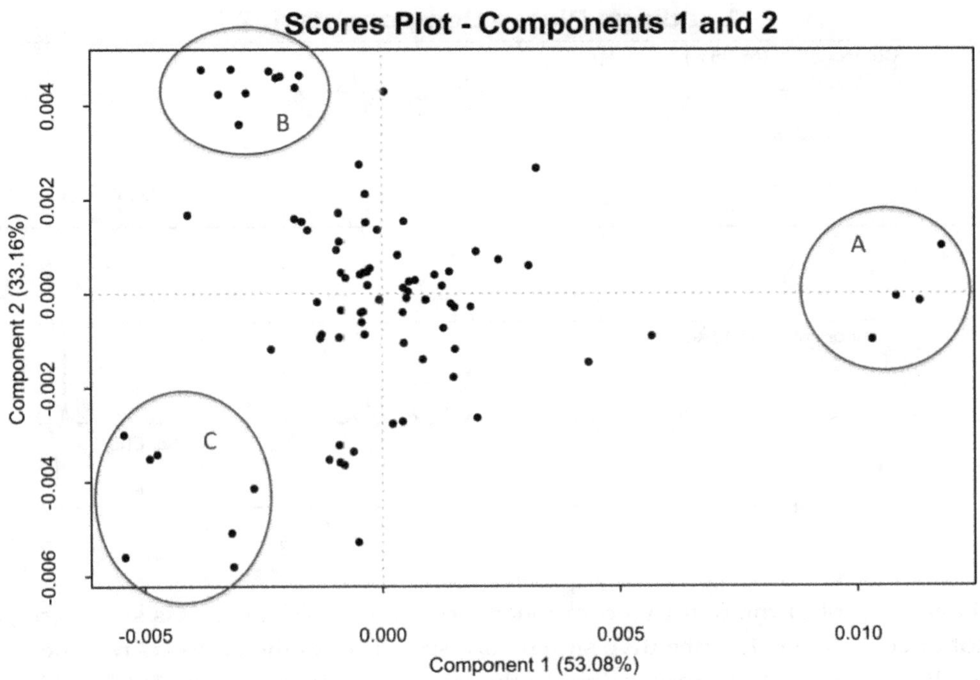

Figure 2. Score plot of the first two components generated by principal component analysis (PCA) of the GAGs signals region of the ^{1}H-NMR spectrum. Most of the samples are centered in the PCA, while there are 21 more peripheral samples: highlighted as A, B, and C.

In the loading plot of the first principal component, the negative signal of the acetyl protons of dermatan sulfate was observed (Figure 3). By contrast, in the loading of the second principal component, signals belonging to the trisulfated disaccharide (corresponding to the most abundant dissacharide of heparin chains) are positive, while the other heparin and chondroitin acetyl signals are negative. The analysis of the loading plots suggested that samples having a positive score in component 1 (Figure 2, group A) contain a low amount of dermatan sulfate, while those having negative score in component 2 (Figure 2, group C) contain highly acetylated heparin with a larger amount of chondroitin. The samples contained within the group B have instead a higher degree of sulfation, together with a large amount of dermatan. The proton spectra of the samples belonging to these groups confirm what was observed by PCA, showing that the spectra of samples belonging to the group A, in the absence of dermatan and chondroitin acetyl signals, match with those of purified heparin (Figure 1).

Since the major differences among the crude samples defined by PCA are due to the content of galactosaminoglycan and the acetylation degree of the heparin component, the PCA was performed also on part of the anomeric region of the proton spectra (5.75–4.94 ppm). In this region, with the exclusion of the weak H1 of I2S of dermatan sulfate (5.18 ppm), no signals belonging to dermatan and chondroitin are present. Before the PCA analysis, the selected region of the proton spectra was aligned with a custom algorithm (Table S14 and Figure S9), because without alignment the shift effect was dominant in the loading plot of the first principal component. After the alignment, PCA differentiates samples on the basis of the sulfation pattern of the heparin/heparan sulfate components. The score plot generated by the PCA of this spectral region is shown in Figure 4. No evident clusters are visible, and the loading plot of the first principal component (Figure S3) can be interpreted in terms of the degree of sulfation of the samples, where the samples positioned in the negative score of the first principal component are more highly sulfated. Although the loading plot of the second component is difficult to interpret, the negative signals corresponding to the H1 of GlcNS,6OH and I2S linked to GlcNS,6OH indicate that the samples with lower 6-*O*-sulfation are located in the negative score of the second principal component (Figure S3).

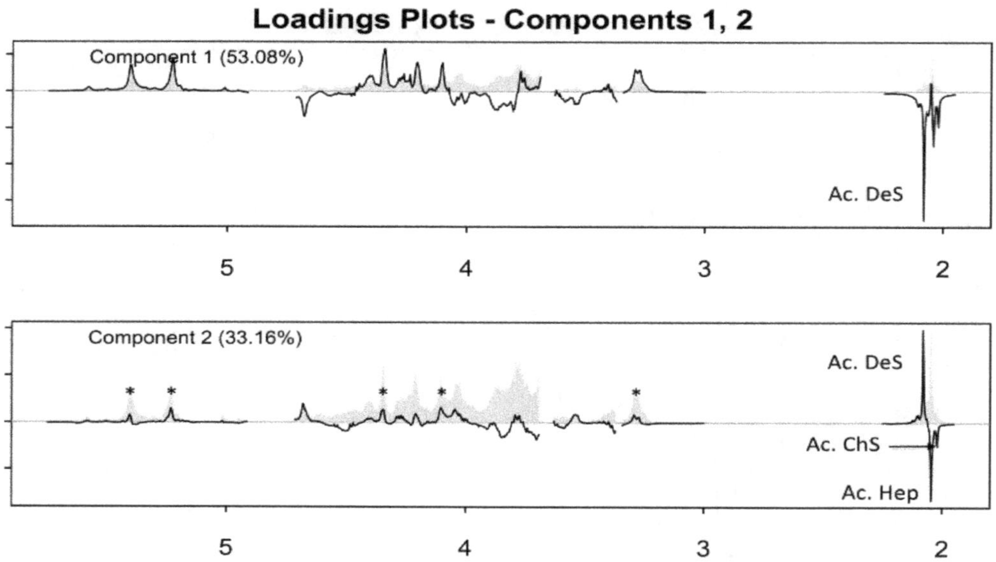

Figure 3. Loading plot of the first two components of the PCA of the GAGs signals region. In the loading plot of component 1, a negative signal corresponding to the *N*-acetyl residue of dermatan is observed. Positive signals corresponding to the trisulfated disaccharide (*) (-I2S-GlcNS,6S-) and negative signals corresponding to the *N*-acetyl residue of glucosamine (Hep) and galatosamine (ChS) are observed in the loading plot of component 2.

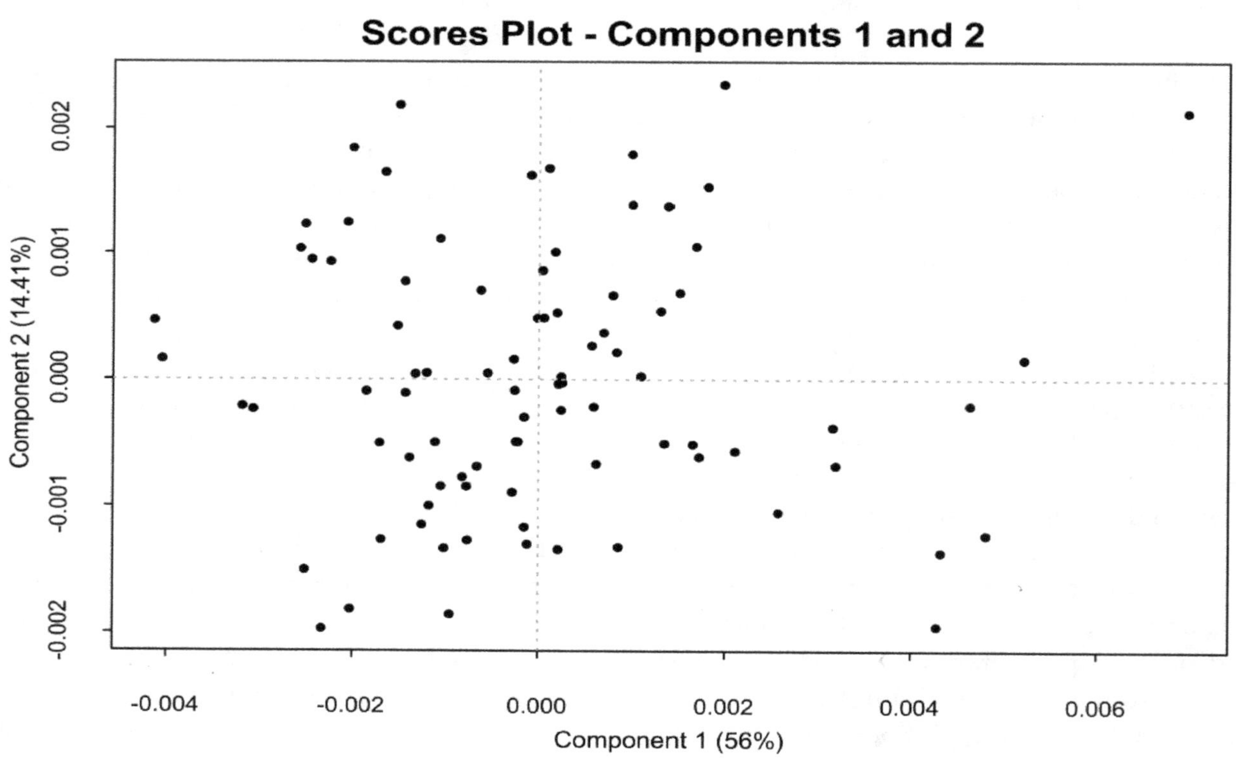

Figure 4. Score plot of the first two components generated by PCA of part of anomeric signals region. No clusters are defined. Only one sample appears isolated in the upper-right of the figure.

2.3. *SAX-HPLC Analysis*

To confirm the results of the NMR chemometric analysis data, the purity of the crude heparin samples was analyzed with a lower resolution method; SAX-HPLC. The SAX-HPLC method applied here separates heparin (~2.5 sulfates per disaccharide) from less sulfated (e.g., ~1 sulfate per disaccaride,

DS/CSA/heparan) or more sulfated (e.g., 4 sulfates per disaccharide, over sulfated chondroitin sulfate (OSCS)) GAGs based on negative charge [9,14]. As shown in Figure 5, the crude heparins in group A were the most pure, with the majority of the signal eluting at ~20.5 min consistent with heparin sodium API. For group B, two major peaks (17.0 and 20.4 min) of similar intensity were observed and attributed to primarily DeS and heparin, respectively. For group C, three major peaks were observed (14.5, 16.6, and 20.5 min), with the intensity of the 14.5 and the 16.6 peaks being much higher than the heparin peak at 20.5 min. These group C peaks are attributed to DNA/RNA, heparan/CSA, DeS, and heparin sulfate. Thus, group C samples contain DNA/RNA impurities as well as more less sulfated GAGs (i.e., CSA/heparan/DeS) than the group B or group A samples (Figure S4). Overall, the chemometric analysis of the NMR data and the visual examination of the SAX-HPLC chromatograms of the crude heparin samples can be used to order the crudes from highest (A) to lowest purity (C) as A, B, and C, respectively.

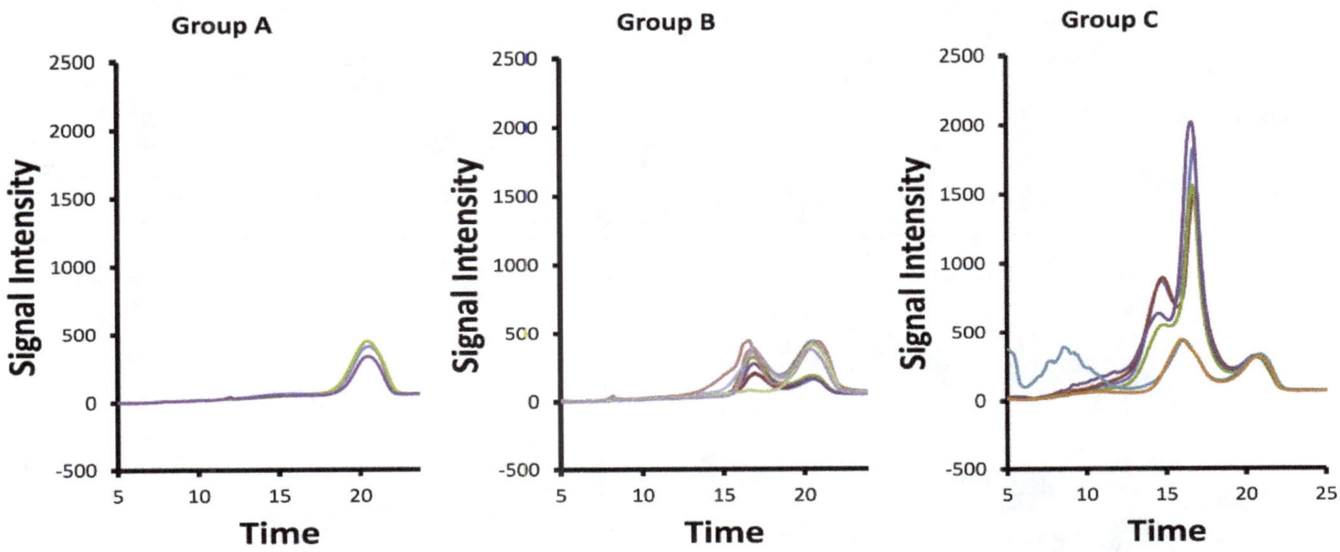

Figure 5. The 5 min to 25 min portion of the strong anion exchange HPLC (SAX-HPLC) chromatograms with UV detection at 215 nm of crudes differentiated into groups A, B, and C by NMR data as shown in Figure 2. Generally, the lower resolution HPLC method shows these groups have increasing levels of different impurities, going from group A to B to C, respectively.

2.4. HSQC Analysis

Quantitative HSQC was recently applied to heparin and low molecular weight heparins (LMWHs). The ^{1}H,^{13}C-HSQC data acquired on heparin APIs were used for calculating the percentage of mono- and disaccharides by normalizing volumes with reference to the sum of volumes of signals corresponding to each monosaccharide type (glucosamines or uronic acids) and the same carbon-proton pair type (e.g., anomeric or C2 position pairs) [10,15–17]. In the HSQC spectra collected here, signals belonging to high molecular weight species, mainly DNA and RNA, were not detected, presumably due to the increased linewidths associated with these slower tumbling larger molecules.

The HSQC spectrum of crude heparin also contains signals belonging to galactosaminoglycan components (DS and CSA), which partially overlap with those of the heparin/heparan sulfate (HS) components. By contrast, in the H2/C2 region, signals belonging to *N*-acetyl-glucosamine were completely separated from those of the *N*-acetyl-galactosamine residues (3.90 ppm/56.0–56.6 ppm and 4.02 ppm/53.8–54.6 ppm, respectively; Figure S5). Thus, the percentage of glucosamine and galactosamino residues could be calculated by the integration of the corresponding residues (Table 2). In addition, the uronic acid components of the galactosaminoglycans were well separated in the anomeric region of the crude heparins (Figure 6). Beside the major IdoA-GalNAc,4S sequences, DeS contains about 10% of disulfated disaccharide sequences, mostly consisting of IdoA2S-GalNAc,4S [18]. The anomeric signals of IdoA and IdoA2S of dermatan sulfate, at 4.88/106.1 ppm and 5.18/103.4 ppm, respectively, could be integrated to determine the IdoA2S/IdoA ratio. Similarly, the anomeric signal of the glucuronic acid of the chondroitin presents distinct chemical shift values on the basis of the position of the sulfate group of the following *N*-Acetyl-galactosamine residue (Figure 6) (4.47/106.6 ppm and 4.50/107.1 ppm for the ChS4S or ChS6S, respectively) [19], allowing the evaluation of the GalNAc,6S/GalNAc,4S ratio. Unfortunately, the anomeric signals of the DeS and ChS *N*-acetyl-galactosamine residues partially overlap with the anomeric signal of heparin glucuronic acid. In particular, if chondroitin is present, the amount of glucuronic acid linked to trisulfated glucosamine (G-$A_{NS,3S,6X}$) could be overestimated.

Table 2. Molar average composition of 88 crude heparin samples. PMHC = pig mucosa heparin crude; Hep = Heparin; DeS = Dermatan sulfate; ChS = Chondroitin sulfate; A = Glucosamine; I = Iduronic acid; G = Glucuronic acid; X = SO_3^- or H; SDEG = Heparin disaccharide degree of sulfation.

PMHC	Hep	DeS	ChS	ANH26X	ANAc6X	ANS3S6X	A6S	G2OH	G2S	I2OH	I2S	SDEG
average	89.3	8.6	2.4	1.8	16.3	4.5	73.3	18.0	0.01	10.5	71.5	2.31
median	89.2	8.7	2.1	1.9	16.3	4.4	73.7	17.9	0.00	10.6	71.4	2.32
st.dev.	4.1	3.1	1.9	0.7	2.0	0.7	3.4	1.9	0.09	0.9	2.5	0.08
min	79.9	0.0	0.0	0.0	11.6	3.1	63.3	14.0	0.00	8.2	65.4	2.13
max	100.0	16.6	7.7	3.0	21.1	5.9	79.8	22.4	0.75	12.4	76.8	2.46

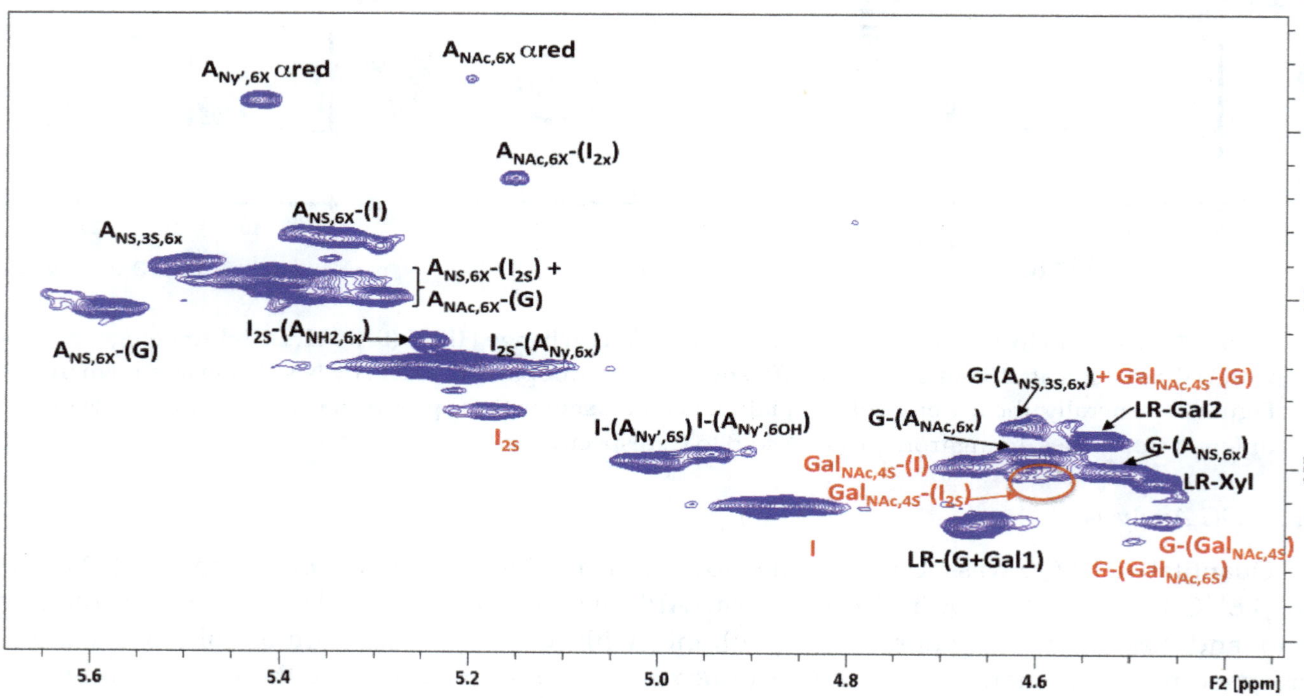

Figure 6. Anomeric region of a crude heparin HSQC spectrum. Signal assignments of heparin and DeS/ChS components are in black and red, respectively.

Finally, the composition of the heparin fraction was obtained as for the API product [10]. Tables S2 and S3 show the signals assignment and the detailed formulas for the calculations. The precision of the method was evaluated using a crude sample positioned close to the origin (0) of the PCA scores plot of Figure 2, therefore having an average composition in DeS/ChS comparable with the whole library of 88 samples. The intermediate precision was determined combining two operators and two spectrometers operating at 500 and 600 MHz (Tables S7–S9). Using a reasonable experimental time (6 h at 600 MHz and 8 h at 500 MHz) it was possible to quantify with sufficient precision all of the fragments above 3%, compared to 2% for API heparin with 2 h at 600 MHz and $3\frac{1}{2}$ h at 500 MHz [10]. This was considered a good result also in view of the fact that the concentration in the NMR tube was limited to 20 mg/0.6 mL compared to 35 mg/0.6 mL for API heparin. Clearly, the limit of quantification (LOQ) of heparin fragments might change according to the dermatan and chondroitin content. It was verified that a reliable estimation of the LOQ is given by the formula

$$\text{LOQ} = 2000 \times \text{VOL}/(\text{VOL\_SUM} \times \text{SNR}) \quad (1)$$

where VOL_SUM is the sum of all heparin anomeric signals, while VOL and SNR are the volume and signal to noise ratio of the anomeric signal of I-($A_{NY',6S}$) or I-($A_{NY',6OH}$) (Figure 6; both residues give comparable values for LOQ). If the LOQ is too high, the spectrum can be acquired again with more scans (NS) for better SNR, as the SNR term is proportional to the square root of NS. The robustness of the method was also evaluated by identifying the most critical parameters of the analytical method: pH of buffer, sample concentration, acquisition temperature, and spectrum phasing. These four parameters where studied at two levels in a Plucket–Burman design (Tables S4–S6). The heparin fragment quantification showed good robustness with respect to all of the parameters. The GAGs content was sensitive to variations of temperature, probably due to the different mobility of the heparin, DeS, and ChS chains.

A summary and the details of the obtained composition of a series of 75 out of 88 crude heparin samples are shown in Table 2 and Tables S10–S13, respectively.

As already observed in the PCA, crude heparin samples are characterized by a large variation in galactosaminoglycan content (0–20%), while the heparin component varies in *N*-acetylation, 6-*O*-sulfation, and nonsulfated uronic acid content (11–21%, 63–79%, and 23–35% respectively). Notably, the serine of the linkage region is almost exclusively present in its intact form (CHα at 4.00/57.4 ppm; Figure S5). However, the oxidized form of serine [20] was detected in the samples of group A by the reduction or absence of the CHα signal and the presence of the anomeric signal of xylose linked to oxidized serine residue (4.48/105.5 ppm; Figure S6). The presence of the oxidized forms in the linkage region suggests that crude heparin has been subject to an oxidizing process; usually, such a step is applied during the purification of crude to API heparin. In fact, the monosaccharide composition of the samples present in group A of the PCA results is compatible with a semi purified product. In addition to showing serine in the oxidized form, their spectra do not contain signals belonging to galactosaminoglycan or DNA/RNA impurities, making the whole spectral profile similar to that of an API product (Figure S6).

2.5. *Crude of Different Origin*

As porcine, bovine, and ovine API heparins differ in many aspects of their structure and activity [21–25], it is important to verify if their structural differences can be observed in the corresponding crude. Six heparin crude samples from bovine intestinal mucosa (BMHC), two from bovine lung (BLHC) and three from ovine intestinal mucosa (OMHC) were characterized by proton and HSQC analysis. The PCA of the GAGs signals region of proton spectra of these samples against the library of porcine crude heparin was not able to differentiate samples according their origin (Figure S7). In spite of the structural differences between the heparins in these crudes, the galactosaminoglycan content mostly contributes to the samples' separation in component 1 (Figure 3). By contrast, PCA performed exclusively on the anomeric region was able to group samples on the basis of their origin, separating them in function of their sulfation pattern in component 1 and of the 6-*O*-sulfation in component 3 (Figure 7 and Figure S8). Indeed, BMHC and PMHC are not fully separated in components 1 and 2 because of their similar degree of sulfation, while in component 3 BMHC are fully distinguished from other crude heparin (Figure 7).

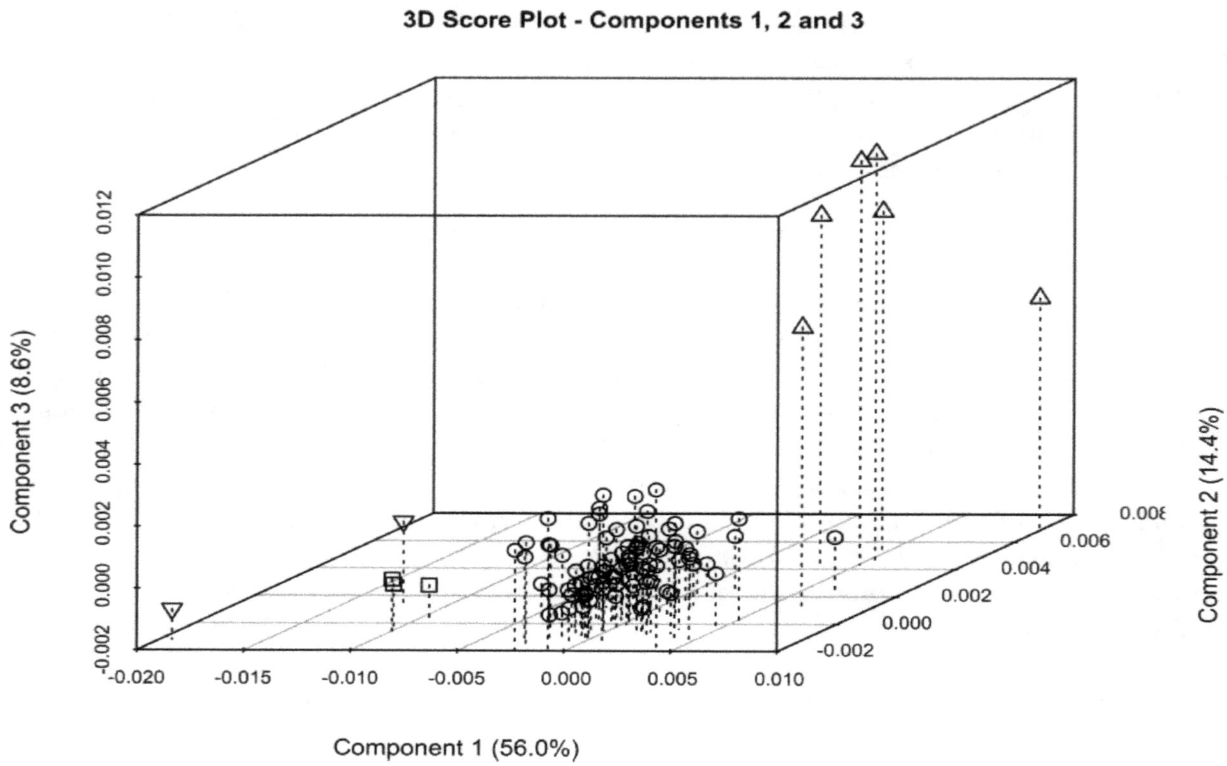

Figure 7. Three-dimensional (3D) Score plot generated by PCA of part of the anomeric signals region. Sample clusters corresponding to the different families of crude heparin are defined. BMHC (above pointing triangles), OMHC (squares) and BLHC (below pointing triangles), against the library of PMHC (circles).

The monosaccharide composition of each crude family was determined by HSQC analysis (Tables 2 and 3). The bovine lung crude shows the highest degree of sulfation and lowest content of acetylation and nonsulfated uronic acid. The lower 6-*O*-sulfation of the bovine mucosa crude agree with those observed in the corresponding API [25], while the degree of sulfation and amount of *N*-acetylation measured for the ovine crude samples is intermediate to that of bovine lung and porcine mucosa heparin, as also observed by the integration of C13 spectra of the purified heparin samples [24]. The greater structural detail obtained applying the HSQC method allows the detection of minor residues in crude heparin, such as G2S, that is more abundant in BMHC compared to ovine or porcine heparins [25].

Table 3. Molar average composition of crude heparin of different species/organ.

BMHC	Hep	DeS	ChS	ANH26X	ANAc6X	ANS3S6X	A6S	G2OH	G2S	I2OH	I2S	SDEG
average	94.7	4.2	0.4	1.5	10.6	2.0	51.7	14.1	1.5	6.8	77.1	2.20
median	98.1	1.1	0.0	1.9	9.6	1.8	52.4	13.8	2.0	6.3	76.9	2.19
st.dev.	5.9	5.8	0.9	1.2	3.3	0.7	4.0	2.0	1.2	1.2	2.8	0.07
min	85.3	0.0	0.0	0.0	8.2	1.3	47.1	11.9	0.0	6.0	73.4	2.12
max	98.8	12.5	2.1	2.6	17.2	3.5	57.2	17.4	2.5	9.2	81.0	2.31
BLHC	**Hep**	**DeS**	**ChS**	**ANH26X**	**ANAc6X**	**ANS3S6X**	**A6S**	**G2OH**	**G2S**	**I2OH**	**I2S**	**SDEG**
Sample 1	94.7	4.2	0.4	1.9	6.6	2.8	85.8	7.8	0.0	4.6	87.6	2.68
Sample 2	98.1	1.1	0.0	0.0	1.6	2.5	90.2	2.3	0.5	2.8	93.4	2.85
OMHC	**Hep**	**DeS**	**ChS**	**ANH26X**	**ANAc6X**	**ANS3S6X**	**A6S**	**G2OH**	**G2S**	**I2OH**	**I2S**	**SDEG**
Sample 1	98.9	1.1	0.0	1.5	8.8	5.0	80.5	10.2	0.0	7.0	82.8	2.58
Sample 2	97.7	2.3	0.0	1.8	8.8	4.7	82.2	10.5	0.0	7.2	82.3	2.59
Sample 3	98.7	1.3	0.0	1.6	7.8	5.3	82.2	9.7	0.0	7.0	83.4	2.61

3. Discussion

The major goals in the analysis of a large number of porcine crude heparins and a range of crude heparin from different animal or tissue sources were: (1) to establish reliable test methods to differentiate them at the crude stage of manufacturing; and (2) to propose a definition for crude heparins as a key intermediate in drug manufacturing. Similar tests can be used to assure the quality of the porcine heparin or bovine heparin API used clinically. Importantly, by checking heparin quality earlier in the supply chain, contaminated material can be prevented from reaching the active pharmaceutical ingredient purification processes, which are often performed under cGMP in U.S. based plants. Because the supply chain for heparin is complex and a global one, controlling the quality of this widely used drug, its intermediates, and starting materials (at least as early as the crude heparin warehouse) solely through cGMP inspection is insufficient and often impractical, in part due to the limited resources that the regulatory authorities have. Thus, there is a need to develop strong analytics and appropriate specifications for crude heparin to ensure the consistent high quality of the final heparin drug substance. For this reason, the tests and the data obtained by applying them will help assure the quality of heparin sodium and LMWH drug products by improving the quality of the entire global heparin supply chain.

In this work, strong anion exchange HPLC (SAX-HPLC) and NMR spectroscopy coupled with chemometrics was demonstrated to be a feasible strategy to characterize crude heparin samples. The proton NMR and HPLC data clearly show that crude heparins vary in terms of glycosaminoglycan composition, amount of DNA/RNA, and other impurities. Proton spectra, when the samples were properly prepared, could be analyzed by PCA, grouping samples based on their composition (relative amount of dermatan, chondroitin, and heparin) or structural properties (degree of sulfation). The presence in the library of some samples that were almost free from galactosaminoglycans and DNA/RNA components suggests that some batches have undergone different levels of purification treatments consistent with the known differences in the way heparins are manufactured by different companies. Quantitative HSQC analysis, recently applied to determine the mono- and disaccharide composition of heparin and LMWH [10], can be extended to crude heparin, allowing an in-depth study of the structural features of samples. Particularly, the degree of sulfation can vary starting from 2.1 to 2.4, the latter value is typical of the purified porcine heparin. Notably, the group of samples that lacked dermatan and chondroitin also contained oxidized serine, suggesting that the products were treated with oxidizing agents, such as those typically used during the production of API. Overall, PCA and HSQC analyses were able to distinguish between crude heparins of different animal and organ sources and manufactured by different processes.

4. Methods

4.1. Reagents and Starting Material

Deuterium oxide 99.9%, sodium dihydrogenphosphate hydrate (NaH2PO4 H2O), disodium hydrogen phosphate dihydrate ($Na_2HPO_4 \cdot H_2O_2$), and 3-(trimethylsilyl)propionic-2,2,3,3-d4 acid sodium salt (TSP) were purchased from Sigma-Aldrich (Milan, Italy). Deuterated EDTA d-16 98% was obtained from Product Cambridge Isotope Laboratories, Inc.

The crude heparin samples were dissolved in phosphate buffer solution, which was prepared as follows: 49.7 mg of sodium dihydrogenphosphate hydrate (0.36 mmol), 202.9 mg of disodium hydrogen phosphate dihydrate (1.14 mmol), and 9.2 mg deuterated EDTA d-16 (0.03 mmol) were dissolved in 10 mL of water. The pH was checked at 7.1. The solution was distributed into 1.3 mL aliquots and then lyophilized. Each aliquot was dissolved in 0.2 mL of D_2O and lyophilized again. Finally, the buffer was dissolved in 1.3 mL deuterium oxide with 0.002% TSP (12 mM).

4.2. Strong Anion Exchange HPLC:

Solutions of crude heparin were prepared as described in Keire et al. [9]. SAX-HPLC separations were performed on a Dionex IonPac® AS11-HC (250 mm × 4 mm) column (Dionex, Sunnyvale, CA, USA). The AS11-HC column's characteristics are: a bead diameter of 9 m with a 2000 Å pore size, particles made of a divinylbenzene/ethylvinylbenzene polymer cross-linked at 55%, coated with microporous latex (DVB/EVB 6% cross-linked) 70 nm particles with hydroxyalkyl quaternary ammonium functional groups, and capacity of 290 equiv./4 mm × 250 mm column. A column temperature of 35 °C was used. The mobile phase was MilliQ water (buffer A) and 2.5 M NaCl with 20 mM TRIS adjusted to pH 3.0 by addition of phosphoric acid (buffer B). The gradient was 0–2 min at 95% A with 5% B, followed by a linear gradient to 100% B at 26 min, a hold at 100% B until 31 min, a linear gradient to 95% A with 5% B at 32 min, and a hold until end of run at 40 min. The flow rate was constant at 0.8 mL/min. The UV detector was set at 215 nm. A 40 L injection volume was used. The liquid chromatography system consisted of Agilent HPLC with a G1314A variable wavelength detector, G1322A degasser, G1311A quaternary pump, column thermostat, and G1313A autosampler.

4.3. Sample Preparation

A 60 mg aliquot of each sample was dissolved in 1.5 mL of D_2O. After two hours, the samples were centrifuged for 4′ at 12,000 rpm, and the supernatant was separated from the precipitated pellet. The supernatant and precipitated pellet were lyophilized. A 20 mg aliquot of the lyophilized supernatant powder was dissolved in 0.6 mL of phosphate buffer solution and transferred to a 5 mm NMR tube.

4.4. ^{1}H-NMR

NMR spectra were measured on a Bruker AVANCE III 600 MHz spectrometer (Karlsruhe, Germany) equipped with TCI 5 mm cryogenic probe. The experiments were acquired with a constant presaturation power of 7 Hz at 298 K, and the following acquisition parameters were used: number scan 32, dummy scan 8, relaxation delay 12 s, spectra width 18 ppm, transmitter offset 4.7 ppm. After exponential multiplication (line broadening of 0.3 Hz), the spectra were Fourier transformed, phased, baseline corrected, and calibrated on the TSP signal.

4.5. HSQC-NMR

The 2D-^{1}H,^{13}C-HSQC spectra were measured on a Bruker AVANCE III 600 MHz spectrometer or on a Bruker AVANCE III HD 500 MHz spectrometer (Karlsruhe, Germany), equipped with TCI 5 mm cryogenic probes, using the Bruker library hsqcetgpsisp2.2 pulse sequence.

The experiments were recorded at 298 K using the following acquisition parameters: number of scan 24 (600 MHz) or 40 (500MHz), dummy scan 16, relaxation delay 2.5 s (600 MHz) or 2 s (500 MHz), spectral width 8 ppm (F2) and 80 ppm (F1), transmitter offset 4.7 ppm (F2) and 80 ppm (F1), 1JC-H = 150 Hz. The chosen processing parameters are: zero filling to 4k in F2; linear prediction to 640 points and zero filling to 1k in F1; and apodization by a 90° shifted squared sine bell function in both dimensions. The spectra were processed and integrated using Topsin software version 3.5 (Bruker BioSpin, Rheinstetten, Germany).

4.6. PCA

Proton NMR spectra were imported into R (R Core Team (2016). R: A language and environment for statistical computing. R Foundation for Statistical Computing, Vienna, Austria. URL https://www.R-project.org/) (R version 3.3.1) and cut according to the chosen spectral region (GAGs signals region: 1.95–2.25, 3.0–3.345, 3.37–3.63, 3.69–4.714, and 4.912–5.75 ppm regions, or part of the anomeric signals region: 4.938–5.75 ppm region). Bucketing was then applied (16 points for GAGs region and 8 points for Heparin/HS region). Spectra were normalized for total area, in the Heparin/HS region case aligned (details in Table S14 and Figure S9), and mean centered. Principal Components Analysis (PCA) was performed using the prcomp function from the R stats package.

Acknowledgments: In part this study was supported by the FDA Critical Path Program and Ronzoni Foundation funds.

Author Contributions: M.G. and D.A.K. drew up the study plan and discussed it with L.M. R.E.K. and M.K. L.M., M.M. and G.M. performed NMR experiments; L.M. performed chemometric studies and organized NMR results; R.E.K. and M.K. performed HPLC study. M.G., D.A.K. and L.M. wrote the paper and revised the manuscript.

References

1. Lever, R.; Mulloy, B.; Page, C.P. (Eds.) *Heparin—A Century of Progress*, 1st ed.; Springer: Berlin/Heidelberg, Germany, 2012.
2. Casu, B. Structure and active domains of heparin. In *Chemistry and Biology of Heparin and Heparan Sulphate*, 1st ed.; Garg, H.G., Linhardt, R.J., Hales, C.A., Eds.; Elsevier Ltd: Oxford, UK, 2005; pp. 1–28.
3. Keire, D.; Mulloy, B.; Chase, C.; Al-Hakim, A.; Cairatti, D.; Gray, E.; Hogwood, J.; Morris, T.; Mourão, P.; Da Luz Carvalho Soares, M.; et al. Diversifying the Global Heparin Supply Chain: Reintroduction of Bovine Heparin in the United States? *Pharm. Technol.* **2015**, *11*, 2–9.
4. Guerrini, M.; Beccati, D.; Shriver, Z.; Naggi, A.; Viswanathan, K.; Bisio, A.; Capila, I.; Lansing, J.C.; Guglieri, S.; Fraser, B.; et al. Oversulfated chondroitinsulfate is a contaminant in heparin associated with adverse clinical events. *Nat. Biotechnol.* **2008**, *26*, 669–675. [CrossRef] [PubMed]
5. Liu, H.; Zhanga, Z.; Linhardt, R.J. Lessons learned from the contamination of heparin. *Nat. Prod. Rep.* **2008**, *26*, 313–321. [CrossRef] [PubMed]
6. Linhardt, R.J.; Gunay, N.S. Production and chemical processing of low molecular weight heparins. *Semin. Thromb. Hemost.* **1999**, *25*, 5–16. [PubMed]
7. U.S. Department of Health and Human Services. Food and Drug Administration. *Guidance for Industry: Heparin for Drug and Medical Device Use: Monitoring Crude Heparin for Quality*; FDA: Silver Spring, MD, USA, 2013. Available online: https://www.fda.gov/downloads/Drugs/GuidanceComplianceRegulatoryInformation/Guidances/UCM291390.png (accessed on 24 April 2017).
8. Sommers, C.D.; Mans, D.J.; Mecker, L.C.; Keire, D.A. Sensitive detection of oversulfated chondroitin sulfate in heparin sodium or crude heparin with a colorimetric microplate based assay. *Anal. Chem.* **2011**, *83*, 3422–3430. [CrossRef] [PubMed]
9. Keire, D.A.; Trehy, M.L.; Reepmeyer, J.C.; Kolinski, R.E.; Ye, W.; Dunn, J.; Westenberger, B.J.; Buhse, L.F. Analysis of crude heparin by ^{1}H-NMR, capillary electrophoresis, and strong-anion-exchange-HPLC for contamination by over sulfated chondroitin sulfate. *J. Pharm. Biomed. Anal.* **2010**, *11*, 921–926. [CrossRef] [PubMed]
10. Mauri, L.; Boccardi, G.; Torri, G.; Karfunkle, M.; Macchi, E.; Muzi, L.; Keire, D.; Guerrini, M. Qualification of HSQC methods for quantitative composition of heparin and low molecular weight heparins. *J. Pharm. Biomed. Anal.* **2017**, *136*, 92–105. [CrossRef] [PubMed]
11. Gatti, G.; Casu, B.; Hamer, G.K.; Perlin, A.S. Studies on the conformation of heparin by ^{1}H and ^{13}C NMR spectroscopy. *Macromolecules* **1979**, *12*, 1001–1007. [CrossRef]
12. Nguyen, K.; Rabenstein, D.L. Determination of the primary structure and carboxyl pKAs of heparin-derived oligosaccharides by band-selective homonuclear-decoupled two-dimensional ^{1}H-NMR. *Anal. Bioanal. Chem.* **2011**, *399*, 663–671. [CrossRef] [PubMed]
13. Jolliffe, I.T. *Principal Component Analysis*, 2nd ed.; Bickel, P., Diggle, P., Fienberg, S., Krickeberg, K., Olkin, I., Wermuth, N., Zeger, S., Eds.; Springer: New York, NY, USA, 2002.
14. Keire, D.A.; Mans, D.J.; Ye, H.; Kolinski, R.E.; Buhse, L.F. Assay of possible economically motivated additives or native impurities levels in heparin by ^{1}H-NMR, SAX-HPLC, and anticoagulation time approaches. *J. Pharm. Biomed. Anal.* **2010**, *52*, 656–664. [CrossRef] [PubMed]
15. Guerrini, M.; Naggi, A.; Guglieri, S.; Santarsiero, R.; Torri, G. Complex glycosaminoglycans: Profiling substitution patterns by two dimensional NMR spectroscopy. *Anal. Biochem.* **2005**, *337*, 35–47. [CrossRef] [PubMed]

16. Guerrini, M.; Guglieri, S.; Naggi, A.; Torri, G. LMWHs: Structural differentiation by bidimensional NMR spectroscopy. *Semin. Thromb. Hemost.* **2007**, *33*, 478–487. [CrossRef] [PubMed]
17. Keire, D.; Buhse, L.F.; al-Hakim, A. Characterization of currently marketed heparin products: Composition analysis by 2D-NMR. *Anal. Methods* **2013**, *5*, 2984–2994. [CrossRef]
18. Mascellani, G.; Liverani, L.; Prete, A.; Bergonzini, G.; Bianchini, P.; Torri, G.; Guerrini, M.; Casu, B. Quantitation of dermatan sulfate active site for the heparin cofactor II by ^{1}H Nuclear Magnetic Resonance spectroscopy. *Anal. Biochem.* **1994**, *223*, 135–141. [CrossRef] [PubMed]
19. Mucci, A.; Schenetti, L.; Volpi, N. ^{1}H and ^{13}C nuclear magnetic resonance identification and characterization of components of chondroitin sulfates of various origin. *Carbohydr. Polym.* **2000**, *41*, 37–45. [CrossRef]
20. Mourier, P.; Anger, P.; Martinez, C.; Herman, F.; Viskov, C. Quantitative compositional analysis of heparin using exhaustive heparinase digestion and strong anion exchange chromatography. *Anal. Chem. Res.* **2015**, *3*, 46–53. [CrossRef]
21. Casu, B.; Guerrini, M.; Naggi, A.; Torri, G.; De-Ambrosi, L.; Boveri, G.; Gonella, S. Differentiation of beef and pig mucosal heparins by NMR spectroscopy. *Thromb. Haemost.* **1995**, *74*, 1205. [PubMed]
22. Watt, D.K.; Yorke, S.C.; Slimb, G.C. Comparison of ovine, bovine and porcine mucosal heparins and low molecular weight heparins by disaccharide analyses and ^{13}C NMR. *Carbohydr. Polym.* **1997**, *33*, 5–11. [CrossRef]
23. Tovar, A.M.F.; Teixeira, A.C.; Rembold, S.M.; Leite, M., Jr.; Lugon, J.R.; Mourão, P.A.S. Bovine and porcine heparins: Different drugs with similar effects on human haemodialysis. *BMC Res. Notes* **2013**, *6*, 230–237. [CrossRef] [PubMed]
24. Fu, L.; Li, G.; Yang, B.; Onishi, A.; Li, L.; Sun, P.; Zhang, F.; Linhardt, R.J. Structural Characterization of Pharmaceutical Heparins Prepared from Different Animal Tissues. *J. Pharm. Sci.* **2013**, *102*, 1447–1457. [CrossRef] [PubMed]
25. Naggi, A.; Gardini, C.; Pedrinola, P.; Mauri, L.; Urso, E.; Alekseeva, A.; Casu, B.; Cassinelli, G.; Guerrini, M.; Iacomini, M.; et al. Structural peculiarity andantithrombin binding region profile of mucosal bovine and porcine heparins. *J. Pharm. Bioanal. Anal.* **2016**, *118*, 52–63. [CrossRef] [PubMed]

7

New Applications of Heparin and Other Glycosaminoglycans

Marcelo Lima [1,2,*], Timothy Rudd [2,3,*] and Edwin Yates [1,2,*]

1. Department of Biochemistry, Federal University of São Paulo (UNIFESP), Vila Clementino, São Paulo, S.P. 04044-020, Brazil
2. Department of Biochemistry, Institute of Integrative Biology, University of Liverpool, Crown Street, Liverpool L69 7ZB, UK
3. National Institute of Biological Standards and Controls (NIBSC), Blanche Lane, Potters Bar, Herts EN6 3QG, UK

* Correspondence: mlima@unifesp.br (M.L.); tim.rudd@nibsc.org (T.R.); eayates@liverpool.ac.uk (E.Y.)

Academic Editor: Giangiacomo Torri

Abstract: Heparin, the widely used pharmaceutical anticoagulant, has been in clinical use for well over half a century. Its introduction reduced clotting risks substantially and subsequent developments, including the introduction of low-molecular-weight heparin, made possible many major surgical interventions that today make heparin an indispensable drug. There has been a recent burgeoning of interest in heparin and related glycosaminoglycan (GAG) polysaccharides, such as chondroitin sulfates, heparan sulfate, and hyaluronate, as potential agents in various applications. This ability arises mainly from the ability of GAGs to interact with, and alter the activity of, a wide range of proteins. Here, we review new developments (since 2010) in the application of heparin and related GAGs across diverse fields ranging from thrombosis and neurodegenerative disorders to microbiology and biotechnology.

Keywords: heparin; glycosaminoglycans; chondroitin sulfate

---

1. Introduction

Heparin, a member of the glycosaminoglycan (GAG) family of sulfated polysaccharides, is one of the most widely used pharmaceuticals, whose major role is in the inhibition of clot formation and thrombi, especially during surgery or following trauma. Beyond referring to some important historical literature, this review will attempt to survey recent (by which we mean from ca. 2010 to 2017) applications for this important and widely used drug, and will include other GAG members, which are being explored increasingly for other potential uses.

Heparin has been an established anticoagulant drug for more than 60 years for the prevention and control of thrombotic events owing to its interaction with a number of proteins of the blood clotting cascade, notably antithrombin and thrombin [1]. It consists of a linear, highly sulfated polysaccharide chain of various lengths varying from 2000 to 40,000 Da [2–4], composed of repeating disaccharide units of 1,4 linked α-L-iduronic or β-D-glucuronic acid (D-GlcA), and α-D-glucosamine (D-GlcN). The predominant substitution pattern comprises 2-*O*-sulfation of the iduronate residues and *N*- and 6-*O*-sulfation of the glucosamine residues [5]. Heparin is also closely related structurally to heparan sulfate (HS), which is present on cell surfaces and in the extracellular matrix. HS is generally less sulfated than heparin and is often considered to have a defined domain structure [6–8] and a lower proportion of L-iduronate residues. There are also D-GlcA and N-acetylated glucosamine (D-GlcNAc) residues, as well as variations in sulfation, including a small proportion of 3-*O*-sulfates on glucosamine residues. Hyaluronic acid (HA) is the only member of the GAG family that is not sulfated, being a homo-polymer consisting of beta (1→4) linked disaccharides of D-GlcA β (1→3) D-GlcNAc. Chondroitin sulfate (CS) encompasses various structures, based on repeating β (1-4) linked disaccharides of GlcA β (1→3) GalNAc containing 6-(Chondroitin sulfate-C: CS-C) and 4-sulfates (CS-A), sulfation at position-2 of the GlcA residues (GlcA2S β (1→3) GalNAc6S) (CS-D), and 4,6-di-sulfated GalNAc (GlcA β (1→3) GalNAc4, 6diS (in CS-E). The polysaccharide, dermatan sulfate (DS), which was formerly known as CS-B, contains repeating →4) L-IdoA β (1→3) D-GalNAc β (1→ units with 4-*O*-sulfation on the GalNAc moiety. GAG-like structures from non-mammalian sources, often marine, have become the focus of attention recently, and these, while possessing similar backbone structures, often include branches of fucose units [9], which can include non-reducing terminal fucose with sulfation at positions-2 and -3 [10].

The discovery and development of heparin as an anticoagulant agent had a tremendous impact on health because major surgical procedures became possible, especially those in which cardiopulmonary bypass (CPB), which was first demonstrated in animals in 1939 [11], were necessary. Another important medical procedure that is only possible due to the anticoagulant properties of heparin is dialysis. Indeed, unfractionated (full-length) heparin (UFH) named heparin sodium, its antidote, protamine sulfate [12], as well as a form of low-molecular-weight heparin (LMWH) [13] all appear in the World Health Organization's (WHO) List of Essential Medicines. The pharmacological activity of heparin results mainly from its ability to bind and accelerate the AT activity, thereby considerably enhancing the inhibition of coagulation factors Xa and IIa, although it interacts in concert with AT and other members of the blood clotting cascade as well, including factor IXa, XIa, and XIIa [14]. In a biological rather than a clinical context though, heparin action is more closely linked to defense against exogenous pathogens [15] and responses following tissue damage. Heparin alters cytokine levels [16], and one of its biological roles may be to dampen the effects of the sudden release of large numbers of cytokines following infection or sudden trauma.

In recent times, the majority of pharmaceutical heparin has been sourced from the intestine of pigs, and detailed studies of the sequence of heparin have involved laborious separation techniques. Recent advances in the biosynthesis of heparin-related structures employing recombinant enzymes and synthetic uridine-diphosphate-monosaccharide donors have been developed by Liu and Linhardt, allowing not only for the production of heparin sequences but also for the systematic and controlled preparation of heparin (and HS) analogues, which will be suitable for a wide-range of experimental purposes and applications [17].

2. Applications in Anticoagulation and Cancer Treatments

In current clinical use, one of the most important forms of heparin is low-molecular-weight heparin (LMWH) which consists of a complex mixture of fragments ranging from tetra to hexadecasaccharides and somewhat higher oligosaccharides [18–20] obtained by various chemical and enzymatic depolymerization processes. The main advantages of LMWHs over UFH are improved bioavailability and higher anti-factor Xa/anti-factor IIa activity ratios, with decreased hemorrhagic risk during prolonged treatments [21]. While UFH can be monitored effectively and reversed in patients undergoing surgery with extracorporeal circulation, LMWHs cannot, because neutralization with protamine sulfate is ineffective. The development of new anticoagulant agents with the beneficial properties of both UFH and LMWH is therefore still pursued and is an important area in which biosynthetic structures are being applied [22,23].

Aside from the well-known anticoagulant activities of heparin and related GAGs or GAG mixtures, such as sulodexide (a mixture of LMWH and DS in the ratio 80:20), heparin is also active in a wide range of activities in which the naturally occurring cell surface polysaccharide, heparan sulfate (HS), is a participant. Many of the proteins with which heparin interacts originate in the extracellular matrix, the best studied of which belong to the fibroblast growth factor (FGF) family. The potential use of heparin to interfere with aberrant cell–cell signaling by this route has been investigated and the relationship between sequence and activity sought [24–27].

The importance of the FGF signaling system to development and regulation, and hence when its function is impaired or altered, also to disease is one obvious area in which heparins, acting in this case as analogues for HS, can be applied. One area in which modulating FGF signaling would be desirable is cancer treatment. However, it is noteworthy that cancer-related thrombotic disorders are also well known and were first described as long ago as 1865, when the clinical association between thrombosis and an initially undiagnosed cancer was noted. Unfractionated heparin and LMWHs have been used successfully for the prophylaxis and treatment of cancer-related hemostatic disorders; however, since cancer patients have an increased risk of bleeding [28], LMWHs have gained significant ground since they produce a more predictable anticoagulant response, display improved subcutaneous bioavailability, and exhibit an extended half-life. Furthermore, heparin-induced thrombocytopenia (HIT) incidence is lower when LMWHs and the synthetic pentasaccharide, Fondaparinux, are used. Novel oral anticoagulants are under development, but their efficacy and safety in cancer-patients has yet to be proved. Despite being well recognized now, the pathogenesis is complex and results from the combination of several factors, but the expression of tumor cell-associated clotting factors is a shared characteristic. The prevention and treatment of these conditions extends beyond the ease of symptoms, it has a direct impact in cancer patient survival [29], and there are some known beneficial effects of heparin, but elucidating these is hampered by the complexity of the systems involved. The widespread use of heparin as a treatment is hindered by unwanted anticoagulant side-effects [30] (see also review by Afratis et al. [31]); however, the possibility of correcting signaling defects caused by altered HS structure (e.g., by sulf enzyme activity) in cancer [32,33] or the direct inhibition of the sulf enzymes with heparin or heparin analogues is an area of potential interest. Of direct relevance to the progression of the disease is the inhibition of a mammalian heparanase enzyme [34], while other routes are thought to influence metastasis, acting via P- and L-selections [35–37], inhibiting galectins [38], inhibiting tumorogenesis and angiogenesis through cellular receptors such as CD44 and growth factor receptors [39], or, in the case of the use of heparin as a means of ameliorating resistance to cisplatin treatment, acting through as-yet unidentified mechanisms [40], all of which are affected by heparin or heparin analogues. Among other GAGs, an example of the treatment of cancer is the use of the non-sulfated GAG, hyaluronate (HA) in pancreatic ductal adenocarcinoma [41].

3. Recovery from Nervous System Damage

Recent work shows that, while CS inhibits the regeneration of neurites in the CNS, CS-bound HB-GAM (pleiotrophin) activates them, inducing dendrite regeneration in adult cerebral cortex and axonal regeneration in adult spinal cord [42]. Chondroitin sulfate forms a barrier following nerve injury [43], but can be digested by enzymes to improve repair [44–47]. Chondroitin sulfate-E (CS-E), containing unusual 4,6 di-sulfated GalNAc residues and 4-sulfated CS in aggrecan, have been shown to be inhibitory to neurite outgrowth [48], and CS-E mediates estrogen-induced osteoanabolism [49], suggesting several potential future applications for CS and its derivatives.

4. Respiratory Diseases

GAGs and heparin in particular have been suggested as playing a protective roles in the inflammation response [50], which has been interpreted as involving (among other things) the inhibition of elastase and the interaction with several cytokines [51]. Heparin and its analogues have been proposed for the application to elastase inhibition for cystic fibrosis treatment (or other conditions, such as acute respiratory distress syndrome (ARDS). Although they do not originate from a conventional mammalian GAG, oligosaccharide fragments of the fucosylated GAG structures from the sea cucumber (*Holothuria forskali*) [9] were shown to lower neutrophil infiltration by reducing selectin interactions.

5. Neurodegenerative Diseases

There is an emerging role in Parkinson's Disease for heparin acting via cathepsin-d activity affecting α-synuclein accumulation [52], while, in Alzheimer's Disease, the inhibition of BACE-1, the key protease responsible for the generation of toxic Aβ fragments (1–42) is inhibited by heparin and its derivatives [53,54], some of which have been engineered to possess very low anticoagulant activity [55,56]. Furthermore, it is known that heparin modulates fibril formation [57], and understanding the mechanisms underlying such events may open new routes for the prevention, for instance, of toxic fibril formation and deposition.

6. Roles as Antimicrobial Agents

6.1. Viruses

GAGs might be expected, on the basis of their universal presence on cell surfaces, to serve as a broad spectrum and relatively non-specific receptors for virus binding [58]; [see also an earlier review: [59]]. Such interactions are not unexpected, since virus envelope proteins present patches of positively charged amino acids. While GAGs have been shown to attach to filoviruses [60] and CS-E, but not CS-D, and inhibit dengue virus infection [61], it is clear that GAGs are indeed of relevance to the mechanisms of viral attachment and invasion. The ability of viruses to bind cell surface HSs and, by extension, bind heparin under experimental conditions has long been known in the case of herpes simplex (HSV) and dengue (DENV) viruses. Heparin as a potential inhibitor of viral attachment follows naturally from these observations and has been demonstrated for DENV [62]. What is less clear is whether and how this knowledge can be exploited to enable GAGs to be applied as inhibitors of attachment, a process that may be able to be exploited for the well-known property of multivalency to increase the avidity of the binding of the viral particles to the GAG, perhaps immobilized in some device, or attached to multidentate ligands in a nanotechnology format (see also a review of this field: [63]). The potential importance of such applications is difficult to over-emphasize, however. Recently, viral attachment to GAGs was reported for IFNα/βBP from variola (smallpox virus), monkeypox viruses [64], and GAGs have been shown to prevent measles virus infection in cell lines via hemagglutinin protein [65]. Other viruses, including hepatitis B, have been found to bind to heparin [66] as has Japanese encephalitis virus (JEV) [67]. Thus, the interest in GAG-based intervention seems set to increase.

Heparin and derivatives have been shown to be effective in preventing the infection of cells by the influenza virus, strain H5N1 [68], and to have effects on ZIKV-induced cell death that are independent of adhesion and invasion [69]. In this case, heparin has only a modest ability to protect infection by analogy with dengue virus, which is also of the flavivirus family, and which interacts with heparin through the envelope glycoproteins [70]. Rather, heparin may be acting to protect infected cells from cytotoxic effects and cell death via the activation of cell survival signaling pathways. The ability of heparin to protect cells from programmed cell death had already been observed in human cells (non-infected) [71], and this may form an interesting new avenue for the application of GAG derivatives in itself.

6.2. Parasites

The involvement of GAGs in a parasitic disease has been studied relatively little. However, the potential for the application of GAGs remains high in cases where GAGs form a major part of the means of attachment and invasion, especially where there is the possibility of topical application. The ability of heparin and derivatives to inhibit rosetting of parasite infected erythrocytes has been noted [72] and, recently, effective inhibitors (comprising fucosylated CS (FucCS)) of cytoadherence (the process of adhesion of infected red blood cells to vascular epithelia) derived from sea cucumber have been reported [73]. Heparin is known to alter the activity of a cysteine protease in the parasite, *L. mexicana*, that causes Leishmaniasis [74] and interacts with a metalloprotease from *L.(v). braziliensis* [75]. Heparin has also been shown to accelerate protein degradation by human neutrophil elastase [76]. Several heparin-binding proteins have also been identified in *T. cruzi*, where some of them are implicated in parasite adhesion to midgut epithelial cells [77].

6.3. Bacteria

Binding of GAGs facilitates Streptococcal entry into the CNS of *Drosophila* [78] and determines disease progression [79]. In relation to the phenomenon of shock, GAGs seem to be elevated overall, perhaps originating from damaged tissue, but they also seem to neutralize antimicrobial peptides [80]. Glycosaminoglycans were studied en masse, however, without paying attention to the individual types involved. Heparin use in sepsis patients, where crosstalk between thrombosis and inflammation plays a critical role, has also been recognized. The use of heparin prevents the development of microthromboembolic disease during sepsis, impairing tissue hypoxygenation and further organ damage and dysfunction [81]. There is also literature pointing to the use of heparin-coated stents for the prevention of bacterial biofilm formation and subsequent microbe attachment [82].

7. Panceatitis

Acute pancreatitis has been reported independently by several groups to benefit from treatment with heparin [83] in rats and in patients [84–86]. Furthermore, LMW heparin has also been shown to be effective [87].

8. Roles in Rheumatoid Arthritis (RA)

Naturally occurring autoantibodies to GAGs are markers in rheumatoid arthritis [88]. The level of IgM type Ab for CS-C in serum correlates with RA, although GAG concentration alone is not a good indicator in knee injury [89] in agreement with earlier findings in horses [90].

9. Inflammation Reduction

Many of the applications of heparin mentioned in this review may stem, at least in part, from the ability of heparin to moderate inflammation. This topic has itself been reviewed in 2013 [91] and, in general, heparin is perceived as acting via several routes, which include interaction with cytokines and as an inhibitor of heparanase, to achieve reduced leukocyte recruitment.

Applications in which these properties may be important include the treatment of burns [92] and the proposed use of heparin in asthma treatment [93]. The potential, based on a projection of the ability of heparin to inhibit bacterial infection and reduce inflammation, to improve the symptoms of cystic fibrosis has also been investigated [94] but no marked improvement at low doses (50,000 IU) has been shown.

While cystic fibrosis applications acting to reduce inflammation assist sputum clearance, inhibit elastase, or act as an inhibitor of microbial attachment or growth have not been convincing, heparin derivatives were shown to be capable of acting at several points in the inflammatory process [51].

10. Alternative Sources of GAG-Like Structures with Potentially Useful Activities

This review attempts to cover not only new applications for heparin but also potential new sources of active agents among the GAGs for both old and new applications. Although not all of these structures correspond to GAGs according to the classical definitions of mammalian GAGs provided above, GAG-like structures are found in a wide range of organisms, including *Cnidaria*, *Arthropoda*, *Mollusca*, *Echinodermata*, and *Chordata* [95]. A host of polysaccharides, either GAGs in the conventional sense or polysaccharides with structural features closely resembling GAGs, usually bearing additional ramifications have been identified and linked to a variety of biological activities. These include Sea cucumber (*S. hermanni*) as an antiinflammatory [95], marine GAG analogues [96], fish cartilage as an antitumor and anti-pathognic agent [97], GAGs from starfish with antithrombotic and anti-inflammatory activities [95], and mussels (*Perna canaliculis*) as an anti-inflammatory agent [98].

11. Biotechnological and Other Applications

An emerging use of GAGs is in biotechnological applications, particularly in the field of embryonic stem cells, for the regulation of differentiation [reviewed in [99]] and neural speciation in mouse embryonic stem cells [100]. The successful fractionation of a cell population by HS epitopes has also been reported [101]. The prospect of incorporating GAGs into electrospun meshes for the purpose of supporting stem cell applications has also been undertaken [102]. A possible role is emerging in muscular dystrophy, following signs of involvement of HS sulfation in the disease process and ageing, acting via FGF-2 [103].

12. Concluding Remarks

Many a student textbook of biochemistry once dismissed the role of GAGs as merely structural; decades of intensive research led to a burgeoning of the biological roles ascribed to them and potential practical applications. The precise nature of the relationship between their structure and function remains a matter of debate, a fact that stems not only from their structural complexity, but also the difficulty of analysis, which may also indicate that new approaches are required. These approaches may need to be sensitive to as yet undefined properties, and one such property is their large-scale vibrational modes [104]. Nevertheless, even without this detailed information, it is clear that the number of roles of these versatile materials seem to set to increase in the future.

References

1. Barrowcliffe, T.W. History of heparin. *Handb. Exp. Pharmacol.* **2012**, *207*, 3–22.
2. Nader, H.B.; McDuffie, N.M.; Dietrich, C.P. Heparin fractionation by electrofocusing: presence of 21 components of different molecular weights. *Biochem. Biophys. Res. Commun.* **1974**, *57*, 488–493. [CrossRef]
3. McDuffie, N.M.; Dietrich, C.P.; Nader, H.B. Electrofocusing of heparin: Fractionation of heparin into 21 components distinguishable from other acidic mucopolysaccharides. *Biopolymers* **1975**, *14*, 1473–1486. [CrossRef] [PubMed]
4. Dietrich, C.P.; Nader, H.B.; Mcduffie, N.N. Electrofocusing of heparin: Presence of 21 monomeric and dimeric molecular species in heparin preparations. *An. Acad. Bras. Cienc.* **1975**, *47*, 301–309. [PubMed]
5. Perlin, A.S.; Mackie, D.M.; Dietrich, C.P. Evidence for a (1→4)-linked 4-*O*-(α-L-idopyranosyluronic acid 2-sulfate)-(2-deoxy-2-sulfoamino-D-glucopyranosyl 6-sulfate) sequence in heparin. *Carbohydr. Res.* **1971**, *18*, 185–194. [CrossRef]
6. Turnbull, J.E.; Gallagher, J.T. Distribution of iduronate 2-sulphate residues in heparan sulphate. Evidence for an ordered polymeric structure. *Biochem. J.* **1991**, *273*, 553–559. [CrossRef] [PubMed]
7. Maccarana, M.; Sakura, Y.; Tawada, A.; Yoshida, K.; Lindahl, U. Domain structure of heparan sulfates from bovine organs. *J. Biol. Chem.* **1996**, *271*, 17804–17810. [CrossRef] [PubMed]
8. Merry, C.L.; Lyon, M.; Deakin, J.A.; Hopwood, J.J.; Gallagher, J.T. Highly sensitive sequencing of the sulfated domains of heparan sulfate. *J. Biol. Chem.* **1999**, *274*, 18455–18462. [CrossRef] [PubMed]
9. Panagos, C.G.; Thomson, D.S.; Moss, C.; Hughes, A.D.; Kelly, M.S.; Liu, Y.; Chai, W.; Venkatasamy, R.; Spina, D.; Page, C.P.; et al. Fucosylated chondroitin sulfates from the body wall of the sea cucumber Holothuria forskali: Conformation, selectin binding, and biological activity. *J. Biol. Chem.* **2014**, *289*, 28284–28298. [CrossRef] [PubMed]
10. Pomin, V.H. Holothurian fucosylated chondroitin sulfate. *Mar. Drugs* **2014**, *12*, 232–254. [CrossRef] [PubMed]
11. Gibbon, J.G., Jr. The maintenance of life during experimental occlusion of the pulmonary artery followed by survival. *Surg Gynecol Obs.* **1939**, *69*, 602–614.
12. Warkentin, T.E.; Crowther, M.A. Reversing anticoagulants both old and new. *Can. J. Anaesth.* **2002**, *49*, S11–S25. [PubMed]

13. Johnson, E.A.; Kirkwood, T.B.; Stirling, Y.; Perez-Requejo, J.L.; Ingram, G.I.; Bangham, D.R.; Brozović, M. Four heparin preparations: Anti-Xa potentiating effect of heparin after subcutaneous injection. *Thromb. Haemost.* **1976**, *35*, 586–591. [PubMed]
14. Beeler, D.L.; Marcum, J.A.; Schiffman, S.; Rosenberg, R.D. Interaction of factor XIa and antithrombin in the presence and absence of heparin. *Blood* **1986**, *67*, 1488–1492. [PubMed]
15. Straus, A.H.; Sant'anna, O.A.; Nader, H.B.; Dietrich, C.P. An inverse relationship between heparin content and antibody response in genetically selected mice. Sex effect and evidence of a polygenic control for skin heparin concentration. *Biochem. J.* **1984**, *220*, 625–630. [CrossRef] [PubMed]
16. Call, D.R.; Remick, D.G. Low molecular weight heparin is associated with greater cytokine production in a stimulated whole blood model. *Shock* **1998**, *10*, 192–197. [CrossRef] [PubMed]
17. Liu, J.; Linhardt, R.J. Chemoenzymatic synthesis of heparan sulfate and heparin. *Nat. Prod. Rep.* **2014**, *31*, 1676–1685. [CrossRef] [PubMed]
18. Viskov, C.; Just, M.; Laux, V.; Mourier, P.; Lorenz, M. Description of the chemical and pharmacological characteristics of a new hemisynthetic ultra-low-molecular-weight heparin, AVE5026. *J. Thromb. Haemost.* **2009**, *7*, 1143–1151. [CrossRef] [PubMed]
19. Bisio, A.; Vecchietti, D.; Citterio, L.; Guerrini, M.; Raman, R.; Bertini, S.; Eisele, G.; Naggi, A.; Sasisekharan, R.; Torri, G. Structural features of low-molecular-weight heparins affecting their affinity to antithrombin. *Thromb. Haemost.* **2009**, *102*, 865–873. [CrossRef] [PubMed]
20. Zhang, Z.; Weïwer, M.; Li, B.; Kemp, M.M.; Daman, T.H.; Linhardt, R.J. Oversulfated chondroitin sulfate: Impact of a heparin impurity, associated with adverse clinical events, on low-molecular-weight heparin preparation. *J. Med. Chem.* **2008**, *51*, 5498–5501. [CrossRef] [PubMed]
21. Hoppensteadt, D.; Iqbal, O.; Fareed, J. Chapter 21—Basic and clinical differences of heparin and low molecular weight heparin treatment. *Chem. Biol. Heparin Heparan Sulfate* **2005**, *1*, 583–606.
22. Xu, Y.; Wang, Z.; Liu, R.; Bridges, A.S.; Huang, X.; Liu, J. Directing the biological activities of heparan sulfate oligosaccharides using a chemoenzymatic approach. *Glycobiology* **2012**, *22*, 96–106. [CrossRef] [PubMed]
23. Xu, Y.; Pempe, E.H.; Liu, J. Chemoenzymatic synthesis of heparin oligosaccharides with both anti-factor Xa and anti-factor IIa activities. *J. Biol. Chem.* **2012**, *287*, 29054–29061. [CrossRef] [PubMed]
24. Xu, R.; Ori, A.; Rudd, T.R.; Uniewicz, K.A.; Ahmed, Y.A.; Guimond, S.E.; Skidmore, M.A.; Siligardi, G.; Yates, E.A.; Fernig, D.G. Diversification of the structural determinants of fibroblast growth factor-heparin interactions: Implications for binding specificity. *J. Biol. Chem.* **2012**, *287*, 40061–40073. [CrossRef] [PubMed]
25. Li, Y.; Sun, C.; Yates, E.A.; Jiang, C.; Wilkinson, M.C.; Fernig, D.G. Heparin binding preference and structures in the fibroblast growth factor family parallel their evolutionary diversification. *Open Biol.* **2016**, *6*, 150275. [CrossRef] [PubMed]
26. Schultz, V.; Suflita, M.; Liu, X.; Zhang, X.; Yu, Y.; Li, L.; Green, D.E.; Xu, Y.; Zhang, F.; DeAngelis, P.L.; et al. Heparan sulfate domains required for fibroblast growth factor 1 and 2 signaling through fibroblast growth factor receptor 1c. *J. Biol. Chem.* **2017**, *292*, 2495–2509. [CrossRef] [PubMed]
27. Theodoraki, A.; Hu, Y.; Poopalasundaram, S.; Oosterhof, A.; Guimond, S.E.; Disterer, P.; Khoo, B.; Hauge-Evans, A.C.; Jones, P.M.; Turnbull, J.E.; et al. Distinct patterns of heparan sulphate in pancreatic islets suggest novel roles in paracrine islet regulation. *Mol. Cell. Endocrinol.* **2015**, *399*, 296–310. [CrossRef] [PubMed]
28. Rickles, F.R.; Falanga, A. Molecular basis for the relationship between thrombosis and cancer. *Thromb. Res.* **2001**, *102*, V215–V224. [CrossRef]
29. Nishioka, J.; Goodin, S. Low-molecular-weight heparin in cancer-associated thrombosis: Treatment, secondary prevention, and survival. *J. Oncol. Pharm. Pract.* **2007**, *13*, 85–97. [CrossRef] [PubMed]
30. Solari, V.; Jesudason, E.C.; Turnbull, J.E.; Yates, E.A. Determining the anti-coagulant-independent anti-cancer effects of heparin. *Br. J. Cancer* **2010**, *103*, 593–594. [CrossRef] [PubMed]
31. Afratis, N.; Gialeli, C.; Nikitovic, D.; Tsegenidis, T.; Karousou, E.; Theocharis, A.D.; Pavão, M.S.; Tzanakakis, G.N.; Karamanos, N.K. Glycosaminoglycans: Key players in cancer cell biology and treatment. *FEBS J.* **2012**, *279*, 1177–1197. [CrossRef] [PubMed]
32. Solari, V.; Borriello, L.; Turcatel, G.; Shimada, H.; Sposto, R.; Fernandez, G.E.; Asgharzadeh, S.; Yates, E.A.; Turnbull, J.E.; DeClerck, Y.A. MYCN-dependent expression of sulfatase-2 regulates neuroblastoma cell survival. *Cancer Res.* **2014**, *74*, 5999–6009. [CrossRef] [PubMed]

33. Vicente, C.M.; Lima, M.A.; Yates, E.A.; Nader, H.B.; Toma, L. Enhanced tumorigenic potential of colorectal cancer cells by extracellular sulfatases. *Mol. Cancer Res.* **2015**, *13*, 510–523. [CrossRef] [PubMed]
34. Vlodavsky, I.; Elkin, M.; Ilan, N. Impact of heparanase and the tumor microenvironment on cancer metastasis and angiogenesis: Basic aspects and clinical applications. *Rambam Maimonides Med. J.* **2011**, *2*, 1–17. [CrossRef] [PubMed]
35. Laubli, H.; Varki, A.; Borsig, L. Antimetastatic properties of low molecular weight heparin. *J. Clin. Oncol.* **2016**, *34*, 2560–2561. [CrossRef] [PubMed]
36. Borsig, L.; Wong, R.; Feramisco, J.; Nadeau, D.R.; Varki, N.M.; Varki, A. Heparin and cancer revisited: Mechanistic connections involving platelets, P-selectin, carcinoma mucins, and tumor metastasis. *Proc. Natl. Acad. Sci. USA* **2001**, *98*, 3352–3357. [CrossRef] [PubMed]
37. Läubli, H.; Stevenson, J.L.; Varki, A.; Varki, N.M.; Borsig, L. L-selectin facilitation of metastasis involves temporal induction of Fut7-dependent ligands at sites of tumor cell arrest. *Cancer Res.* **2006**, *66*, 1536–1542. [CrossRef] [PubMed]
38. Duckworth, C.A.; Guimond, S.E.; Sindrewicz, P.; Hughes, A.J.; French, N.S.; Lian, L.-Y.; Yates, E.A.; Pritchard, D.M.; Rhodes, J.M.; Turnbull, J.E.; et al. Chemically modified, non-anticoagulant heparin derivatives are potent galectin-3 binding inhibitors and inhibit circulating galectin-3-promoted metastasis. *Oncotarget* **2015**, *6*, 23671–23687. [CrossRef] [PubMed]
39. Karousou, E.; Misra, S.; Ghatak, S.; Dobra, K.; Götte, M.; Vigetti, D.; Passi, A.; Karamanos, N.K.; Skandalis, S.S. Roles and targeting of the HAS/hyaluronan/CD44 molecular system in cancer. *Matrix Biol.* **2016**, *59*, 1–20. [CrossRef] [PubMed]
40. Pfankuchen, D.B.; Stölting, D.P.; Schlesinger, M.; Royer, H.-D.; Bendas, G.; Bastian, D.; Philipp, D.; Schlesinger, M.; Royer, H.-D.; Bendas, G. Low molecular weight heparin tinzaparin antagonizes cisplatin resistance of ovarian cancer cells. *Biochem. Pharmacol.* **2015**, *97*, 147–157. [CrossRef] [PubMed]
41. Sato, N.; Cheng, X.-B.; Kohi, S.; Koga, A.; Hirata, K. Targeting hyaluronan for the treatment of pancreatic ductal adenocarcinoma. *Acta Pharm. Sin. B* **2016**, *6*, 101–105. [CrossRef] [PubMed]
42. Paveliev, M.; Fenrich, K.K.; Kislin, M.; Kuja-Panula, J.; Kulesskiy, E.; Varjosalo, M.; Kajander, T.; Mugantseva, E.; Ahonen-Bishopp, A.; Khiroug, L.; et al. HB-GAM (pleiotrophin) reverses inhibition of neural regeneration by the CNS extracellular matrix. *Nat. Publ. Gr.* **2016**, *6*, 33916. [CrossRef] [PubMed]
43. Siebert, J.R.; Conta Steencken, A.; Osterhout, D.J. Chondroitin Sulfate Proteoglycans in the Nervous System: Inhibitors to Repair. *Biomed Res. Int.* **2014**, *2014*, 845323. [CrossRef] [PubMed]
44. Kwok, J.C.F.; Yang, S.; Fawcett, J.W. Neural ECM in regeneration and rehabilitation. *Prog. Brain Res.* **2014**, *214*, 179–192.
45. Dick, G.; Liktan, C.; Alves, J.N.; Ehlert, E.M.E.; Miller, G.M.; Hsieh-Wilson, L.C.; Sugahara, K.; Oosterhof, A.; Van Kuppevelt, T.H.; Verhaagen, J.; et al. Semaphorin 3A binds to the perineuronal nets via chondroitin sulfate type E motifs in rodent brains. *J. Biol. Chem.* **2013**, *288*, 27384–27395. [CrossRef] [PubMed]
46. Orlando, C.; Ster, J.; Gerber, U.; Fawcett, J.W.; Raineteau, O. Perisynaptic chondroitin sulfate proteoglycans restrict structural plasticity in an integrin-dependent manner. *J. Neurosci.* **2012**, *32*, 18009–18017. [CrossRef] [PubMed]
47. Wang, D.; Ichiyama, R.M.; Zhao, R.; Andrews, M.R.; Fawcett, J.W. Chondroitinase Combined with Rehabilitation Promotes Recovery of Forelimb Function in Rats with Chronic Spinal Cord Injury. *J. Neurosci.* **2011**, *31*, 9332–9344. [CrossRef] [PubMed]
48. Gilbert, R.J.; McKeon, R.J.; Darr, A.; Calabro, A.; Hascall, V.C.; Bellamkonda, R. V CS-4,6 is differentially upregulated in glial scar and is a potent inhibitor of neurite extension. *Mol. Cell. Neurosci.* **2005**, *29*, 545–558. [CrossRef] [PubMed]
49. Koike, T.; Mikami, T.; Shida, M.; Habuchi, O.; Kitagawa, H. Chondroitin sulfate-E mediates estrogen-induced osteoanabolism. *Sci. Rep.* **2015**, *5*, 8994. [CrossRef] [PubMed]
50. Li, L.; Ling, Y.; Huang, M.; Yin, T.; Gou, S.M.; Zhan, N.Y.; Xiong, J.X.; Wu, H.S.; Yang, Z.Y.; Wang, C.Y. Heparin inhibits the inflammatory response induced by LPS and HMGB1 by blocking the binding of HMGB1 to the surface of macrophages. *Cytokine* **2015**, *72*, 36–42. [CrossRef] [PubMed]
51. Veraldi, N.; Hughes, A.J.; Rudd, T.R.; Thomas, H.B.; Edwards, S.W.; Hadfield, L.; Skidmore, M.A.; Siligardi, G.; Cosentino, C.; Shute, J.K.; et al. Heparin derivatives for the targeting of multiple activities in the inflammatory response. *Carbohydr. Polym.* **2015**, *117*, 400–407. [CrossRef] [PubMed]

52. Lehri-Boufala, S.; Ouidja, M.O.; Barbier-Chassefière, V.; Hénault, E.; Raisman-Vozari, R.; Garrigue-Antar, L.; Papy-Garcia, D.; Morin, C. New roles of glycosaminoglycans in α-synuclein aggregation in a cellular model of Parkinson disease. *PLoS ONE* **2015**, *10*, e0116641. [CrossRef] [PubMed]
53. Scholefield, Z.; Yates, E.A.; Wayne, G.; Amour, A.; McDowell, W.; Turnbull, J.E. Heparan sulfate regulates amyloid precursor protein processing by BACE1, the Alzheimer's β-secretase. *J. Cell Biol.* **2003**, *163*, 97–107. [CrossRef] [PubMed]
54. Zhang, X.; Zhao, X.; Lang, Y.; Li, Q.; Liu, X.; Cai, C.; Hao, J.; Li, G.; Yu, G. Low anticoagulant heparin oligosaccharides as inhibitors of BACE-1, the Alzheimer's β-secretase. *Carbohydr. Polym.* **2016**, *151*, 51–59. [CrossRef] [PubMed]
55. Patey, S.J.; Edwards, E.A.; Yates, E.A.; Turnbull, J.E. Heparin derivatives as inhibitors of BACE-1, the Alzheimer's β-secretase, with reduced activity against factor Xa and other proteases. *J. Med. Chem.* **2006**, *49*, 6129–6132. [CrossRef] [PubMed]
56. Ma, Q.; Cornelli, U.; Hanin, I.; Jeske, W.P.; Linhardt, R.J.; Walenga, J.M.; Fareed, J.; Lee, J.M. Heparin Oligosaccharides as Potential Therapeutic Agents in Senile Dementia. *Curr Pharm Des.* **2007**, *13*, 1607–1616. [CrossRef] [PubMed]
57. Stewart, K.L.; Hughes, E.; Yates, E.A.; Akien, G.R.; Huang, T.Y.; Lima, M.A.; Rudd, T.R.; Guerrini, M.; Hung, S.C.; Radford, S.E.; Middleton, D.A. Atomic Details of the Interactions of Glycosaminoglycans with Amyloid-β Fibrils. *J. Am. Chem. Soc.* **2016**, *138*, 8328–8331. [CrossRef] [PubMed]
58. Vigant, F.; Santos, N.C.; Lee, B. Broad-spectrum antivirals against viral fusion. *Nat. Rev. Microbiol.* **2015**, *13*, 426–437. [CrossRef] [PubMed]
59. *Nonanticoagulant Actions of Glycosaminoglycans*; Harenberg, J.; Casu, B., Eds.; Springer US: Boston, MA, USA, 2012.
60. Salvador, B.; Sexton, N.R.; Carrion, R.; Nunneley, J.; Patterson, J.L.; Steffen, I.; Lu, K.; Muench, M.O.; Lembo, D.; Simmons, G. Filoviruses utilize glycosaminoglycans for their attachment to target cells. *J. Virol.* **2013**, *87*, 3295–3304. [CrossRef] [PubMed]
61. Kato, D.; Era, S.; Watanabe, I.; Arihara, M.; Sugiura, N.; Kimata, K.; Suzuki, Y.; Morita, K.; Hidari, K.I.P.J.; Suzuki, T. Antiviral activity of chondroitin sulphate E targeting dengue virus envelope protein. *Antiviral Res.* **2010**, *88*, 236–243. [CrossRef] [PubMed]
62. Lin, Y.-L.; Lei, H.-Y.; Lin, Y.-S.; Yeh, T.-M.; Chen, S.-H.; Liu, H.-S. Heparin inhibits dengue-2 virus infection of five human liver cell lines. *Antiviral Res.* **2002**, *56*, 93–96. [CrossRef]
63. Sapsford, K.E.; Algar, W.R.; Berti, L.; Gemmill, K.B.; Casey, B.J.; Oh, E.; Stewart, M.H.; Medintz, I.L. Functionalizing nanoparticles with biological molecules: Developing chemistries that facilitate nanotechnology. *Chem. Rev.* **2013**, *113*, 1904–2074. [CrossRef] [PubMed]
64. Montanuy, I.; Alejo, A.; Alcami, A. Glycosaminoglycans mediate retention of the poxvirus type I interferon binding protein at the cell surface to locally block interferon antiviral responses. *FASEB J.* **2011**, *25*, 1960–1971. [CrossRef] [PubMed]
65. Terao-Muto, Y.; Yoneda, M.; Seki, T.; Watanabe, A.; Tsukiyama-Kohara, K.; Fujita, K.; Kai, C. Heparin-like glycosaminoglycans prevent the infection of measles virus in SLAM-negative cell lines. *Antiviral Res.* **2008**, *80*, 370–376. [CrossRef] [PubMed]
66. Schulze, A.; Gripon, P.; Urban, S. Hepatitis B virus infection initiates with a large surface protein-dependent binding to heparan sulfate proteoglycans. *Hepatology* **2007**, *46*, 1759–1768. [CrossRef] [PubMed]
67. Su, C.M.; Liao, C.L.; Lee, Y.L.; Lin, Y.L. Highly sulfated forms of heparin sulfate are involved in japanese encephalitis virus infection. *Virology* **2001**, *286*, 206–215. [CrossRef] [PubMed]
68. Skidmore, M.A.; Kajaste-Rudnitski, A.; Wells, N.M.; Guimond, S.E.; Rudd, T.R.; Yates, E.A.; Vicenzi, E. Inhibition of influenza H5N1 invasion by modified heparin derivatives. *Med. Chem. Commun.* **2015**, *6*, 640–646. [CrossRef]
69. Ghezzi, S.; Cooper, L.; Rubio, A.; Pagani, I.; Capobianchi, M.R.; Ippolito, G.; Pelletier, J.; Meneghetti, M.C.Z.; Lima, M.A.; Skidmore, M.A.; et al. Heparin prevents Zika virus induced-cytopathic effects in human neural progenitor cells. *Antiviral Res.* **2017**, *140*, 13–17. [CrossRef] [PubMed]
70. Kim, S.Y.; Zhao, J.; Liu, X.; Fraser, K.; Lin, L.; Zhang, X.; Zhang, F.; Dordick, J.S.; Linhardt, R.J. Interaction of Zika Virus Envelope Protein with Glycosaminoglycans. *Biochemistry* **2017**, *56*, 1151–1162. [CrossRef] [PubMed]

71. Hills, F.A.; Abrahams, V.M.; González-Timón, B.; Francis, J.; Cloke, B.; Hinkson, L.; Rai, R.; Mor, G.; Regan, L.; Sullivan, M.; et al. Heparin prevents programmed cell death in human trophoblast. *Mol. Hum. Reprod.* **2006**, *12*, 237–243. [CrossRef] [PubMed]
72. Skidmore, M.A.; Dumax-Vorzet, A.F.; Guimond, S.E.; Rudd, T.R.; Edwards, E.A.; Turnbull, J.E.; Craig, A.G.; Yates, E.A. Disruption of rosetting in Plasmodium falciparum malaria with chemically modified heparin and low molecular weight derivatives possessing reduced anticoagulant and other serine protease inhibition activities. *J. Med. Chem.* **2008**, *51*, 1453–1458. [CrossRef] [PubMed]
73. Bastos, M.F.; Albrecht, L.; Kozlowski, E.O.; Lopes, S.C.P.; Blanco, Y.C.; Carlos, B.C.; Castiñeiras, C.; Vicente, C.P.; Werneck, C.C.; Wunderlich, G.; et al. Fucosylated chondroitin sulfate inhibits Plasmodium falciparum cytoadhesion and merozoite invasion. *Antimicrob. Agents Chemother.* **2014**, *58*, 1862–1871. [CrossRef] [PubMed]
74. Judice, W.A.S.; Manfredi, M.A.; Souza, G.P.; Sansevero, T.M.; Almeida, P.C.; Shida, C.S.; Gesteira, T.F.; Juliano, L.; Westrop, G.D.; Sanderson, S.J.; et al. Heparin modulates the endopeptidase activity of Leishmania mexicana cysteine protease cathepsin L-like rCPB2.8. *PLoS ONE* **2013**, *8*, 602–614. [CrossRef] [PubMed]
75. De Castro Côrtes, L.; de Souza Pereira, M.; da Silva, F.; Pereira, B.A.; de Oliveira Junior, F.; de Araújo Soares, R.; Brazil, R.; Toma, L.; Vicente, C.; Nader, H.; et al. Participation of heparin binding proteins from the surface of Leishmania (Viannia) braziliensis promastigotes in the adhesion of parasites to Lutzomyia longipalpis cells (Lulo) in vitro. *Parasit. Vectors* **2012**, *5*, 142. [CrossRef] [PubMed]
76. Nunes, G.L.C.; Simões, A.; Dyszy, F.H.; Shida, C.S.; Juliano, M.A.; Juliano, L.; Gesteira, T.F.; Nader, H.B.; Murphy, G.; Chaffotte, A.F.; et al. Mechanism of heparin acceleration of tissue inhibitor of metalloproteases-1 (TIMP-1) degradation by the human neutrophil elastase. *PLoS ONE* **2011**, *6*, e21525. [CrossRef] [PubMed]
77. Oliveira, F.O.R.; Alves, C.R.; Souza-Silva, F.; Calvet, C.M.; Côrtes, L.M.C.; Gonzalez, M.S.; Toma, L.; Bouças, R.I.; Nader, H.B.; Pereira, M.C.S. Trypanosoma cruzi heparin-binding proteins mediate the adherence of epimastigotes to the midgut epithelial cells of Rhodnius prolixus. *Parasitology* **2012**, *139*, 735–743. [CrossRef] [PubMed]
78. Chang, Y.C.; Wang, Z.; Flax, L.A.; Xu, D.; Esko, J.D.; Nizet, V.; Baron, M.J. Glycosaminoglycan binding facilitates entry of a bacterial pathogen into central nervous systems. *PLoS Pathog.* **2011**, *7*, e1002082. [CrossRef] [PubMed]
79. Wang, Z.; Flax, L.A.; Kemp, M.M.; Linhardt, R.J.; Baron, M.J. Host and pathogen glycosaminoglycan-binding proteins modulate antimicrobial peptide responses in Drosophila melanogaster. *Infect. Immun.* **2011**, *79*, 606–616. [CrossRef] [PubMed]
80. Nelson, A.; Berkestedt, I.; Schmidtchen, A.; Ljunggren, L.; Bodelsson, M. Increased levels of glycosaminoglycans during septic shock: Relation to mortality and the antibacterial actions of plasma. *Shock* **2008**, *30*, 623–627. [CrossRef] [PubMed]
81. Cornet, A.D.; Smit, E.G.M.; Beishuizen, A.; Groeneveld, A.B.J. The role of heparin and allied compounds in the treatment of sepsis. *Thromb. Haemost.* **2007**, *98*, 579–586. [CrossRef] [PubMed]
82. Tenke, P.; Riedl, C.R.; Jones, G.L.; Williams, G.J.; Stickler, D.; Nagy, E. Bacterial biofilm formation on urologic devices and heparin coating as preventive strategy. *Int. J. Antimicrob. Agents* **2004**, *23*, S67–S74. [CrossRef] [PubMed]
83. Ceranowicz, P.; Dembinski, A.; Warzecha, Z.; Dembinski, M.; Cieszkowski, J.; Rembisz, K.; Konturek, S.J.; Kusnierz-Cabala, B.; Tomaszewska, R.; Pawlik, W.W. Protective and therapeutic effect of heparin in acute pancreatitis. *J. Physiol. Pharmacol.* **2008**, *59*, 103–125. [PubMed]
84. Berger, Z.; Quera, R.; Poniachik, J.; Oksenberg, D.; Guerrero, J. Heparin and insulin treatment of acute pancreatitis caused by hypertriglyceridemia. Experience of 5 cases. *Rev. Med. Chil.* **2001**, *129*, 1373–1378. [CrossRef] [PubMed]
85. Qiu, F.; Lu, X.S.; Huang, Y.K. Protective effect of low-molecular-weight heparin on pancreatic encephalopathy in severe acute pancreatic rats. *Inflamm. Res.* **2012**, *61*, 1203–1209. [CrossRef] [PubMed]
86. Trzaskoma, A.; Kruczek, M.; Rawski, B.; Poniewierka, E.; Kempiński, R. The use of heparin in the treatment of acute pancreatitis. *Pol. Przegl. Chir.* **2013**, *85*, 223–227. [CrossRef] [PubMed]
87. Lu, X.-S.; Qiu, F.; Li, J.-Q.; Fan, Q.-Q.; Zhou, R.-G.; Ai, Y.-H.; Zhang, K.-C.; Li, Y.-X. Low molecular weight heparin in the treatment of severe acute pancreatitis: A multiple centre prospective clinical study. *Asian J. Surg.* **2009**, *32*, 89–94. [PubMed]

88. Gyorgy, B.; Tothfalusi, L.; Nagy, G.; Pasztoi, M.; Geher, P.; Polgar, A.; Rojkovich, B.; Ujfalussy, I.; Misjak, P.; Koncz, A.; Pozsonyi, E.; Fust, G.; Falus, A.; Buzas, E.I. Natural autoantibodies reactive to glycosaminoglycans are disease state markers in rheumatoid arthritis and are associated with HLA. *Ann. Rheum. Dis.* **2010**, *69*, A2. [CrossRef]
89. Larsson, S.; Lohmander, L.S.; Struglics, A. Synovial fluid level of aggrecan ARGS fragments is a more sensitive marker of joint disease than glycosaminoglycan or aggrecan levels: A cross-sectional study. *Arthritis Res. Ther.* **2009**, *11*, R92. [CrossRef] [PubMed]
90. Palmer, J.L.; Bertone, A.L.; McClain, H. Assessment of glycosaminoglycan concentration in equine synovial fluid as a marker of joint disease. *Can. J. Vet. Res.* **1995**, *59*, 205–212. [PubMed]
91. Page, C. Heparin and related drugs: beyond anticoagulant activity. *ISRN Pharmacol.* **2013**, *2013*, 910743. [CrossRef] [PubMed]
92. McIntire, A.M.; Harris, S.A.; Whitten, J.A.; Fritschle-Hilliard, A.C.; Foster, D.R.; Sood, R.; Walroth, T.A. Outcomes Following the Use of Nebulized Heparin for Inhalation Injury (HIHI Study). *J. Burn Care Res.* **2017**, *38*, 45–52. [CrossRef] [PubMed]
93. Shastri, M.D.; Peterson, G.M.; Stewart, N. Non-anticoagulant derivatives of heparin for the management of asthma: Distant dream or close reality? *Expert Opin. Investig. Drugs* **2014**, *23*, 357–373. [CrossRef] [PubMed]
94. Serisier, D.J.; Shute, J.K.; Hockey, P.M.; Higgins, B.; Conway, J.; Carroll, M.P. Inhaled heparin in cystic fibrosis. *Eur. Respir. J.* **2006**, *27*, 354–358. [CrossRef] [PubMed]
95. Kozlowski, E.O.; Gomes, A.M.; Silva, C.S. Structure and Biological Activities of Glycosaminoglycan analogs from marine invertebrates: New therapeutic agents? In *Glycans in Diseases and Therapeutics, Biology of the Extracellular Matrix 158*; Pavão, M.S.G., Ed.; Springer: Berlin/Heidelberg, Germany, 2011; pp. 159–184.
96. Pavão, M.S.G. Glycosaminoglycans analogs from marine invertebrates: Structure, biological effects, and potential as new therapeutics. *Front. Cell. Infect. Microbiol.* **2014**, *4*, 123.
97. Sato, K.; Tsutsumi, M.; Nomura, Y.; Murata, N.; Kondo, N. Proteoglycan Isolated from Cartilaginous Fish and Process for Producing the Same. WO/2004/083257, 30 September 2004.
98. Brosstad, F.; Flengsrud, R.; Skjervold, P.O.; Odegaard, O.R. Glycosaminoglycan Anticoagulants Derived from Fish. US7618652 B2, 22 March 2002.
99. Holley, R.J.; Meade, K.A.; Merry, C.L.R. Using embryonic stem cells to understand how glycosaminoglycans regulate differentiation. *Biochem. Soc. Trans.* **2014**, *42*, 689–695. [CrossRef] [PubMed]
100. Pickford, C.E.; Holley, R.J.; Rushton, G.; Stavridis, M.P.; Ward, C.M.; Merry, C.L.R. Specific glycosaminoglycans modulate neural specification of mouse embryonic stem cells. *Stem Cells* **2011**, *29*, 629–640. [CrossRef] [PubMed]
101. Holley, R.J.; Smith, R.A.; van de Westerlo, E.M.A.; Pickford, C.E.; Merry, C.L.R.; van Kuppevelt, T.H. Use of flow cytometry for characterization and fractionation of cell populations based on their expression of heparan sulfate epitopes. *Methods Mol. Biol.* **2015**, *1229*, 239–251. [PubMed]
102. Meade, K.A.; White, K.J.; Pickford, C.E.; Holley, R.J.; Marson, A.; Tillotson, D.; Van Kuppevelt, T.H.; Whittle, J.D.; Day, A.J.; Merry, C.L.R. Immobilization of heparan sulfate on electrospun meshes to support embryonic stem cell culture and differentiation. *J. Biol. Chem.* **2013**, *288*, 5530–5538. [CrossRef] [PubMed]
103. Ghadiali, R.S.; Guimond, S.E.; Turnbull, J.E.; Pisconti, A. Dynamic changes in heparan sulfate during muscle differentiation and ageing regulate myoblast cell fate and FGF2 signaling. *Matrix Biol.* **2017**, *59*, 54–68. [CrossRef]
104. Holder, G.M.; Bowfield, A.; Surman, M.; Suepfle, M.; Moss, D.; Tucker, C.E.; Rudd, T.R.; Fernig, D.G.; Yates, E.A.; Weightman, P. Fundamental differences in model cell-surface polysaccharides revealed by complementary optical and spectroscopic techniques. *Soft Matter* **2012**, *8*, 6521–6527. [CrossRef]

8

Structure-Activity Relationships of Bioengineered Heparin/Heparan Sulfates Produced in Different Bioreactors

Ha Na Kim, John M. Whitelock and Megan S. Lord *

Graduate School of Biomedical Engineering, University of New South Wales, Sydney, NSW 2052, Australia; h.n.kim@unsw.edu.au (H.N.K.); j.whitelock@unsw.edu.au (J.M.W.)

* Correspondence: m.lord@unsw.edu.au

Academic Editors: Giangiacomo Torri and Jawed Fareed

Abstract: Heparin and heparan sulfate are structurally-related carbohydrates with therapeutic applications in anticoagulation, drug delivery, and regenerative medicine. This study explored the effect of different bioreactor conditions on the production of heparin/heparan sulfate chains via the recombinant expression of serglycin in mammalian cells. Tissue culture flasks and continuously-stirred tank reactors promoted the production of serglycin decorated with heparin/heparan sulfate, as well as chondroitin sulfate, while the serglycin secreted by cells in the tissue culture flasks produced more highly-sulfated heparin/heparan sulfate chains. The serglycin produced in tissue culture flasks was effective in binding and signaling fibroblast growth factor 2, indicating the utility of this molecule in drug delivery and regenerative medicine applications in addition to its well-known anticoagulant activity.

Keywords: heparin; heparan sulfate; serglycin; proteoglycan; recombinant expression; bioreactor

1. Introduction

Heparin is used clinically as an anticoagulant due to its ability to bind anti-thrombin and modulate downstream events in the clotting cascade [1,2]. The large market for clinical heparin, including more than 300,000 doses used per day in the US [3,4], has also enabled researchers to explore its therapeutic application to reduce the thrombogenecity of materials and deliver growth factors for tissue repair [5]. Heparan sulfate is structurally similar to heparin with both being linear polysaccharides composed of repeating disaccharides of hexuronic acid and glucosamine. Heparin contains a higher degree of sulfation than heparan sulfate [6] with, on average, 2.7 sulfate groups per disaccharide, whereas heparan sulfate contains at least one sulfate group per disaccharide [7].

Heparin is only known to be expressed by mast cells in tissues that are in direct contact with the environment, including lung, skin, and intestine, and decorates the protein core of a single intracellular proteoglycan, serglycin [8–11]. Thus, the biological function of heparin is unlikely to be the prevention of blood coagulation. Heparan sulfate, however, is ubiquitous on the cell surface and in the extracellular matrix of tissues and decorates the protein core of many cell surface, including syndecans and glypicans, and extracellular matrix, including perlecan, agrin, and type XVIII collagen, proteoglycans and displays tissue-specific sulfation patterns [12,13]. These structural differences account for tissue-specific activities of heparan sulfates in modulating cellular interactions, as well as the binding and activity of enzymes, growth factors and extracellular matrix proteins [14,15]. Thus, there is growing interest in the therapeutic application of heparan sulfates for selective biological activities.

Both heparin and heparan sulfate isolated from tissues vary in composition and sequence between sources due to their synthesis via a non-template-driven process involving the timed activity of approximately twenty enzymes in the Golgi [16], although the regulators of the expression of these enzymes are not fully understood. These enzymes are involved in chain initiation, elongation, epimerization, and sulfation. While this structural heterogeneity provides an opportunity to fine-tune the biological activity for particular applications, the precise identification of structure-function relationships has been challenging [17]. However, certain structural features are known to be required for highly-specific interactions, such as a pentasaccharide structure containing an 3-*O*-sulfated glucosamine for binding to anti-thrombin III [18], whereas other structures are less specific, such as a contiguous string of highly-sulfated disaccharides for binding to fibroblast growth factor (FGF) and downstream growth factor activation [19].

Heparin is sourced predominantly from animal tissues, particularly porcine intestinal mucosa and, to a lesser extent, bovine lung tissues due to concerns over bovine spongiform encephalopathy contamination [20]. Commercially-available heparan sulfates are synthesized as byproducts of heparin production or by selective de-sulfation of heparin [21,22]. The production of heparan sulfate libraries from tissues is time consuming and technically challenging [23]. The growing demand for heparin and heparan sulfates for clinical applications has led researchers to explore alternative methods of production including chemoenzymatic synthesis [24], chemical synthesis [25], sulfation of polysaccharides [26], and metabolic engineering [27]. A bioengineered heparin-like heparan sulfate was recently reported by the authors by expressing serglycin in mammalian cells [1]. This recombinant serglycin was decorated with chondroitin/dermatan sulfate in addition to heparin/heparan sulfate chains [1,28] similar to serglycin isolated from natural sources where it has been shown to be decorated with multiple types of glycosaminoglycan chains covalently attached to its eight glycosaminoglycan attachment sites [8–11].

The aim of this study was to explore the effect of different bioreactor conditions on the yield, structure, and activity of heparin/heparan sulfates produced by expressing serglycin in mammalian cells. Bioreactors, including tissue culture flasks, continuously-stirred tank reactors (CSTR), and shaker flasks, were investigated as each of these have been used for commercial scale production of bioactives [29]. Different bioreactors and culture conditions were found to change the structure of the heparin/heparan sulfate chains produced by the cells with the serglycin produced being effective at binding and signaling FGF-2. This supports the use of these bioreactors and our approach to produce heparin/heparan sulfates for use in the clinic as an anticoagulant, as well as future uses in drug delivery and regenerative medicine applications.

2. Results

2.1. *The Effect of Different Bioreactors on Serglycin Production*

HEK-293 cells expressing serglycin were cultured for three days in different bioreactors, including batch culture in tissue culture flasks, CSTR, and shaker flasks (Figure 1A). The morphology of cells after three days in culture was analyzed by phase contrast microscopy (Figure 1B). Cells cultured in the tissue culture flasks formed a confluent monolayer of cells with the characteristic polygonal morphology of adherent cells (Figure 1B(i)). In contrast, aggregated spheroids of cells were found in both the CSTR and shaker flasks (Figure 1B(ii),(iii)). Cells cultured in the CSTR were stirred at 100 rpm, which produced aggregates in the size range 50–300 μm (Figure 1B(ii)). Cells cultured in the shaker flasks were subjected to constant agitation using an orbital shaker operated at 80 rpm, which induced the formation of uniform cell spheroids that ranged in size from 180–200 μm (Figure 1B(iii)).

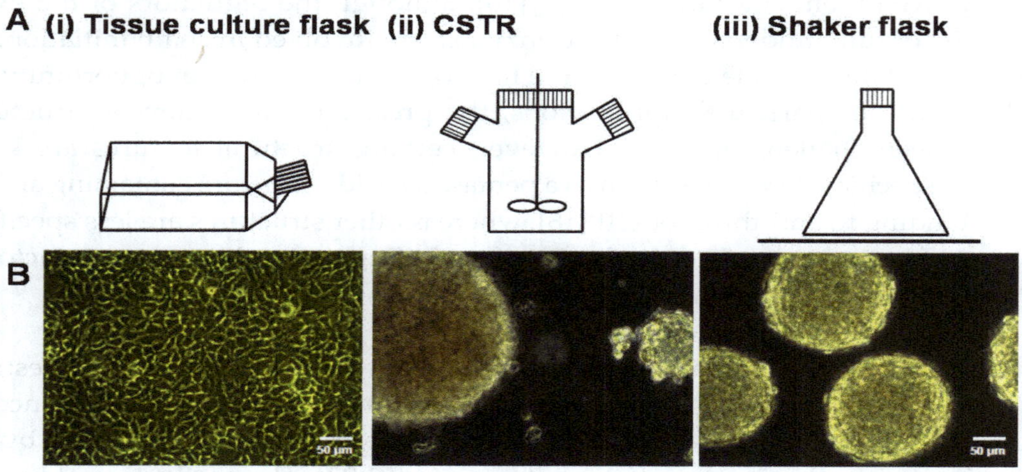

Figure 1. (**A**) Schematic of different bioreactors used to culture the HEK-293 cells expressing serglycin including (**i**) tissue culture flasks, (**ii**) continuously stirred tank reactors (CSTR), and (**iii**) shaker flasks; and (**B**) phase contrast images of cells after three days of culture in the different bioreactor conditions. The scale bar represents 50 μm.

The influence of the different bioreactors on cell proliferation was analyzed over three days (Figure 2). Cells cultured in the tissue culture flasks supported the highest level of cell proliferation. Both the CSTR and shaker flasks supported significantly reduced ($p < 0.05$) cell proliferation compared to the cultures in the tissue culture flasks. The CSTR and shaker flasks induced the formation of spheroid cultures that appeared to have reduced the proliferation of the cells.

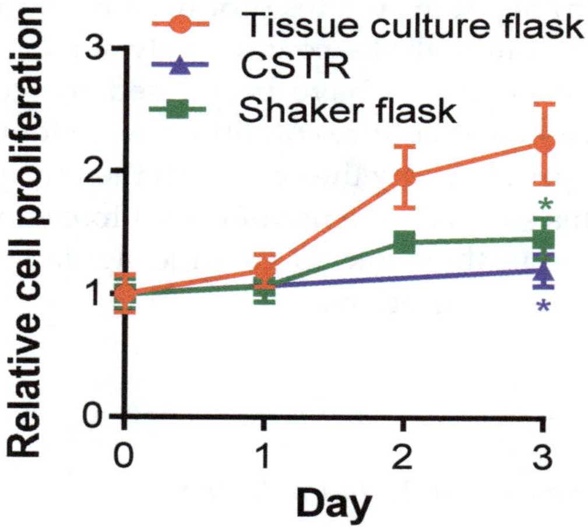

Figure 2. The relative number of cells measured over three days in the different bioreactors, including tissue culture flasks, CSTR, and shaker flasks. Data are presented as means ± standard deviation ($n = 3$). * indicates significant differences ($p < 0.05$) compared to tissue culture flasks at day 3 analyzed by one-way ANOVA.

The influence of the different bioreactors on the cells was also analyzed in terms of yield of proteins and glycosaminoglycans after enrichment of the conditioned medium by anion exchange chromatography for proteoglycans, of which the major proteoglycan produced by these cells was serglycin. The highest yield of proteins was obtained from the tissue culture flasks, followed by the CSTR, and then the shaker flasks, which demonstrated the lowest yield (Figure 3A). The highest yield of glycosaminoglycans was obtained from the CSTR and shaker flasks, and the lowest yield of glycosaminoglycans was obtained from the tissue culture flasks (Figure 3B). Analysis of the ratio of glycosaminoglycan to protein yields indicated that the CSTR and shaker flasks produced the highest amount, and the tissue culture flasks the least (Figure 3C). These data suggest that the spheroid cultures reduced cell proliferation and encouraged glycosaminoglycan decoration of the serglycin protein core to a greater extent than tissue culture flasks that encouraged cell proliferation and protein production.

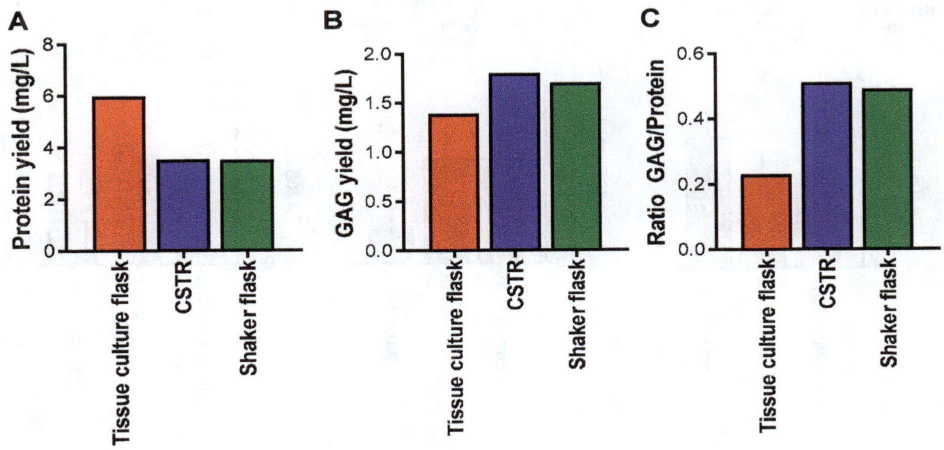

Figure 3. Yield of (**A**) protein; (**B**) glycosaminoglycan (GAG); and (**C**) the ratio of GAG to protein from HEK-293 cells expressing serglycin cultured in different bioreactors over three days and purified by anion exchange chromatography. Protein concentration was measured by Coomassie protein assay and GAG concentration was measured by Dimethylmethylene Blue (DMMB) assay.

The effect of bioreactors on serglycin production and glycosaminoglycan decoration was also explored. There was no difference on the level of serglycin produced by cells in each of the bioreactors (Figure 4A). Tissue culture flasks and the CSTR produced the same level of heparin/heparan sulfate chains as detected by the presence of the HS stub structure that is demonstrated following heparinase III (HepIII) digestion and recognized by the monoclonal antibody 3G10 (Figure 4B). In contrast, the shaker flasks significantly reduced ($p < 0.05$) the level of heparin/heparan sulfate chains (Figure 4B). Unlike heparin/heparan sulfate, which has one stub structure, chondroitin sulfate (CS) has multiple stub structures, following chondroitinase (C'ase) ABC digestion, including the 4- or 6-sulfated stub that can be detected with monoclonal antibodies 2B6 or 3B3, respectively (Figure 4C). While the level of chondroitin sulfate chains with 6-sulfated stub structures was not altered in any of the bioreactors analyzed, the level of 4-sulfated stub structures was significantly reduced in the shaker flasks compared to the tissue culture flask and CSTR (Figure 4C).

The effect of the different bioreactors was further assessed by analyzing the sub-structure of the heparan and chondroitin sulfate chains produced by ELISA (Figure 5). Interestingly, the CSTR promoted the production of heparan sulfate chains containing N-acetylated glucosamine resides, as detected using the heparan sulfate chain antibody, to a significantly greater ($p < 0.05$) extent than either the tissue culture flasks or the shaker flasks (Figure 5A). Together with the data presented in Figure 4B, this indicated that the tissue culture flasks promoted heparan sulfate/heparin chains with a different structure to the CSTR as they exhibited the same level of heparan sulfate/heparin chains. It is speculated that the tissue culture flasks promoted heparan sulfate/heparin chains with sulfated disaccharides, as observed previously [1]. The shaker flasks facilitated minimal heparan sulfate/heparin chain production with no detectable heparan sulfate chains using the heparan sulfate chain antibody (Figure 5A). Both the tissue culture flasks and the CSTR supported the production of chondroitin sulfate containing type A and C disaccharides, while the shaker flask did not support the production of this type of chondroitin sulfate chain (Figure 5B). These data align with the level of 4-sulfated chondroitin sulfate stub structures detected in each of the cultures (Figure 4C).

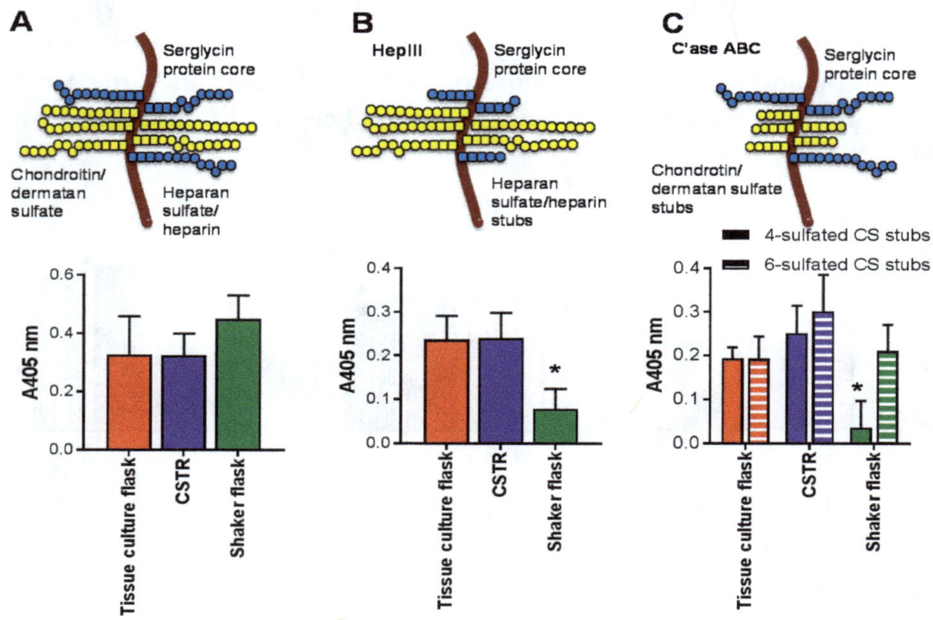

Figure 4. The effect of bioreactors on the production of serglycin, heparin/heparan sulfate and chondroitin sulfate. The schematic indicates the structure of serglycin with eight glycosaminoglycan attachment sites that can be decorated with either chondroitin/dermatan sulfate or heparin/heparan sulfate chains. The effect of glycosaminoglycan lyase digestion on the glycosaminoglycan chains are indicated in panels (**B**,**C**) with HepIII removing heparin/heparan sulfate chains to reveal a single stub structure and chondroitinase ABC (C'ase ABC) removing chondroitin/dermatan sulfate chains to reveal a stub structure. ELISA for the presence of (**A**) serglycin core protein; (**B**) heparin/heparan sulfate stubs detected using anti-heparan sulfate/heparin-stub antibody clone 3G10 following HepIII digestion, and (**C**) chondroitin sulfate stubs detected using anti-4-sulfated chondroitin sulfate stub antibody clone 2B6 and anti-6-sulfated chondroitin sulfate stub antibody clone 3B3 following C'ase ABC digestion. Data are presented as means ± standard deviation ($n = 3$). * indicates significant differences ($p < 0.05$) compared to tissue culture flasks analyzed by one-way ANOVA.

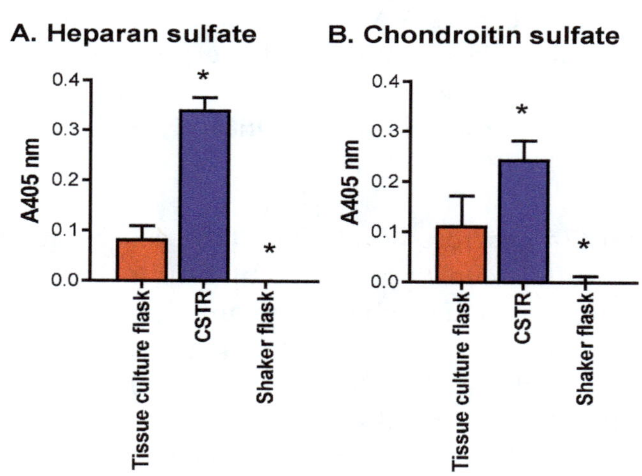

Figure 5. Effect of bioreactors on heparan and chondroitin sulfate structure. ELISA for the presence of (**A**) heparan sulfate chains detected using anti-heparan sulfate chain antibody clone 10E4 and (**B**) chondroitin sulfate chains detected using anti-chondroitin sulfate chain antibody clone CS-56. Data are presented as means ± standard deviation ($n = 3$). * indicates significant differences ($p < 0.05$) compared to batch cultures analyzed by one-way ANOVA.

2.2. The Effect of Different Culture Conditions on Serglycin Production

As the tissue culture flasks promoted the production of heparan sulfate/heparin, this type of bioreactor was explored further over a seven-day batch culture with HEK-293 cells expressing serglycin. Cells were cultured in three different glucose concentrations of 5.5, 25, and 50 mM as a previous study where the cultures that were passaged weekly and fed every three days indicated that the level of glucose in the medium affected heparin/heparan sulfate production [1]. The influence of glucose concentration on the cells was analyzed in terms of serglycin production and glycosaminoglycan decoration after enrichment of the conditioned medium by anion exchange chromatography for serglycin (Figure 6). Increasing the level of glucose in the medium increased the level of serglycin produced (Figure 6A). There was, however, no difference in the level of heparan sulfate/heparin stubs produced by cells in each of the conditions (Figure 6B) and only baseline levels of heparan sulfate chains containing *N*-acetylated glucosamine residues detected in each condition (Figure 6C). It is speculated that cells grown in tissue culture flasks for extended periods, regardless of glucose concentration, promoted heparan sulfate/heparin chains with sulfated disaccharides, as observed previously [1]. In contrast, cells cultured in medium containing 5.5 mM glucose produced significantly ($p < 0.05$) lower levels of chondroitin sulfate containing type A and C disaccharides compared to cells cultured in medium containing either 25 or 50 mM glucose (Figure 6D).

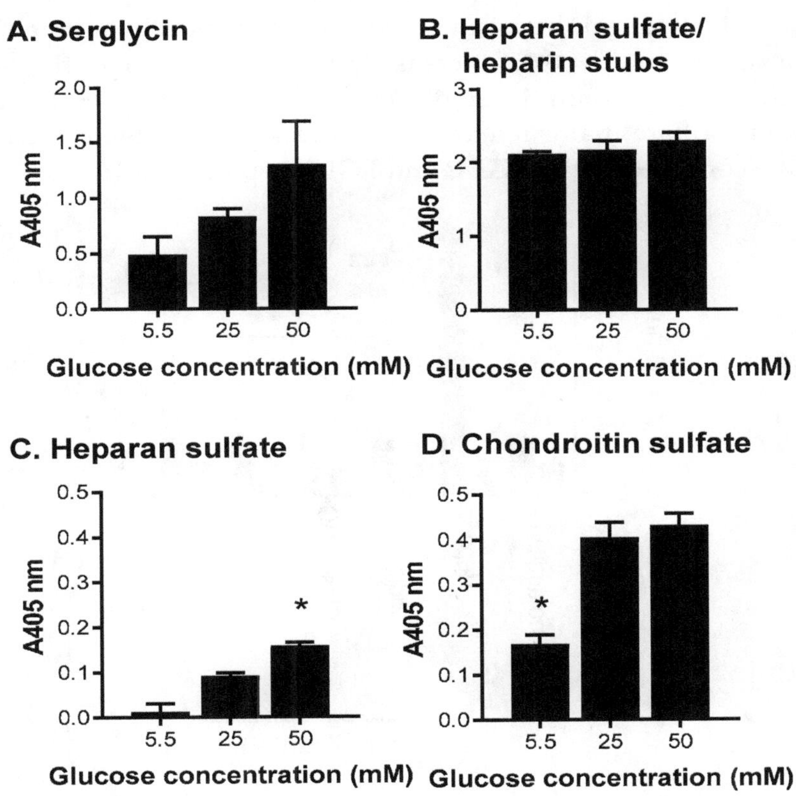

Figure 6. The effects of altering glucose concentrations in media for the production of serglycin, heparan sulfate/heparin and chondroitin sulfate. ELISA for the presence of (**A**) serglycin was detected using a polyclonal anti-serglycin antibody; (**B**) heparan sulfate/heparin stubs were detected using anti-heparan sulfate stub antibody clone 3G10 following HepIII digestion; (**C**) heparan sulfate chains were detected using anti-heparan sulfate antibody clone 10E4; and (**D**) chondroitin sulfate chains were detected using anti- chondroitin sulfate chain antibody clone CS-56. Data are presented as means ± standard deviation ($n = 3$). * indicates significant differences ($p < 0.05$) compared to 25 mM glucose analyzed by one-way ANOVA.

2.3. The Effect of Serglycin Glycosaminoglycan Decoration on Growth Factor Binding and Signaling

One of the major functions of the glycosaminoglycans, such as heparin/heparan sulfate, is to bind and signal growth factors. The production of proteoglycans capable of recapitulating this function in vivo is of therapeutic interest due to the relatively low abundance of naturally-occurring proteoglycans at sites of wound healing. Thus the binding and signaling of the mitogenic growth factor, FGF-2, was analyzed using the BaF32 cell assay. The BaF32 cells proliferate when biologically-active ternary complexes are formed between cell surface FGF receptors, FGF-2 and heparin/heparan sulfate. The positive control for the assay was the FGF receptor type 1c expressing cells exposed to heparin and FGF-2 as shown by the significant ($p < 0.05$) increase in absorbance compared to cells exposed to either heparin or FGF-2 (Figure 7). The addition of serglycin produced by cells cultured for seven days in medium containing 25 mM glucose, as this preparation contained both highly-sulfated heparan sulfate/heparin and chondroitin sulfate, bound and signaled FGF-2 as shown by the significant ($p < 0.05$) increase in cell proliferation compared to cells only exposed to serglycin. Digestion of the chondroitin sulfate chains that decorated serglycin resulted in significantly ($p < 0.05$) greater proliferation of the cells when exposed to FGF-2 compared to cells exposed to undigested serglycin and FGF-2. These data indicated that removal of the chondroitin sulfate chains increased the ability of the heparin/heparan sulfate chains that decorated serglycin to bind and signal FGF-2. Digestion of the heparin/heparan sulfate chains that decorated serglycin resulted in no significant difference in the proliferation of the cells when exposed to FGF-2 compared to cells exposed to undigested serglycin and FGF-2. Digestion of the heparin/heparan sulfate and chondroitin sulfate chains that decorated serglycin resulted in a significant ($p < 0.05$) increase in the proliferation of the cells when exposed to FGF-2 compared to cells exposed to undigested serglycin and FGF-2. Together these data suggested that the heparin/heparan sulfate chains released from the serglycin core protein by HepIII digestion were able to form active complexes with FGF-2 and FGF receptor type 1c.

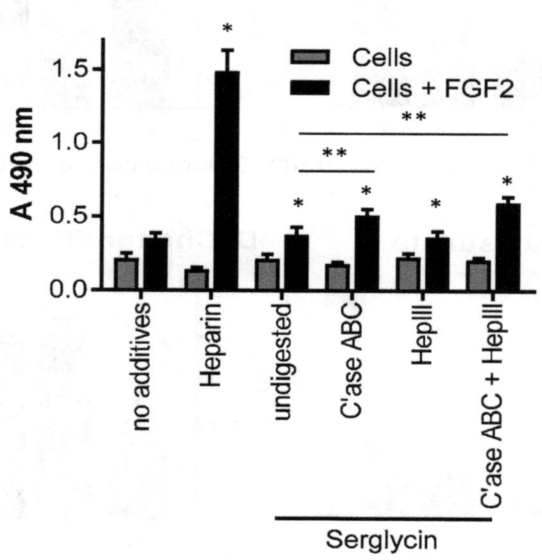

Figure 7. Activity of serglycin with heparin/heparan sulfate and chondroitin sulfate chains determined by the signaling of FGF receptor type 1c expressing BaF32 cells in the presence of FGF-2 as mesured by the MTS assay. Cells in the presence of FGF-2 and heparin were used as a control for the formation of active ternary complexes. Negative controls were cells in the presence of no additives, heparin, or FGF-2. Selected serglycin preparations were digested with either chondroitinase ABC, hepIII or both glycosaminoglycan lysases prior to the assay. Cell proliferation was measured after 72 h. * indicated significant differences ($p < 0.05$) within treatments for cells and FGF-2 compared to cells only as determined by a one-way ANOVA; ** indicated significant differences ($p < 0.05$) as determined by two-way ANOVA.

3. Discussion

This study explored the production of recombinant serglycin in different bioreactors including tissue culture flasks, CSTR, and shaker flasks. Bioreactors that maintain cells in a suspension culture are widely used in industry enabling scale-up of bioactive production [29]. The HEK-293 cells used in this study that had been transfected to stably express serglycin are an adherent cell line, so it was of interest to subject them to the CSTR and shaker flask bioreactors that did not provide conditions for cell adhesion and explore their ability to proliferate and express serglycin. Interestingly, the cells cultured in these bioreactors proliferated, albeit at reduced levels compared to the cells grown in tissue culture flasks. In addition, the cells in both the CSTR and shaker flasks formed spheroids similar to what can be achieved with packed bed bioreactors, however, without an adhesive bead matrix to support cell adhesion [30]. The cell spheroids formed in the CSTR and shaker flasks indicated that the cells under these conditions, formed stable cell-cell contacts providing a different microenvironment to cells grown in the tissue culture flasks.

The microenvironment of cells is known to affect the type and structure of glycosaminoglycans that decorate proteoglycans leading to tissue-specific sulfation patterns [12,13]. The authors recently reported that mast cells cultured in different microenvironments change the type of glycosaminoglycans that they produce [31]. Thus, it was not surprising to discover in this study that the type of bioreactor used to produce proteoglycans altered the production of heparin/heparan and chondroitin sulfate chains. Interestingly, while there were differences in the extent and type of glycosaminoglycans produced, there was no change in the level of serglycin produced in each of the bioreactors. It was interesting to note that while the CSTR and shaker flask bioreactors both induced cell spheroid cultures, albeit of different sized spheroids, the cells produced a similar level of glycosaminoglycan decoration of the protein cores, but with different structures. This finding further supports the concept that the microenvironment plays a key role in determining the type and structure of glycosaminoglycans.

The level of glucose in the culture medium has been reported to affect cell proliferation [32], as well as protein production and glycosylation [33–36]. A comparison of the results of this study and a previous study by the authors indicated that changes in the method of culture in tissue culture flasks is sufficient to alter both serglycin protein core production and the type of glycosaminoglycans [1]. Previously, the cells were cultured for seven days in tissue culture flasks in medium containing 5.5, 25, or 50 mM glucose, passaged weekly and fed every three days. These conditions indicated that the level of glucose in the medium affected both serglycin and heparin/heparan sulfate production [1]. In contrast, this study, cells were grown for three days in tissue culture flasks in medium containing 5.5, 25, or 50 mM glucose prior to passaging, demonstrated that the level of glucose in the medium also affected chondroitin sulfate production.

As the recombinant serglycin produced in this study was decorated with heparin/heparan sulfate chains, it was of interest to determine its ability to bind and signal growth factors. Heparin/heparan sulfate chains are known to bind FGF-2 involving regions of high sulfation called S-domains [19,37]. Thus the serglycin preparation containing sulfated heparan sulfate/heparin and chondroitin sulfate was explored for FGF-2 signaling. This study found that the serglycin bound and signaled FGF-2 through its heparin/heparan sulfate chains both when attached to the serglycin protein core and following HepIII digestion. HepIII depolymerizes heparan sulfate by elimination of hexuronic acids acting next to *N*-sulfated or *N*-acetated residues without sulfation, or with low levels of O-sulfation [38]. Thus HepIII has a limited ability to depolymerize heparin. The heparin/heparan sulfate chains attached to serglycin used in this assay were found to contain highly-sulfated disaccharides, thus, treatment with HepIII would have released heparin/highly-sulfated heparan sulfated oligomers accounting for the FGF-2 activity of the heparin/heparan sulfate chains in solution in addition to when presented on the protein core of serglycin. While chondroitin sulfate is not involved in FGF-2 signaling [39], removal of the chondroitin sulfate chains from serglycin in this study was able to enhance the binding and signaling of the heparin/heparan sulfate bound to serglycin. This is likely due to the close proximity of the eight glycosaminoglycan attachment sites within the central region of the serglycin protein core. Removal of the chondroitin sulfate chains from the protein core of serglycin is likely to have enabled increased flexibility of the heparin/heparan sulfate chains attached to serglycin. A similar phenomenon has been observed for perlecan decorated with both heparan and chondroitin sulfate [40].

In conclusion, this study demonstrated that different bioreactors, including tissue culture flasks, CSTRs, and shaker flasks, in addition to different levels of glucose in the media, produced unique microenvironments that differentially decorated serglycin with heparin/heparan sulfate, as well as chondroitin sulfate. The serglycin produced bound and signaled FGF 2 via its heparin/heparan sulfate chains both when presented as a proteoglycan or as isolated glycosaminoglycan chains. These data demonstrate that the recombinant expression of serglycin is a promising approach for the production of tailored glycosaminoglycan structures with broad applications in drug delivery and regenerative medicine.

4. Materials and Methods

4.1. Culture of Mammalian Cells Expressing Serglycin

Human embryonic kidney (HEK-293) cell were transfected to stably express serglycin, as previously described [1]. Cells were maintained with DMEM culture medium containing 25 mM glucose, 10% (*v*/*v*) fetal bovine serum (FBS) and 100 μg/mL penicillin and streptomycin at 37 °C, 5% CO_2 in a humidified incubator. Cells seeded at 2×10^5 cells/mL were cultured in standard T75 culture flasks (reactor volume of 10 mL), a continuously-stirred tank reactor (CSTR) operated at 100 rpm, or a conical shaker flask on an orbital shaker operated at 80 rpm, each with a reactor volume of 250 mL. The speed of rotation of the CSTR and shaker flasks was determined with reference to previous studies using suspension cells [31]. Each of the bioreactors was operated in batch mode over three days. Additionally, cells were cultured in DMEM culture medium containing 5.5, 25, or 50 mM glucose, 10% (*v*/*v*) FBS and 100 μg/mL penicillin and streptomycin at 37 °C, 5% CO_2 in a humidified incubator in standard T75 culture flasks in batch mode for seven days.

4.2. Cell Proliferation Assay

At each time point 50 μL of cell suspension was removed from the CSTR and shaker flasks and the number of viable cells analyzed using a hemocytometer and the trypan blue exclusion dye. For the tissue culture flasks, cell proliferation was analyzed by setting up parallel conditions in a 96 well tissue culture plate seeded with 2×10^5 cells/mL and the number of cells at each time point was analyzed by the MTS assay using Cell Titer 96 Aqueous One Solution Reagent (Promega, Madison, WI, USA) and absorbance was measured at 490 nm.

4.3. Isolation of Serglycin

Serglycin was isolated from the conditioned medium by anion exchange chromatography. The diethylaminoethyl (DEAE) column was equilibrated at 1 mL/min with running buffer (250 mM NaCl, 20 mM Tris, 10 mM EDTA, pH 7.5) before the addition of medium conditioned by cells and the baseline absorbance was re-established with running buffer. Serglycin was eluted using an eluting buffer (1 M NaCl, 20 mM Tris, 10 mM EDTA, pH 7.5) and concentrated. Serglycin-enriched fractions were subsequently concentrated and analyzed for protein concentration using a Coomassie Blue protein assay (Thermo Scientific, Scoresby, Australia). Glycosaminoglycan concentration was determined using the Dimethylmethylene Blue assay (DMMB) as previously described [41].

4.4. Glycosaminoglycan Digestion

Samples were digested with 50 mU/mL proteinase-free chondroitinase (C'ase) ABC (EC 4.2.2.4) purified from *Proteus vulgaris* in 0.1 M Tris acetate, pH 8 at 37 °C for 16 h to confirm the presence of CS/DS. Samples were digested with 10 mU/mL of heparinase (Hep) III (EC 4.2.2.8) purified from

Flavobacterium heparinum (Seikagaku Corp., Tokyo, Japan) diluted in 10 mM Tris-HCl, pH 7.4 at 37 °C for 16 h to determine the presence of heparin/HS.

4.5. ELISA

Serglycin-enriched samples (10 µg based on Coomassie protein assay) with and without glycosaminoglycan lyase digestion were coated onto high-binding 96-well ELISA plates (Greiner, Frickenhausen, Germany) for 2 h at 25 °C. Wells were rinsed twice with Dulbecco's phosphate-buffered saline, pH 7.4 (DPBS) followed by blocking with 0.1% (*w*/*v*) casein in DPBS for 1 h at 25 °C. Wells were rinsed twice with DPBS with 1% (*v*/*v*) Tween 20 (PBST) followed by incubation with primary antibodies diluted in 0.1% (*w*/*v*) casein in DPBS for 2 h at 25 °C. Primary antibodies used included a rabbit polyclonal anti-serglycin antibody (ascites 1:5000), mouse monoclonal anti-4-sulfated chondroitin sulfate stub antibody (clone 2B6, gift from Prof Bruce Caterson, Cardiff University, conditioned medium 1:1000), mouse monoclonal anti-6-sulfated chondroitin sulfate stub antibody (clone 3B3, gift from Prof Bruce Caterson, Cardiff University, conditioned medium 1:1000), mouse monoclonal anti-heparan sulfate stub antibody (clone 3G10, Seikagaku, 1 µg/mL), mouse monoclonal anti-chondroitin sulfate type A and C antibody (clone CS-56, ascites 1:2500), and mouse monoclonal anti-heparan sulfate antibody (clone 10E4, Seikagaku Corp., 1 µg/mL). Wells were rinsed twice with PBST, followed by incubation with biotinylated secondary antibodies (1:1000) diluted in 0.1% (*w*/*v*) casein in DPBS for 1 h at 25 °C, rinsed twice again with PBST, and then incubated with streptavidin-HRP (1:500) for 30 min at 25 °C. Binding of the antibodies to the samples was detected using the colorimetric substrate, 2,2-azinodi-(3-ethylbenzthiazoline sulfonic acid), and absorbance was measured at 405 nm.

4.6. Growth Factor Binding and Signaling of FGF-2

BaF32 cells were derived from an IL-3-dependent and heparan sulfate proteoglycan-deficient myeloid B cell line that has been stably transfected with fibroblast growth factor receptor (FGFR) 1c [42]. BaF32 cells represent a model system developed to identify heparin/heparan sulfate structures that interact with FGFs and their receptors. The readout of this assay is cell proliferation which indicated the formation of ternary complexes on the cell surface between heparin/heparan sulfate, FGF-2 and FGFR1c. BaF32 cells were maintained in RPMI 1640 medium containing 10% (*v*/*v*) FBS, 10% (*v*/*v*) WEHI-3BD conditioned medium, 100 µg/mL penicillin, and streptomycin. WEHI-3BD cells were maintained in RPMI 1640 medium supplemented with 2 g/L sodium bicarbonate, 10% (*v*/*v*) FBS, 100 µg/mL penicillin, and streptomycin, and the conditioned medium was collected three times per week and stored at −20 °C until it was required. For the mitogenic assays, the BaF32 cells were transferred into IL-3 depleted medium for 24 h prior to experimentation and seeded into 96-well plates at a density of 2×10^4 cells/well in the presence of medium only, 120 nM heparin, 0.5 µg/mL serglycin either in the presence or absence of 0.03 nM FGF-2. To analyze the role of the different glycosaminoglycans that decorated recombinant serglycin, serglycin was also treated with C'ase ABC and/or HepIII prior to use in the assay. Cells exposed to heparin and FGF-2 were used as a positive control for the assay, as this combination is known to induce cell proliferation, while cells exposed to each of the treatments in the absence of FGF-2 were used as a negative control. Background absorbance readings were also obtained for each of the treatments in the absence of cells. Cells were incubated for 72 h in 5% CO_2 at 37 °C, and the number of cells present was assessed using the MTS assay. The MTS reagent (Promega, Madison, WI, USA) was added to the cell cultures 6 h prior to measurement of the absorbance at 490 nm.

Acknowledgments: The authors thank Achilles Theocharis (University of Patras, Greece) for the rabbit polyclonal anti-serglycin antibody. The authors acknowledge Phoebe Lingat for technical assistance. The authors acknowledge grant support from the Australian Research Council Linkage Project Scheme.

Author Contributions: H.N.K., J.M.W., and M.S.L. conceived and designed the experiments, analyzed the data and wrote the paper; and H.N.K. performed the experiments.

References

1. Lord, M.S.; Cheng, B.; Tang, F.; Lyons, J.G.; Rnjak-Kovacina, J.; Whitelock, J.M. Bioengineered human heparin with anticoagulant activity. *Metab. Eng.* **2016**, *38*, 105–114. [CrossRef] [PubMed]
2. Lindahl, U.; Backstrom, G.; Hook, M.; Thunberg, L.; Fransson, L.A.; Linker, A. Structure of the antithrombin-binding site in heparin. *Proc. Natl. Acad. Sci. USA* **1979**, *76*, 3198–3202. [CrossRef] [PubMed]
3. Linhardt, R.J. 2003 Claude S. Hudson Award address in carbohydrate chemistry. Heparin: Structure and activity. *J. Med. Chem.* **2003**, *46*, 2551–2564. [CrossRef] [PubMed]
4. Bhaskar, U.; Sterner, E.; Hickey, A.M.; Onishi, A.; Zhang, F.; Dordick, J.S.; Linhardt, R.J. Engineering of routes to heparin and related polysaccharides. *Appl. Microbiol. Biotechnol.* **2012**, *93*, 1–16. [CrossRef] [PubMed]
5. Sakiyama-Elbert, S.E. Incorporation of heparin into biomaterials. *Acta Biomater.* **2014**, *10*, 1581–1587. [CrossRef] [PubMed]
6. Lever, R.; Page, C.P. Novel drug development opportunities for heparin. *Nat. Rev. Drug Discov.* **2002**, *1*, 140–148. [CrossRef] [PubMed]
7. Toida, T.; Yoshida, H.; Toyoda, H.; Koshiishi, I.; Imanari, T.; Hileman, R.E.; Fromm, J.R.; Linhardt, R.J. Structural differences and the presence of unsubstituted amino groups in heparan sulphates from different tissues and species. *Biochem. J.* **1997**, *322*, 499–506. [CrossRef] [PubMed]
8. Kolset, S.O.; Gallagher, J. Proteoglycans in haemopoietic cells. *Biochim. Biophys. Acta* **1990**, *1032*, 191–221. [CrossRef]
9. Kolset, S.O.; Mann, D.M.; Uhlin-Hansen, L.; Winberg, J.O.; Ruoslahti, E. Serglycin-binding proteins in activated macrophages and platelets. *J. Leukoc. Biol.* **1996**, *59*, 545–554. [PubMed]
10. Kolset, S.O.; Pejler, G. Serglycin: A structural and functional chameleon with wide impact on immune cells. *J. Immunol.* **2011**, *187*, 4927–4933. [CrossRef] [PubMed]
11. Kolset, S.O.; Tveit, H. Serglycin—Structure and biology. *Cell. Mol. Life Sci.* **2008**, *65*, 1073–1085. [CrossRef] [PubMed]
12. Kato, M.; Wang, H.; Bernfield, M.; Gallagher, J.T.; Turnbull, J.E. Cell surface syndecan-1 on distinct cell types differs in fine structure and ligand binding of its heparan sulfate chains. *J. Biol. Chem.* **1994**, *269*, 18881–18890. [PubMed]
13. Iozzo, R.V.; Schaefer, L. Proteoglycan form and function: A comprehensive nomenclature of proteoglycans. *Matrix Biol.* **2015**, *42*, 11–55. [CrossRef] [PubMed]
14. Bernfield, M.; Gotte, M.; Park, P.W.; Reizes, O.; Fitzgerald, M.L.; Lincecum, J.; Zako, M. Functions of cell surface heparan sulfate proteoglycans. *Annu. Rev. Biochem.* **1999**, *68*, 729–777. [CrossRef] [PubMed]
15. Lin, X. Fuctions of heparan sulfate proteoglycans in cell signaling during development. *Development* **2004**, *131*, 6009–6021. [CrossRef] [PubMed]
16. Salmivirta, M.; Lidholt, K.; Linhadl, U. Heparan sulfate: A piece of information. *FASEB J.* **1996**, *10*, 1270–1279. [PubMed]
17. Turnbull, J.E. Heparan sulfate glycomics: Towards systems biology strategies. *Biochem. Soc. Trans.* **2010**, *38*, 1356–1360. [CrossRef] [PubMed]
18. Rosenberg, R.D.; Shworak, N.W.; Liu, J.; Schwartz, J.J.; Zhang, L. Heparan sulfate proteoglycans of the cardiovascular system. Specific structures emerge but how is synthesis regulated? *J. Clin. Investig.* **1997**, *99*, 2062–2070. [CrossRef] [PubMed]
19. Kreuger, J.; Salmivirta, M.; Sturiale, L.; Gimenez-Gallego, G.; Lindahl, U. Sequence analysis of heparan sulfate epitopes with graded affinities for fibroblast growth factors 1 and 2. *J. Biol. Chem.* **2001**, *276*, 30744–30752. [CrossRef] [PubMed]
20. Linhardt, R.J.; Gunay, N.S. Production and chemical processing of low molecular weight heparins. *Semin. Thromb. Hemost.* **1999**, *25*, 5–16. [PubMed]
21. Ashikari-Hada, S.; Habuchi, H.; Kariya, Y.; Itoh, N.; Reddi, A.H.; Kimata, K. Characterization of growth factor-binding structures in heparin/heparan sulfate using an octasaccharide library. *J. Biol. Chem.* **2004**, *279*, 12346–12354. [CrossRef] [PubMed]
22. Yates, E.A.; Guimond, S.E.; Turnbull, J.E. Highly diverse heparan sulfate analogue libraries: Providing access to expanded areas of sequence space for bioactivity screening. *J. Med. Chem.* **2004**, *47*, 277–280. [CrossRef] [PubMed]
23. Powell, A.K.; Ahmed, Y.A.; Yates, E.A.; Turnbull, J.E. Generating heparan sulfate saccharide libraries for glycomics applications. *Nat. Protoc.* **2010**, *5*, 821–833. [CrossRef] [PubMed]

24. DeAngelis, P.L.; Liu, J.; Linhardt, R.J. Chemoenzymatic synthesis of glycosaminoglycans: Re-creating, re-modeling and re-designing nature's longest or most complex carbohydrate chains. *Glycobiology* **2013**, *23*, 764–777. [CrossRef] [PubMed]
25. Choay, J.; Petitou, M.; Lormeau, J.C.; Sinaÿ, P.; Casu, B.; Gatti, G. Structure-activity relationship in heparin: A synthetic pentasaccharide with high affinity for antithrombin III and eliciting high anti-factor Xa activity. *Biochem. Biophys. Res. Commun.* **1983**, *116*, 492–499. [CrossRef]
26. Farrugia, B.L.; Lord, M.S.; Melrose, J.; Whitelock, J.M. Can we produce heparin/heparan sulfate biomimetics using 'mother-nature' as the gold standard? *Molecules* **2015**, *20*, 4254–4276. [CrossRef] [PubMed]
27. Baik, J.Y.; Gasimli, L.; Yang, B.; Datta, P.; Zhang, F.; Glass, C.A.; Esko, J.D.; Linhardt, R.J.; Sharfstein, S.T. Metabolic engineering of Chinese hamster ovary cells: Towards a bioengineered heparin. *Metab. Eng.* **2012**, *14*, 81–90. [CrossRef] [PubMed]
28. Lord, M.S.; Cheng, B.; Farrugia, B.L.; McCarthy, S.; Whitelock, J.M. Platelet factor 4 binds to vascular proteoglycans and controls both growth factor activities and platelet activation. *J. Biol. Chem.* **2017**, *292*, 4054–4063. [CrossRef] [PubMed]
29. Eibl, R.; Kaiser, S.; Lombriser, R.; Eibl, D. Disposble bioreactors: The current state-of-the-art and recommended applications in biotechnology. *Appl. Microbiol. Biotechnol.* **2010**, *86*, 41–49. [CrossRef] [PubMed]
30. Meuwly, F.; Ruffieux, P.A.; Kadouri, A.; von Stockar, U. Packed-bed bioreactors for mammalian cell culture: Bioprocess and biomedical applications. *Biotechnol. Adv.* **2007**, *25*, 45–56. [CrossRef] [PubMed]
31. Lord, M.S.; Jung, M.; Whitelock, J.M. Optimization of bioengineered heparin/heparan sulfate production for therapeutic applications. *Bioengineered* **2017**, *10*, 1–4. [CrossRef] [PubMed]
32. Sugiura, T. Effects of glucose on the production of recombinant protein C in mammalian cell culture. *Biotechnol. Bioeng.* **1992**, *39*, 953–959. [CrossRef] [PubMed]
33. Whitford, W.G. Fed-batch mammalian cell culture in bioproduction. *BioProcess. Int.* **2006**, *4*, 30–40.
34. Cechowska-Pasko, M.; Bańkowski, E. Glucose deficiency inhibits glycosaminoglycans synthesis in fibroblast cultures. *Biochimie* **2010**, *92*, 806–813. [CrossRef] [PubMed]
35. Wang, A.; Midura, R.J.; Vasanji, A.; Wang, A.J.; Hascall, V.C. Hyperglycemia diverts dividing osteoblastic precursor cells to an adipogenic pathway and induces synthesis of a hyaluronan matrix that is adhesive for monocytes. *J. Biol. Chem.* **2014**, *289*, 11410–11420. [CrossRef] [PubMed]
36. Vogl-Willis, C.A.; Edwards, I.J. High-glucose-induced structural changes in the heparan sulfate proteoglycan, perlecan, of cultured human aortic endothelial cells. *Biochim. Biophys. Acta* **2004**, *1672*, 36–45. [CrossRef] [PubMed]
37. Gallagher, J.T. Heparan sulfate: Growth control with a restricted sequence menu. *J. Clin. Investig.* **2001**, *108*, 357–361. [CrossRef] [PubMed]
38. Wei, Z.; Lyon, M.; Gallagher, J.T. Distinct substrate specificities of bacterial heparinases against *N*-unsubstituted glucosamine residues in heparan sulfate. *J. Biol. Chem.* **2005**, *280*, 15742–15748. [CrossRef] [PubMed]
39. Chuang, C.Y.; Lord, M.S.; Melrose, J.; Rees, M.D.; Knox, S.M.; Freeman, C.; Iozzo, R.V.; Whitelock, J.M. Heparan sulfate dependent signaling of fibroblast growth factor (FGF) 18 by chondrocyte-derived perlecan. *Biochemistry* **2010**, *49*, 5524–5532. [CrossRef] [PubMed]
40. Smith, S.M.L.; West, L.A.; Govindraj, P.; Zhang, X.; Ornitz, D.M.; Hassell, J.R. Heparan and chondroitin sulfate on growth plate perlecan mediate binding and delivery of FGF-2 to FGF receptors. *Matrix Biol.* **2007**, *26*, 175–184. [CrossRef] [PubMed]
41. Davies, N.P.; Roubin, R.H.; Whitelock, J.M. Characterization and purification of glycosaminoglycans from crude biological samples. *J. Agric. Food Chem.* **2008**, *56*, 343–348. [CrossRef] [PubMed]
42. Ornitz, D.M.; Yayon, A.; Flanagan, J.G.; Svahn, C.M.; Levi, E.; Leder, P. Heparin is required for cell-free binding of basic fibroblast growth factor to a soluble receptor and for mitogenesis in whole cells. *Mol. Cell Biol.* **1992**, *12*, 240–247. [CrossRef] [PubMed]

9

Albumin and Hyaluronic Acid-Coated Superparamagnetic Iron Oxide Nanoparticles Loaded with Paclitaxel for Biomedical Applications

Elena Vismara [1,*], Chiara Bongio [1], Alessia Coletti [1], Ravit Edelman [2], Andrea Serafini [1], Michele Mauri [3], Roberto Simonutti [3], Sabrina Bertini [4], Elena Urso [4], Yehuda G. Assaraf [5] and Yoav D. Livney [2,*]

1 Department of Chemistry, Materials and Chemical Engineering "G. Natta", Politecnico di Milano, 20131 Milano, Italy; chiara.bongio@polimi.it (C.B.); alessia.coletti08@gmail.com (A.C.); andrea.serafini@polimi.it (A.S.)
2 Biotechnology and Food Engineering Department, Technion-Israel Institute of Technology, Haifa 3200000, Israel; sravitm@gmail.com (R.E.); roberto.simonutti@unimib.it (R.S.)
3 Department of Materials Science, University of Milan Bicocca, 20125 Milano, Italy; michele.mauri@mater.unimib.it
4 Istituto scientifico di chimica e biochimica "G. Ronzoni", 20133 Milano, Italy; bertini@ronzoni.it (S.B.); urso@ronzoni.it (E.U.)
5 Biology Department, Technion-Israel Institute of Technology, Haifa 3200000, Israel; assaraf@technion.ac.il
* Correspondence: elena.vismara@polimi.it (E.V.); livney@technion.ac.il (Y.D.L.)

Academic Editors: Jawed Fareed, Giangiacomo Torri and Diego Muñoz-Torrero

Abstract: Super paramagnetic iron oxide nanoparticles (SPION) were augmented by both hyaluronic acid (HA) and bovine serum albumin (BSA), each covalently conjugated to dopamine (DA) enabling their anchoring to the SPION. HA and BSA were found to simultaneously serve as stabilizing polymers of Fe_3O_4·DA-BSA/HA in water. Fe_3O_4·DA-BSA/HA efficiently entrapped and released the hydrophobic cytotoxic drug paclitaxel (PTX). The relative amount of HA and BSA modulates not only the total solubility but also the paramagnetic relaxation properties of the preparation. The entrapping of PTX did not influence the paramagnetic relaxation properties of Fe_3O_4·DA-BSA. Thus, by tuning the surface structure and loading, we can tune the theranostic properties of the system.

Keywords: super paramagnetic iron oxide nanoparticles (SPION); hyaluronic acid (HA); bovine serum albumin (BSA); Fe_3O_4·DA-BSA/HA; paclitaxel (PTX); magnetic resonance imaging (MRI)

---

1. Introduction

Nanotechnology has opened the way to an incredibly high number of new composite materials. As part of the growing field of nanomedicine [1], composite nanoscale biomaterials are based on assembling nanoparticles with biomolecules. The palette of available nanoparticles is large and matched by an equally large number of biomolecules [2]. Iron oxide nanoparticles are among the most extensively studied types of nanoparticles (NPs) [3]. Superparamagnetic iron oxides nanoparticles (SPIONs), composed by magnetite (Fe_3O_4) or maghemite (γ-Fe_2O_3), have been explored in view of their potentiality in biomedical applications [4]. In fact, a key advantage of iron oxide nanoparticles in comparison to other heavy metal-based NPs is their natural integration into tissue physiology. They can be part of superparamagnetic materials, whose suspensions are generally referred to as ferrofluids, clinically investigated as MRI contrast agents [5,6]. An overview has been published both on the many possibilities to prepare SPIONs suitable for enhancing with biomolecules and for potentially engineering for biomedical applications [7]. The authors of reference [8] have already described the logic of SPION-developed biomedical applications in recent years. SPION-appropriate surface coatings can be studied for various biomedical applications, such as magnetic resonance imaging, hyperthermia, drug delivery, tissue repair, cell and tissue targeting, and transfection. Development of coated and loaded SPIONs is a promising theranostic approach. In fact, following a quite similar approach, we pursued multitasking nanostructures—using cyclodextrin as a vector of antitumor drugs and low molecular weight heparins, covalently linked to cyclodextrin—that were thought to target the nanostructures to the tumor mass, according to heparanase and growth factors inhibition mechanisms [9]. We then progressed to iron oxide and heparin-based materials to introduce the diagnostic functionality [10,11]. Since 2005, magnetic NPs have been considered of great interest for biomedical applications, and, among them, iron oxide NPs have been considered the more promising [12]. Additionally, depending on particle size, positive or negative contrast agents can be prepared [13,14]. Even though SPIONs have been clinically approved metal oxide NPs, the potential toxicity of SPION has been thoroughly investigated [14]. Although there is no intrinsic risk associated with SPION per se, adverse biological effects and safety issues could be associated with specific SPIONs. Ref. [15] argues about issues that need be addressed by the scientific community prior to approving their clinical use. We already cited that SPION-appropriate surface coatings divert SPION towards different biomedical applications. In advance, SPION coating has been used to modulate their biocompatibility and to reduce their toxicity. This is the case of Bovine Serum Albumin (BSA) protein [16]. The same authors from Reference [16] are working today on human serum albumin, for better biocompatibility, thus supporting the crucial role that protein corona can play [17].

The common challenge of engineered SPION for biomedical applications is that the material used for surface coating of the magnetic particles must not only be nontoxic and biocompatible but also enable selective targeted delivery of the particles to the location of the disease. Passive targeting of long circulating nanoparticles via the enhanced permeability and retention (EPR) effect is one of the mechanisms by which such coated nanoparticles can reach solid tumors. Decoration of engineered magnetic nanoparticles with targeting molecules that selectively bind to target proteins overexpressed on the target cells could significantly enhance the selectivity of their targeting to these cells [18,19]. Magnetic nanoparticles can deliver drugs and an external magnetic field can be applied to guide them to the target site. Different polymers/molecules have been used for nanoparticle coating to stabilize the suspensions of magnetic nanoparticles under in vitro and in vivo situation and selected proteins/targeting ligands have been used for derivatizing magnetic nanoparticles. It is noteworthy that magnetic drug targeting employing nanoparticles as carriers is a promising cancer theranostic treatment, avoiding the side effects of conventional chemotherapy [3]. Molecular imaging is one of the most promising applications of targeted iron oxide nanoparticles, and various applications using targeted iron oxide nanoparticles have been evaluated in vitro and in animal experiments [20]. Looking forward, the fact that targeted superparamagnetic iron oxide nanoparticles can be used for early detection of cancer has to be considered a plus [21]. On the other hand, the challenges associated with penetration of nanoparticles across cell and tissue barriers have been recently reviewed [22]. Therefore, current understanding led us to the conclusion that the combination of a diagnostic imaging aid along with a targeted therapeutic compound loaded onto the same NP systems is a promising route of drug delivery.

The challenge of our study was to design and build new theranostic SPION systems starting from a magnetic iron oxide core decorated with bovine serum albumin (BSA) and hyaluronic acid (HA), where each component was selected to play its peculiar role and where the SPION systems could include paclitaxel (PTX) as a drug. Hyaluronic acid (HA) is a natural linear anionic glycosaminoglycan (molecular weight (MW) 5–10^4 kDa), composed of repeating disaccharide units of D-glucuronic acid and *N*-acetyl-D-glucosamine linked via alternating β-1,4 and β-1,3 glycosidic bonds. Owing to its biocompatibility and biodegradability, HA has been extensively investigated for medical applications. In particular, HA can specifically bind to various cancer cells that overexpress CD44 receptors.

In this regard, different considerations concerning the utile length of HA oligomers must be reported. Selecting HA oligosaccharides long enough to bind to more than one CD44 receptor but too short to bind to the hyaluronic acid receptor for endocytosis (HARE) receptors in the liver (preferably <10 kDa) may enable the formation of an HA-based CD44-targeted carrier that avoids hepatic elimination while achieving tumor targeting [23]. Recently, this enhanced tumor-targeting ability as well as higher therapeutic efficacy compared to free anti-cancer agents has been reported [24]. Therefore, several HA-conjugates containing anticancer agents (such as paclitaxel or doxorubicin) have already been designed [25]. Over the years, ever new functions of the CD44 protein have been found, but the main one for our purposes is the recognition of hyaluronic acid as a component of the extracellular matrix in particular areas, such as embryonic connective tissues and the outline of invasive cancerous lesions. Most HA-drug conjugates have been developed for cancer chemotherapy as macromolecular prodrugs. HA has also been conjugated onto various drug-loaded nanoparticles for use as a targeting moiety. Hyaluronic acid was bound to the initially dextran-coated SPIONs by esterification [26].

Bovine serum albumin (BSA) protein was used to improve the colloidal stability of the nanoparticles. BSA has been one of the most extensively studied proteins because of its sequence and structural homology with human serum albumin (HSA). HSA could be considered the most suitable protein for biocompatible coating of nanoparticles for biomedical applications. Herein we used BSA as a model for HSA, with the aim of ultimately using HSA for future clinical stages. BSA is an abundant serum protein with a MW of ~66 kDa. The primary physiological function of serum albumin (SA) is to transport lipids and metabolites present in blood plasma; hence, it is a suitable carrier for hydrophobic drugs. Due to the high protein binding of various drugs, it could be used for effective incorporation of these compounds. It has an extraordinary ligand binding capacity, providing a depot for a wide variety of compounds with favorable monovalent reversible binding characteristics for transport in the body and release at the cell surface. Folate–bovine serum albumin-functionalized polymeric micelles loaded with superparamagnetic iron oxide nanoparticles have been proposed for tumor targeting and magnetic resonance imaging [27,28]. Ultrasound-triggered BSA/SPION hybrid nanoclusters investigated for liver-specific magnetic resonance imaging support the interest in the use of SA in the field of nanomedicine [29].

Paclitaxel (PTX) is a medication used to treat a number of types of cancer, including ovarian cancer, breast cancer, lung cancer, and pancreatic cancer, among others. Its clinical application is hampered by poor solubility in water and other pharmaceutically acceptable solvents (<2 μg/mL). To increase its bioavaibility, various alternative formulation approaches have been explored, including emulsions, nanoparticles, polymeric micelles, cyclodextrins, liposomes, etc. [30]. Of note, hyaluronic acid-anchored PTX nanocrystals have been found to improve chemotherapeutic efficacy and inhibit lung metastasis in tumor-bearing rat models [31].

The aim of this study was to design and develop a new theranostic nanosystem, named Fe_3O_4·DA-BSA/HA, suitable for loading PTX (see Scheme 1). The iron core and HA were selected according to the specific roles they can play in therapy, diagnosis and targeting, while BSA could make stable, biocompatible and non-toxic the hybrid Fe_3O_4·DA-BSA/HA system. The iron core was decorated irreversibly by BSA and HA [32]. This is the reason why dopamine (DA) is a fundamental part of the system. Covalent linkage of both BSA and HA with DA was built up, DA being identified as the specific anchoring molecule to the inorganic core. BSA-DA and HA-DA were both linked to the surface of the iron core, in order to obtain a strong interaction between the bioorganic layer and the inorganic core. Scheme 1 summarizes the schematic protocol to Fe_3O_4·DA-BSA/HA that was thought to be as simple as possible, reproducible, and suitable for scaling up. The choice of HA and BSA was also in agreement with the final challenge of the work, that is the loading of Fe_3O_4·DA-BSA/HA with the real anticancer PTX drug. The rational of the PTX Fe_3O_4·DA-BSA/HA inclusion can also be supported by the fact that, on 6 September 2013, the Food and Drug Administration (FDA) approved PTX albumin-stabilized nanoparticle formulation and also partially by Ref. [31].

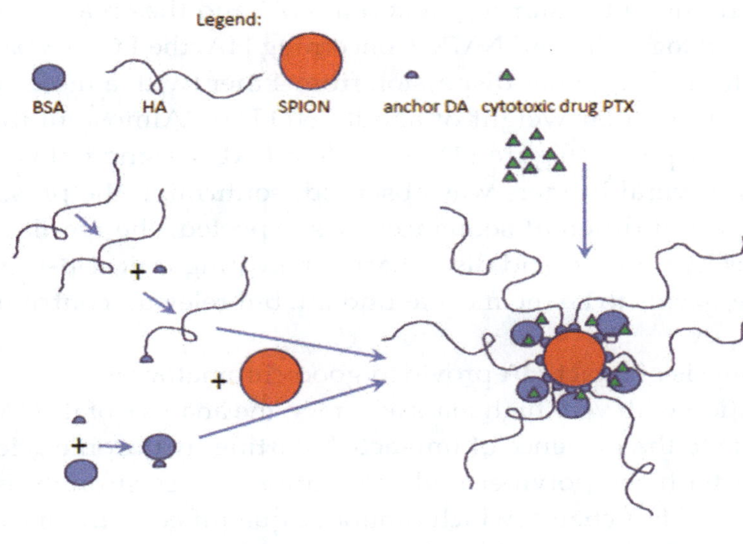

Scheme 1. A schematic protocol of the envisioned Fe_3O_4·DA-BSA/HA nanoparticle, where DA means dopamine, loaded with paclitaxel (PTX), BSA—bovine serum albumin; HA—hyaluronic acid.

2. Results

2.1. Preparation and Characterization

2.1.1. Synthesis of BSA-DA Adduct

Since DA and BSA respectively possess amine and carboxylic moieties, the common carbodimmide cross-linker chemistry was explored. The condensation between DA and BSA was performed by employing 1-ethyl-3-(3′-dimethyl-aminopropyl)-carbodiimide (EDC).

The DA:BSA degree of substitution was evaluated by means of MALDI–TOF analysis (Figure 1). The spectrum shows a large peak at mass-to-charge (*m/z*) values of about 70,000 Da, corresponding to the medium average derivatization of 20:1 (20 molecules of DA for each molecule of BSA).

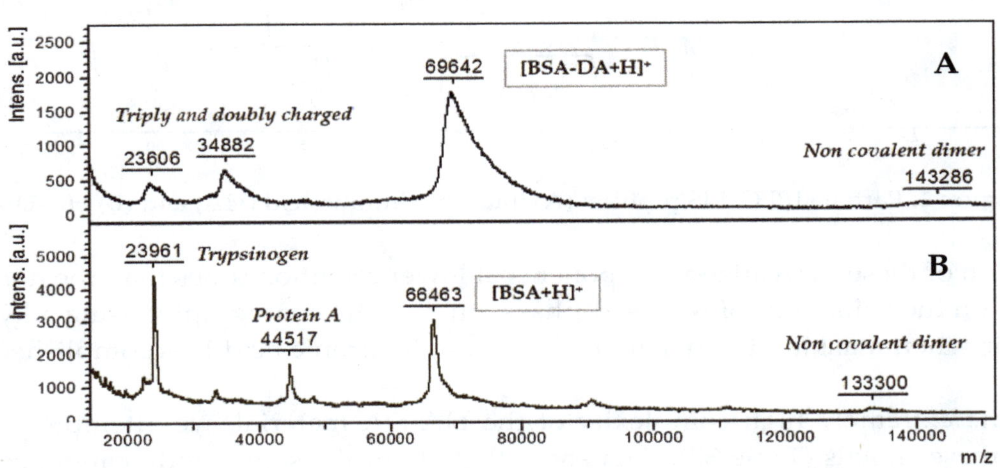

Figure 1. Matrix-assisted laser desorption/ionization (MALDI)-time of flight (TOF) spectra of (**A**) bovine serum albumin-dopamine (BSA-DA) and (**B**) BSA protein, protein A and trypsinogen.

2.1.2. Synthesis of HA-DA Adduct

Commercial low molecular weight hyaluronic acid (HA, 5400 Da) and dopamine hydrochloride were reacted to form HA-DA conjugates using EDC as the activating agent of carboxyl groups of the HA chain. The crude HA-DA was dialyzed before characterization.

Structural characterization of the starting material (HA) and the obtained HA-DA adduct was performed by LC–MS chromatography and NMR. Concerning HA, the LC–MS based method allowed the elution and identification of oligomer dispersion from 4 mer (with a molecular weight of about 700 Da) to 40 mer (with a molecular weight of about 7600 Da). Almost all the species eluting in the labelled chromatographic peaks (Figure S1) were identified; assignment is reported in Table S1. At any rate, the elution of several isomers was observed, confirming the presence of species with the same molecular weight but different sequences. As expected, the regular chains distribution on $(G\text{-}ANAc)_n$, that means hyaluronic acid disaccharide repeating unit, 4-β-D-glucuronic acid (1–3) *N*-acetyl β-D-glucosamine, seems to be the most abundant, but relevant contribution arises from the other species.

While the LC–MS analysis of intact HA provided good chromatographic separation of numerous species and their identification with very high mass accuracy, the analysis of its DA conjugate (HA-DA) showed several issues, due to the presence of unreacted starting hyaluronic acid, eventual reagents carried by the interaction with the polymer and the elution of less strongly retained derivatized oligomers under the unreacted HA chains, which cannot be quantified with this technique. Expanded portions of the chromatograms (Figure 2) allow for detecting the appearance of several mass signals corresponding to derivatized HA chains observed in the extracted ion chromatograms (Figure 3).

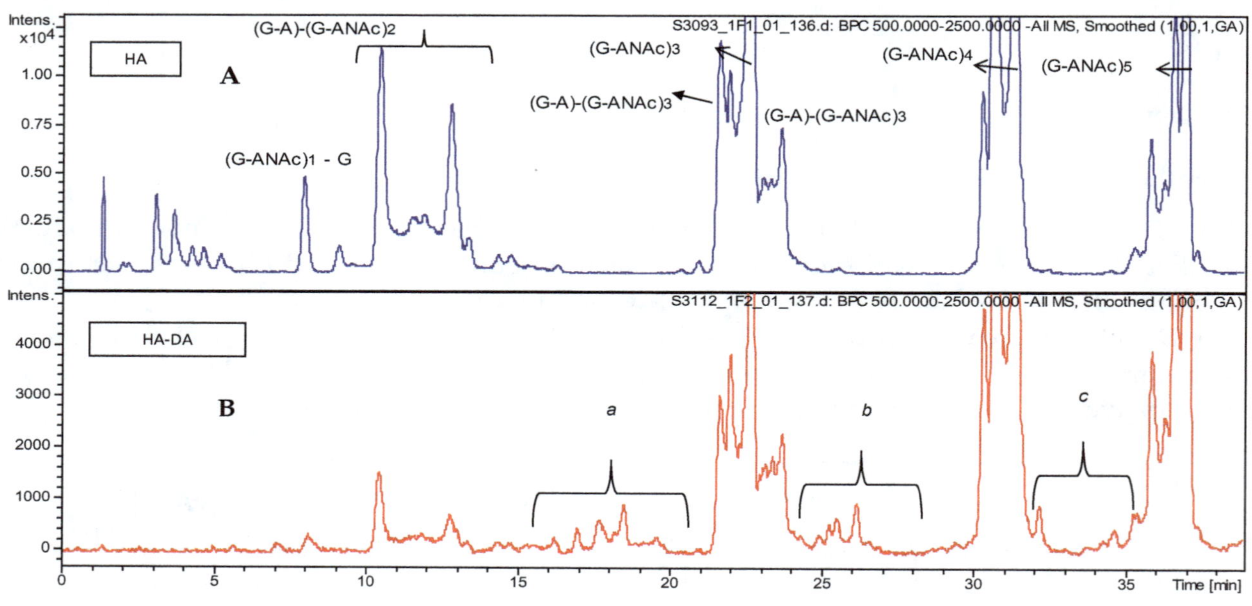

Figure 2. Partial HPLC–MS profiles: (**A**) intact hyaluronic acid (HA) and (**B**) HA-DA.

The elution of these derivatized components at lower retention times than the non-derivatized ones agrees with the behaviour of reversed-phase ion pair chromatography using alkylammonium as the ion pair when masking the negative charge of glucuronic acid is accomplished by reaction with DA.

Due to the extremely high complexity of the HA-DA material, we attempted to assign the structures of these signals (Table S2); data show that about the same modification, corresponding to a mass addition of about 534 Daltons, was observed in all HA components from 5 mer to 20 mer, suggesting the formation of modified HA chains containing at least three DA molecules. This first level of investigation appeared to be enough to confirm the HA derivatization with DA in the HA-DA material, as supported by parallel NMR analysis. No information can be provided via LC–MS analysis about the formation of the non-covalent HA/DA complex.

Structural characterization of HA-DA material was also performed using ^{1}H- and ^{13}C-NMR with mono- and bidimensional techniques such as COSY, TOCSY, DOSY, HSQC, and HMBC. Table 1 shows the chemical shifts and assignments of the signals.

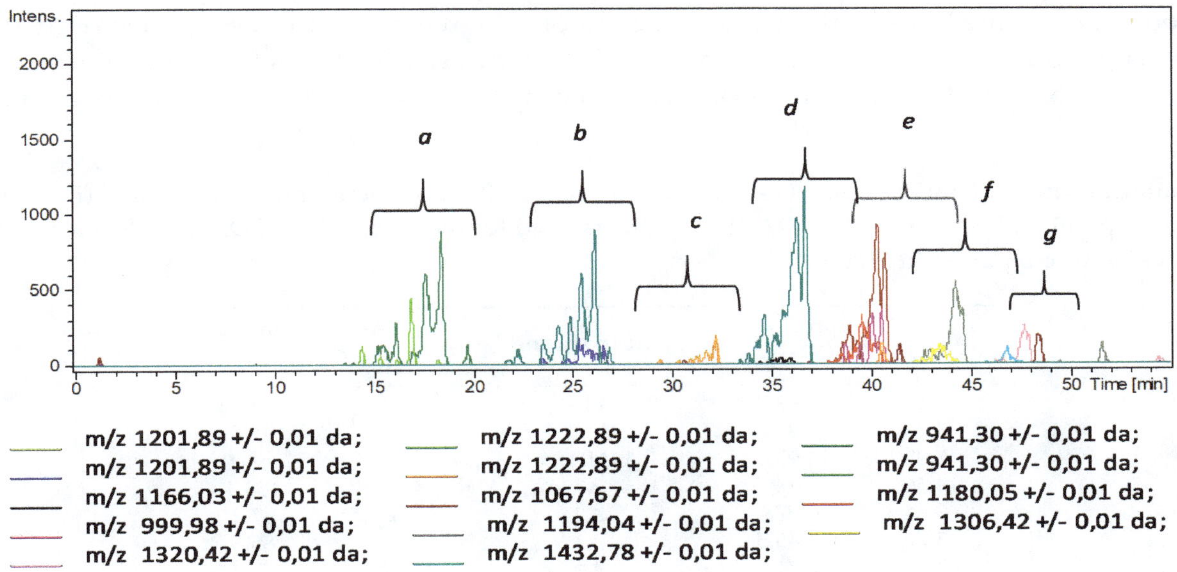

Figure 3. Extracted ion chromatograms (EIC) of mass signals identified as derivatized HA chains (HA-DA) ranging from 5-mer oligomers (Mw ~1500) to 20-mer oligomers (Mw ~4300) (see Table S2).

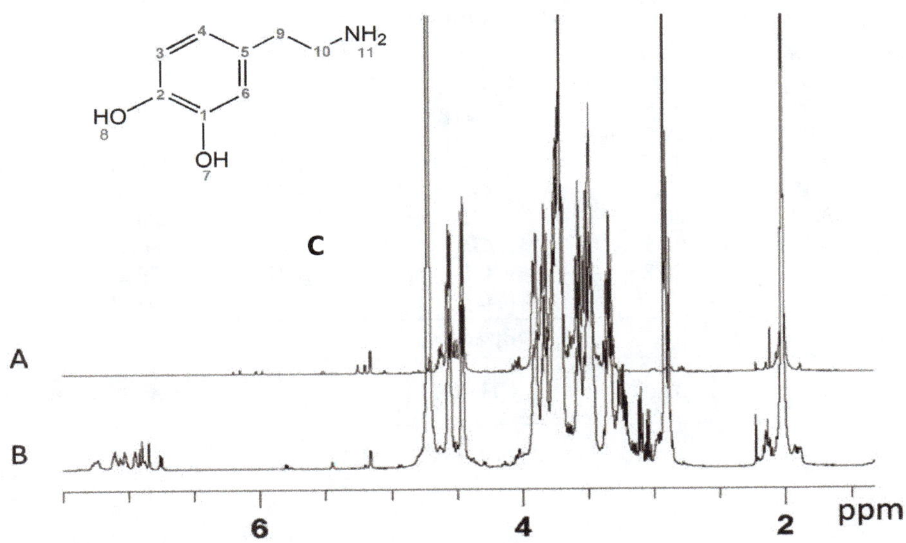

Figure 4. Proton spectra of HA (**A**) and HA-DA (**B**), (**C**) the DA chemical structure.

The HA ^{1}H-NMR (Figure 4A) spectrum signals a low molecular weight structure. The main signals are sharper than the usual polymeric HA ones, while minor signals are due to the reducing and non-reducing terminal chain residues. Both the glucosamine and the glucuronic acid show their terminal reducing residues, suggesting a non-enzymatic chemical degradation. Integration values of easily detectable reduced end signals correspond to an average of chains centred between nine and ten disaccharide units. Free NH_2 glucosamine is also detected, in the range of 1.5%. The spectrum of the product shows traces of minor components.

The HA-DA derivative presents a simplified ^{1}H-NMR spectrum (Figure 4B) with respect to the corresponding HA spectrum induced by the derivatization procedure. The reducing anomeric pattern and other minor signals have disappeared or are significantly lowered, corresponding to a loss of the shortest HA oligomers. The quantification of reducing end anomeric signals is no longer possible due to the occurred derivatization. The main spectrum signals are unmodified, while the new signals in the expected region of the DA signals appear to be minor, in agreement with the planned derivatization degree. The ratio between the aromatic and the anomeric signals allows for estimating an average ratio of 2 DA for each 10 disaccharide building blocks. A high complexity in these spectral regions is observed.

Table 1. Proton ^{1}H and carbon ^{13}C structure-chemical shift assignment of hyaluronic acid (HA) and HA-dopamine (DA). Italics: free DA. The numbers used for the attribution of DA signals refer to the DA structure reported in Figure 4.

HA (ppm)		Glucosamine	HA-DA (ppm)	
^{1}H	^{13}C		^{1}H	^{13}C
5.16	93.8	**A1α**	5.16	93.9
4.71	97.6	**A1β**	4.71	97.6
5.22	95.1	**A1NH$_2\alpha$**	-	-
4.56	103.3	**A1**	4.56	103.4
3.84	57.1	**A2**	3.83	57.2
3.72	85.5	**A3**	3.71	85.5
3.52	71.3	**A4**	3.51	71.3
3.48	78.3	**A5**	3.46	78.3
3.76 3.92	63.4	**A6** **A6′**	3.75 3.90	63.4
2.02	25.4	**ME**	2.02	25.4
-	177.8	**N-CO**	-	177.7
		Glucuronic Acid		
5.26	94.9	**$G1_{red\,\alpha}$**	5.20	94.9
3.01	57.1	**$G2_{red\,\alpha}$**	nd	nd
4.61	98.9	**$G1_{red\,\beta}$**	4.62	99.0
2.77	59.7	**$G2_{red\,\beta}$**	nd	nd
4.46	106.0	**G1**	4.45	105.8
3.45	75.4	**G2**	3.33	75.3
3.58	76.5	**G3**	3.56	76.5
3.74	82.8	**G4**	3.71	85.5
3.71	79.2	**G5**	3.71	79.2
-	176.9	**G6**	-	176.9
		Dopamine		
2.87	32.0	**CH_2 (9)**	2.98–2.93 2.96–2.87	34.8
3.22	40.0	**CH_2-Nr (10)**	3.27 3.23	43.3 39.5
6.75	123.0	**4**	6.88 6.93 6.76	124.7 124.2 124.1
-	130.1	**5**		138.9 141.3 131.9
6.90	117.4	**3**	7.10 7.26 7.23 6.91	130.7 125.8 125.7 119.4
6.85	117.4	**6**	7.02 7.09 6.85	121.2 126.7 119.5
-	145.0 143.8	**1 and 2**		132.1 140.2 149.9 150.7 151.1 147.1 145.9

At least three different structures are detectable at the level of the aromatic signals (Figure S2). One appears with sharp signals, and the chemical shift of the signals corresponds to the free dopamine's surviving the dialysis step, probably because of salt effect with HA. These signals were not considered for quantitative evaluations. The two other observable structures present similar signal patterns, but both show deshielded signals, in different degrees, with respect to the free DA. Furthermore, the signals appear as broad ones, due to their incorporation in a polymeric structure. This interpretation was supported by a DOSY NMR experiment that allows identification of homogeneous molecules through their diffusion coefficients, which depend on the size and shape of the molecule. The experiment shows the polymeric chain signals containing the linked aromatic ones all aligned and having similar low diffusion coefficients, while the small components show different distributions. The discriminating spectrum of the DOSY experiment shows that the free DA component is lost while the DA-HA linked components survive (see Figure 5).

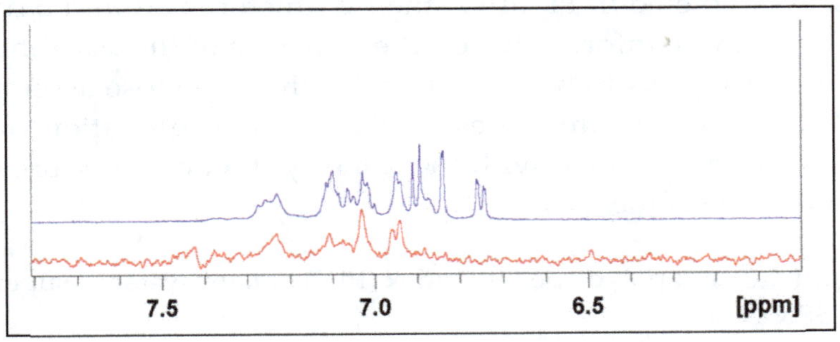

Figure 5. Comparison of aromatic proton sector of normal NMR spectrum (**blue**) with a DOSY section (**red**) taken in the correspondence of the polymeric chain signals.

The ^{13}C spectrum and the multiple bond correlation experiment (HMBC) associated with the heteronuclear correlation (HSQC) was determinant for the identification of the quaternary carbons and their correlations with the protons of the structure. It was possible to identify the correlations, in addition to the HA structural components, of quaternary aromatic carbons of DA substituent (Figure 6) with the aliphatic CH_2 of the linkage sequence $–CH_2–NHR$. They showed chemical shifts between 3.2 and 3.3, while CH_2 linked to the aromatic residue showed values between 2.8 and 3.0 ppm.

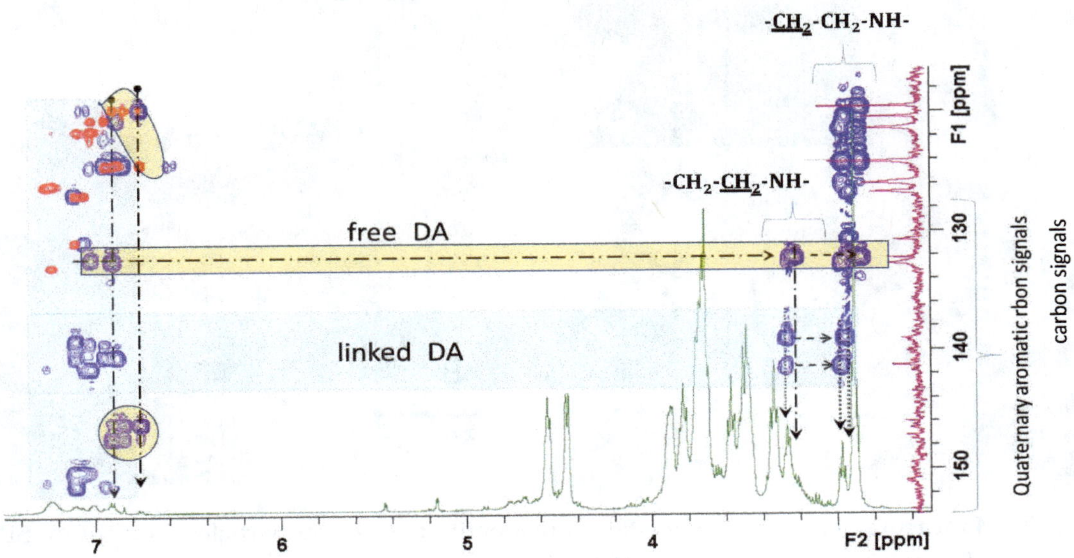

Figure 6. HMBC partial spectrum of HA-DA aromatic quaternary carbon correlation signals (**blue**) superimposed on the HSQC (**red**) and ^{1}H spectrum (**green**). Correlations of the DA polymeric components are underlined in the light blue areas while the free form is evidenced in the yellow area.

2.1.3. Synthesis of Fe_3O_4·OA Nanoparticles

The synthesis of magnetite-oleate nanoparticles (Fe_3O_4·OA, SPION1) was performed according to the following description. The magnetite was prepared by coprecipitation of a Fe^{2+} and Fe^{3+} salt solution ($FeCl_2 \cdot 4H_2O$ and $FeCl_3 \cdot 6H_2O$, respectively) with the introduction of ammonia as an alkaline agent. No post-treatment procedure was required, since the oleic acid was introduced as a reactant during the crystallization. The FTIR spectrum (Figure S3) confirmed the formation of the product due to the presence of the bands typical for the symmetric and antisymmetric stretching vibration of oleate (1407 cm^{-1} and 1520 cm^{-1}, respectively) and the signal at 600 cm^{-1}, which is representative of Fe–O bond in the crystalline lattice of magnetite. Concerning the morphological characterization, dynamic light scattering (DLS) measurements showed that the averaged hydrodynamic diameter (Z_{av}) of obtained oleate-nanocrystals is 31.12 ± 0.41, with a good polydispersity index (PDI) of 0.219 (Table 2). TEM images allow estimation of the size of the iron cores throughout the steps leading to the nanoassemblies. As depicted in Figure 7, their diameter is around 5 nm, and it is conserved in subsequent steps. DLS is more informative on the structure of the assemblies: the solvodynamic diameter of 30 nm of the Fe_3O_4·OA in hexane indicates that the loose assemblies appearing in the dry samples (Figure 7 and Table S3) are representative of the aggregation state seen in dispersion. Furthermore, different samples obtained with the same synthetic procedure over time highlighted good reproducibility of the size values.

Table 2. Zeta average (Z_{av}) and polydispersity index (PDI) of nanosystems, superparamagnetic iron oxide nanoparticle (SPION) 1–5.

Sample	Z_{av} (d. nm)	PDI
SPION1	31.1 ± 0.4	0.22
SPION2	77.5 ± 1.3	0.28
SPION3	83.9 ± 0.9	0.28
SPION5	75.0 ± 1.3	0.29
SPION6	79.4 ± 0.7	0.28

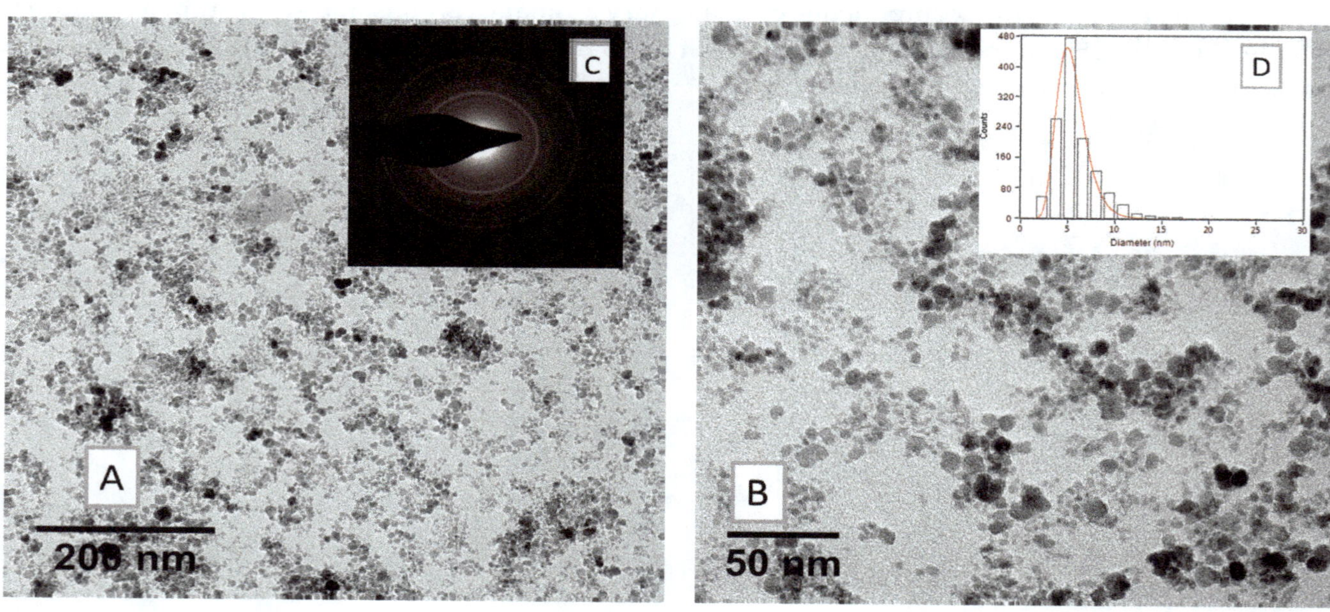

Figure 7. TEM measurements on nanocrystals of magnetite-oleate nanoparticles (Fe_3O_4·OA, SPION1) (**A**) low and (**B**) high magnification bright field micrographs; (**C**) relevant selected-area electron diffraction (SAED) pattern and (**D**) size distribution histogram of the nanoparticles ensemble.

2.1.4. Synthesis of Fe_3O_4·DA-BSA/HA Nanoparticles

Once the BSA-DA and HA-DA adducts were prepared, they were employed in a one-pot reaction procedure by using cetyl trimethylammonium bromide (CTAB), which acts as a phase transfer agent, allowing the dispersion of magnetite-oleate nanoparticles (Fe_3O_4·OA, SPION1) in water and the contemporary ligand exchange reaction with BSA-DA and HA-DA adducts, giving sample SPION2. Figure 8 shows the FTIR spectrum of SPION2, which is representative of all Fe_3O_4·DA-BSA/HA.

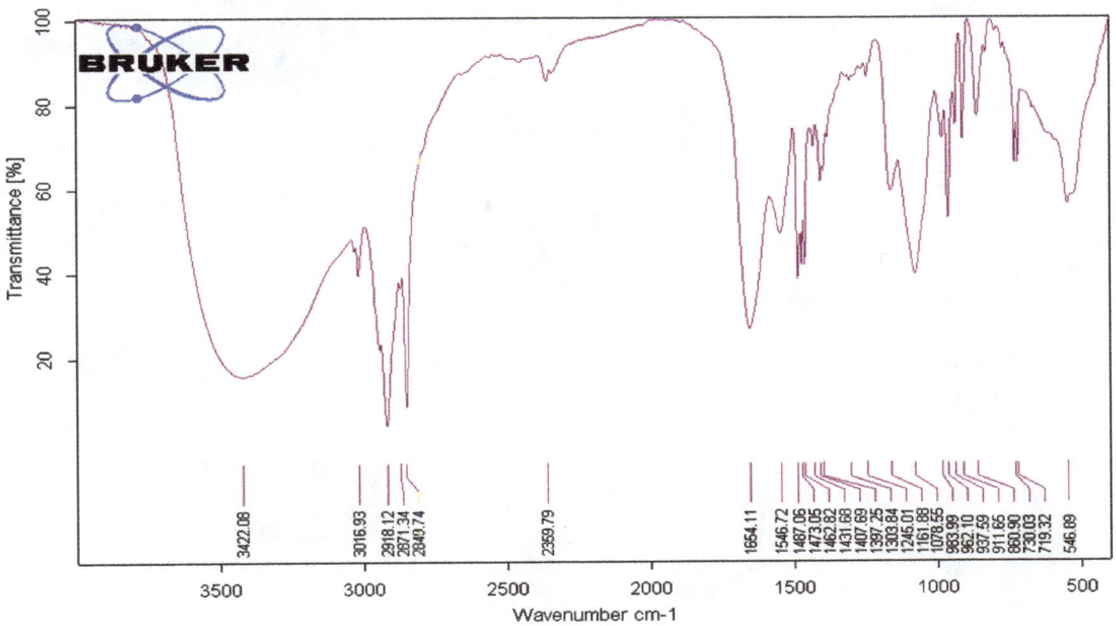

Figure 8. Fourier transform infrared spectroscopy (FTIR) spectrum of SPION2.

It is possible to identify the presence of DA, HA, BSA, and cetyl trimethylammonium cation (CTA) structures and the core Fe–O by diagnostic wavenumbers per every component: ν_{max} cm^{-1}: 3422.08 (O–H sym stretching, N–H stretching amide); 3016.93 (aromatic sym C–H stretching); 2918.1, 2871, 2849 (CH_3 asymmetric stretching and $-N^+(CH_3)_3$ symmetric stretching vibrations, CTA), 1654.11 CONH (C=O stretching); 1546.72 (aromatic sym C–C stretching); 1487.06 (benzene ring vibrations); 1473.05; 1462.82 (CH_2 bending); 1431.68; 1397.25 (aromatic C=C bonds); 1303.84 (aromatic C–O asym bending); 1245.01 (aromatic C–O sym bending); 1161.88 (C–O alcohol); 1078.55 (C–O alcohol) 962.10 (aromatic C–C–H sym bending); 937 (–CH=CH–ring); 730.03 (C–C–C asym bending); 719.32 (C–C–C asym bending); 546.89 (Fe–O).

The bands at 1481, 1333, and 1258 cm^{-1} have been assigned as diagnostic signals in the infrared spectrum of the bidentate ligand catechol bound to TiO_2 [33]. Accordingly, we tentatively assigned the bands at 1487.06, 1397.25, and 1245.01 to the bidentate ligand DA bound to Fe. Bands at 2918.1, 2871, 2849, and 1462.82 were assigned to CTA, in keeping with a very recent article, "Electrochemistry and surface-enhanced Raman spectroscopy of CTAB modulated interactions of magnetic nanoparticles with biomolecules", strictly related to our work [34]. Both TEM (Figure 9) and DLS (Z_{av} = 77.51 ± 1.32, PDI = 0.28, Table 2) depicted a significant change in the morphology of the system. The overall dimensions grew and took the shape of multiple small cores coated by shells of organic material.

Since organic layer size could interfere with MRI detection by shielding the iron core, the amount of HA was decreased, giving SPION3 and SPION4 with different relative amounts of HA and BSA (20% and 10% HA, respectively, in comparison with SPION2): see the TEM images in Figures 10 and 11. The choice to modulate HA content depends on the fact that HA is the real targeting component of Fe_3O_4·DA-BSA/HA. Hence, the availability of SPIONs 2–4 could endow Fe_3O_4·DA-BSA/HA with different targeting properties. Table 3 summarizes the different amounts of BSA and HA.

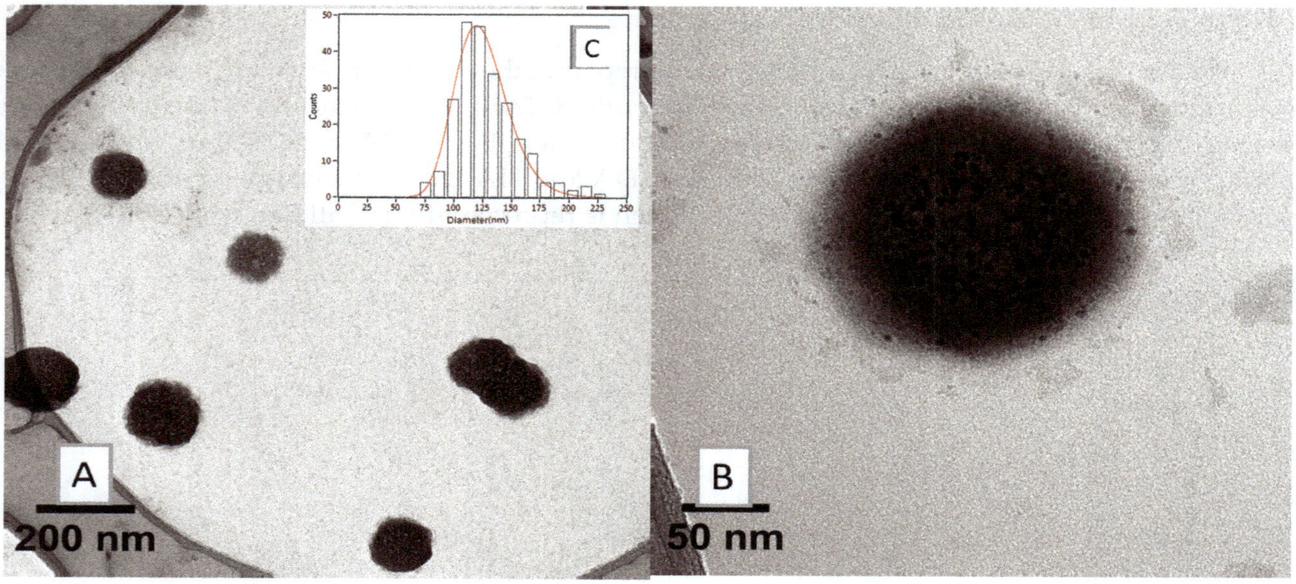

Figure 9. TEM analysis on SPION2: (**A**) low- and (**B**) high-magnification bright field micrographs and (**C**) size distribution histogram of the nanosystems.

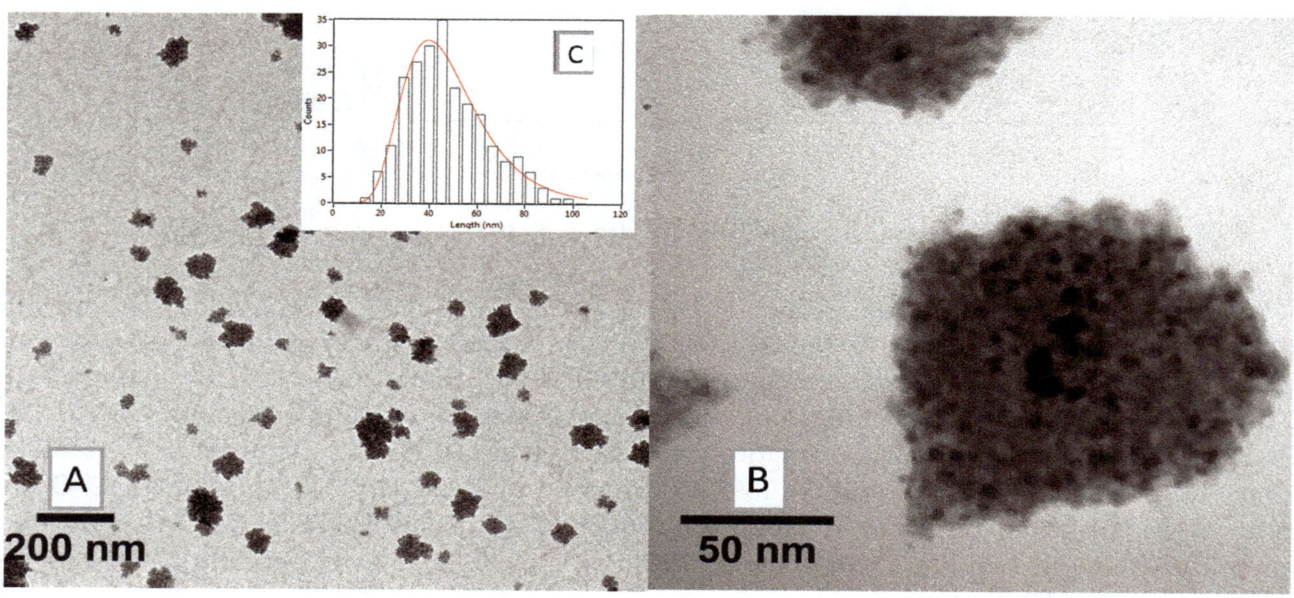

Figure 10. TEM analysis on SPION3: (**A**) low and (**B**) high-magnification bright field micrographs, and (**C**) size distribution histogram of the nanosystems.

Table 3. Different HA amounts (mg) used for the preparation of Fe_3O_4·DA-BSA/HA nanoparticles.

Fe_3O_4·OA (SPION1)	BSA	HA	Samples
		250	SPION2
100	250	50	SPION3
		25	SPION4

The huge decrease of HA organic components appeared to provoke a loss in the homogeneous morphology of SPION4 (as is clearly detectable from the TEM image, Figure 11). For these reasons, SPION4 was discarded for subsequent evaluations. Concerning SPION2 and SPION3, minor differences in nanoparticle size were noticed in DLS measurements (Table 2 and Figure 12).

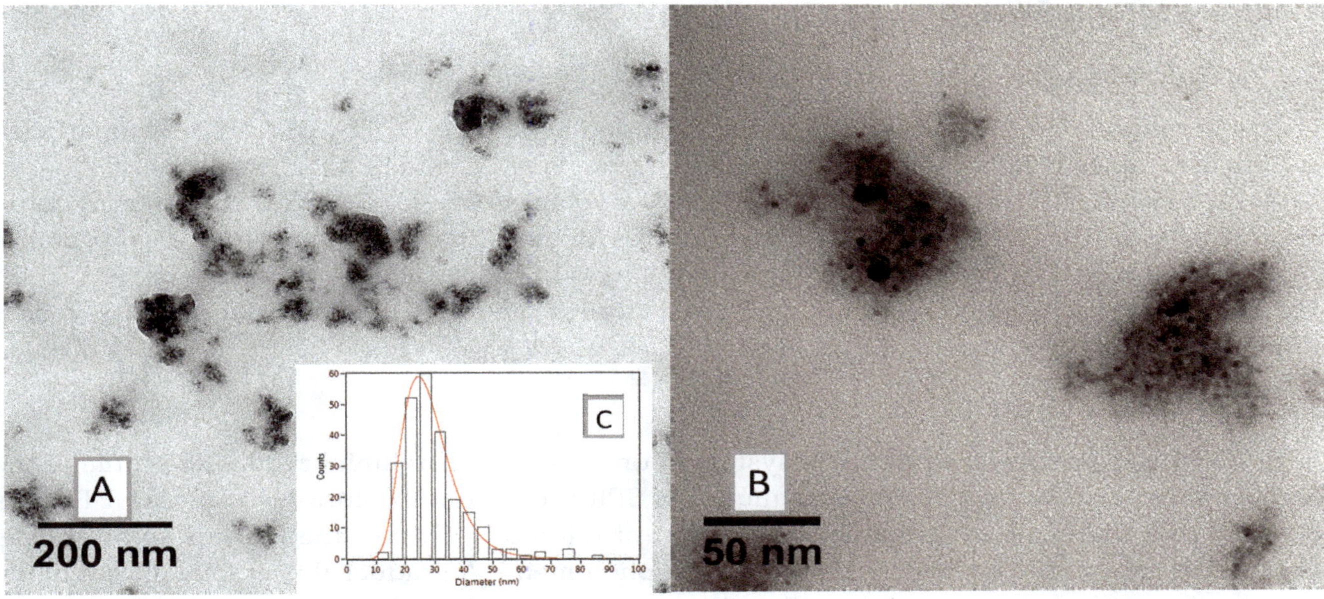

Figure 11. TEM analysis on SPION4: (**A**) low and (**B**) high magnification bright field micrographs, and (**C**) size distribution histogram of the nanosystems.

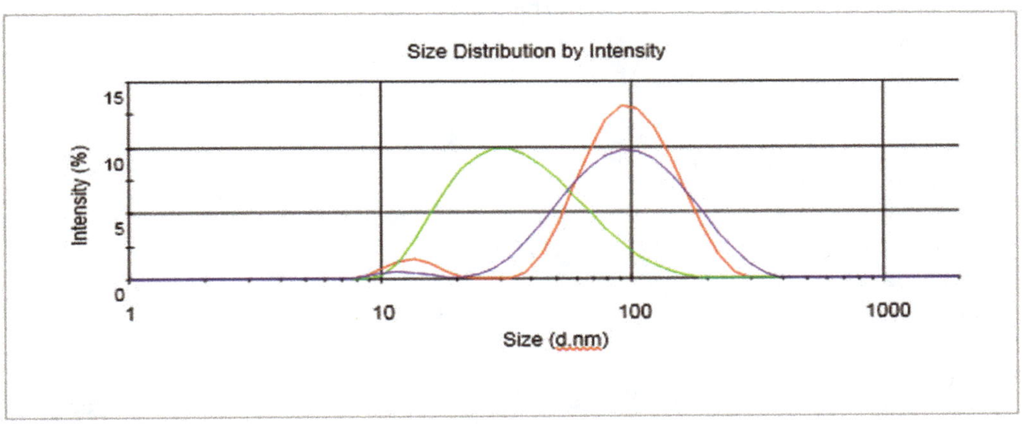

Figure 12. Dynamic light scattering (DLS) profiles of SPION1 (**green**), SPION2 (**red**), and SPION3 (**blue**).

Concerning the evaluation of the surface charges of the nanosystem, Table 4 reports Z potential (ξ) values of different samples. Both of the functional organic molecules (HA and BSA) own an overall negative surface charge, which is slightly decreased as a result of the covalent linkage with dopamine moiety. The positive ξ values of SPIONs depend on the surface charge due to the CTA [34].

Table 4. Zeta potential (ξ) values for HA, BSA, BSA-DA, HA-DA, and SPION2, 3, and 6.

	ξ (mV)
Hyaluronic Acid (HA)	−30.8 ± 1.74
Bovine Serum Albumin (BSA)	−26.4 ± 1.51
BSA-DA	−6.14 ± 1.30
HA-DA	−2.17 ± 0.83
SPION2	+15.3 ± 1.01
SPION3	+19.2 ± 1.16
SPION6	+17.5 ± 2.21

2.2. *Inclusion of Paclitaxel and Drug Release*

2.2.1. Fe_3O_4·DA-BSA/HA Nanoparticles with Paclitaxel (PTX)

The antimitotic drug Paclitaxel (PTX) was included in both Fe_3O_4·DA-BSA/HA nanoparticles, resulting in samples SPION5 and SPION6, obtained from SPION2 and SPION3, respectively.

A dispersion of PTX was slowly added to progressive volumes of Fe_3O_4·DA-BSA/HA nanoparticles in PBS (until 1:3 *v/v*). The efficiency of the entrapment was firstly verified due to the visual disappearance of water-insoluble PTX crystals. No significant changes in the structure of the assemblies (Z_{av} in Table 2 and Figure S7), in their morphology (TEM, Figure S8) and in their superficial electric potential (ξ, Table 4) were observed.

2.2.2. PTX Release Kinetics

SPION6 was used as the pilot nanosystem in order to test a preliminary kinetic profile of the PTX release over time. In particular, an aliquot of SPION6 colloidal solution containing PTX was submitted to a dialysis-based assay. The amount of released PTX into the dialysis solution was monitored by means of quantitative UV-Vis spectrophotometry. A gradual almost total release of the drug was observed, as detectable by plotting the percentage of released PTX versus times (Figure 13). More details are reported in the experimental part (see Section 4.4).

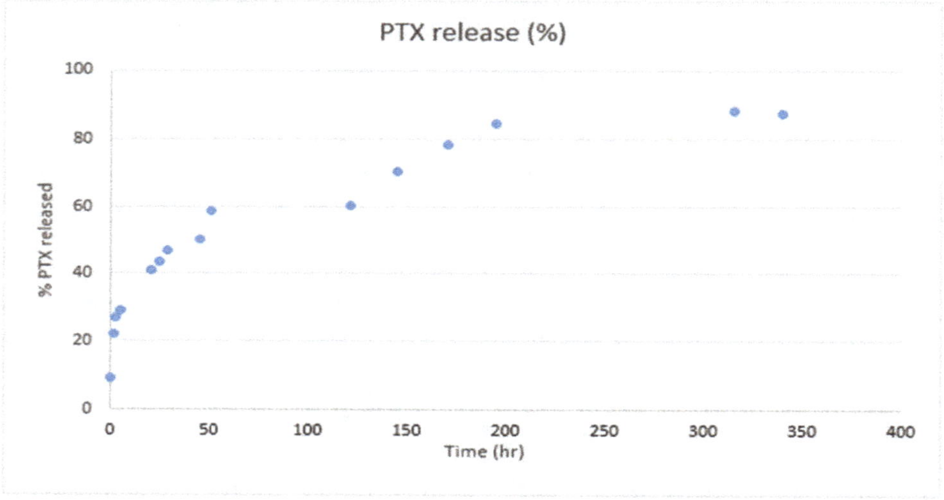

Figure 13. Percentage of released PTX plotted against time (hours). Data were obtained with UV-Vis experiments performed on SPION6 (see Figure S4).

2.3. *Time-domain (TD)-NMR Experiments*

The solution behavior of contrast agents is often used to screen their potential before animal testing [35]. Thus, relaxation times T_1 and T_2 were calculated for all preparations at several different dilutions, starting from saturated dispersions of samples SPION2 and SPION3. Additionally, we tested corresponding preparations where PTX was added. For the base dispersions, we measured the amount of nanoparticles, expressed in weight, by drying. In addition, we determined the Fe atomic content of SPION2 and SPION3 by inductively coupled plasma (ICP) spectrometry. The results, expressed in % wt, are 1.38% and 5.45% for SPION2 and SPION3, respectively. Addition of the PTX was performed by adding 1 mL of PTX solution to 3 mL nanoparticle solution.

All NMR experimental data were well fitted by monomodal decay functions (Figure S5). An absence of multimodal decay indicates the system is in rapid exchange regime, with relaxation averaged by fast molecular motion between bulk solvent and nanoparticle surface. Iron nanoparticles are covered by a HA/BSA layer that makes them compatible with water as well as with each other.

The coexistence of these interactions makes the grafted particles stick together into hierarchical superstructures, as is clearly detectable from TEM images (Figures 10 and 11). Microscopically, they are loose assemblies where water molecules can move easily throughout the soft and hydrophilic particle organic cover, coming in proximity of the paramagnetic iron oxide cores dispersed within with high rate. This is very promising for future study on renal clearance, a desirable goal for nanoparticle design since it avoids iron buildup within the body. This kind of clearance is usually limited to nanoparticles with less than a 5.5 nm hydrodynamic radius [36], a much smaller value than that measured by DLS for the present samples. Still, it is well known that soft and flexible particles can squeeze through the renal nodules [37]. Furthermore, while the present samples are stable in PBS solution, their hierarchical nature provides the opportunity to further tune the surface for stimuli-responsive decomposition [13], ultimately separating component particles which are in the range of 3–5 nm.

Relaxation rates R_1 and R_2, defined as the inverse of relaxation times T_1 and T_2, respectively, were plotted against the molar concentration of Fe, as exemplified by Figure 14A, which shows a comparison between the R_2 values for samples SPION2 and SPION3. The resulting plots were highly linear ($R^2 > 0.99$); thus, molar relaxivities r_1 and r_2 could be calculated as slopes of the linear fitting and are indicated in Table 5. Firstly, the high linearity indicates that the aggregates are stable, since any phenomenon of aggregation or splitting of the nanoassemblies would qualitatively change the interaction with water. The values in Fe molar concentration for the two samples span different ranges because the nanoparticle concentration in the dispersions is the same, but the nanoassemblies prepared with lower amounts of HA have a higher content in Fe cores. This is apparent in Figure 14B, where we instead plot the same relaxivity values against the amount of nanoparticles (not of Fe). Due to the higher Fe loading potential of SPION3, this compound could be the most suitable for medical applications.

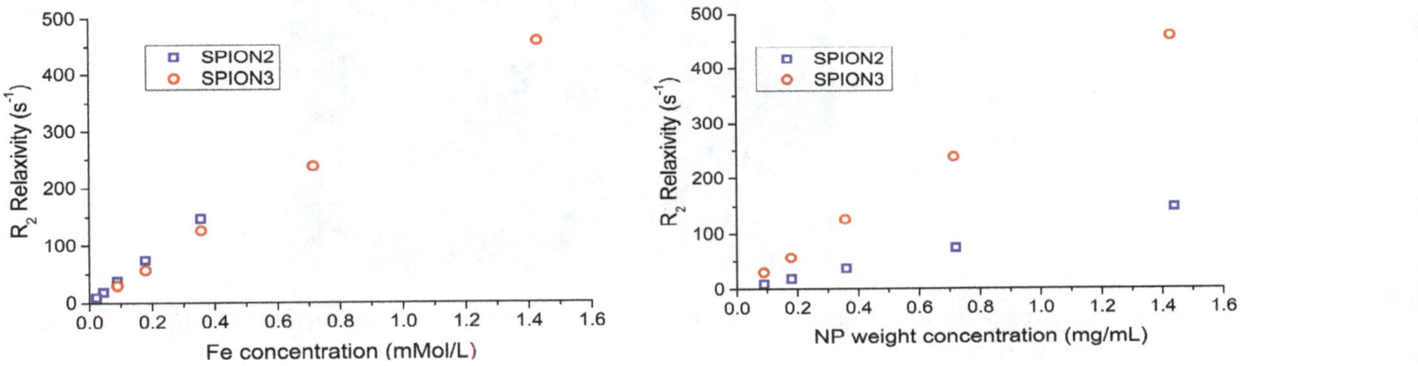

(A) **(B)**

Figure 14. Dependence of R_2 relaxation rates for unloaded NP over **(A)** Fe concentration and **(B)** amount of nanoparticles.

Table 5. Longitudinal relaxation R_1 of SPION2, SPION5, SPION3 and SPION6.

Sample	Composition	$r_1 \pm$ SD (s^{-1} Mm^{-1})	$r_2 \pm$ SD (s^{-1} Mm^{-1})	$r_2/r_1 \pm$ SD
SPION2	Fe_3O_4·DA-BSA/HA	76.8 ± 1.4	414 ± 4	5.41 ± 0.03
SPION5	SPION2 + PTX	81.2 ± 1.4	396 ± 5	4.88 ± 0.04
SPION3	Fe_3O_4·DA-BSA/HA $_{20\%}$	61.1 ± 0.7	321 ± 6	5.26 ± 0.04
SPION6	SPION3 + PTX	62.9 ± 1.2	333 ± 6	5.29 ± 0.005

On the other hand, the similarity of the values plotted against Fe concentration indicates that the particles have fundamentally the same interactions with water regardless of the BSA/HA ratio.

Later, we also verified the effect of the presence of PTX. From the data presented in Table 5 (see also figures), it is apparent that there is no effect. Similar plots were prepared for longitudinal relaxation R_1; those values are also reported in Table 5.

The high molar relaxivity values show high promise for application as an MRI agent, since both the r_1 and r_2 values are comparable to top end commercial contrast agents [38]. In addition, the inclusion of PTX did not significantly influence the relaxometric parameters, suggesting theranostic applications. Since current MRI techniques are based on achieving contrast in different T_1 and T_2 experiments, the R_2/R_1 ratio is often used to evaluate the applicability of a system for use as a black or white contrast agent [39]. The present samples have values of around 5, indicating a preferential usage as a dark contrast agent, but also some possible applications for white contrast, a field currently dominated by Gd contrast agents, which have high effectivity but some well-known side effects including deposition in brain tissue and a risk of nephrogenic fibrosis.

Figure 15 shows that SPIONs have a darkening effect on T2w scans, as expected, dilution of the sample with PBS decreased the signal of the SPIONs as the iron concentration decreased. The concentration of Fe_3O_4 in the samples was insufficient for significant signal because HA unexpectedly caused a lightening effect in the MRI, which counteracted the SPION signal reducing the signal darkening effect. A significant signal darkening was observed for the original samples of SPION3 and SPION4, but, after 50-fold dilution, the signal of SPION3 was dramatically less dark compared to SPION4, which corresponds to the fact that HA concentration of SPION4 was half the concentration of SPION3. We can conclude from this experiment that decreasing HA concentration significantly improved the ability of the SPIONs to serve as good contrast agents in MRI.

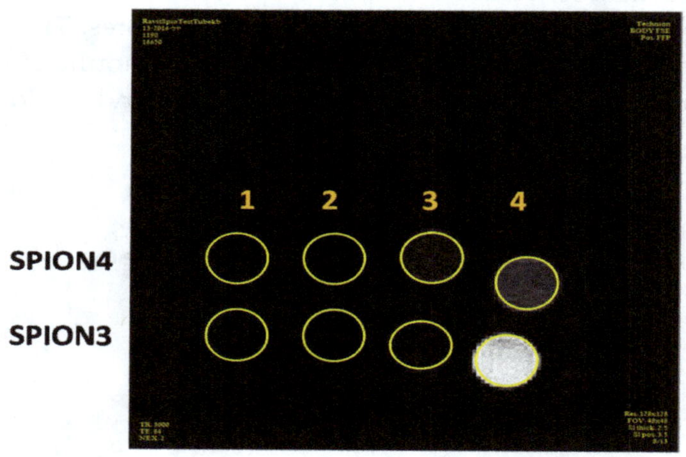

Figure 15. In vitro MRI T2w scans of samples SPION3 and SPION4. (**1**) Original sample; (**2**) 2-fold dilution; (**3**) 10-fold dilution; and (**4**) 50-fold dilution.

3. Discussion

The challenge of this work was to prepare Fe_3O_4·DA-BSA/HA nanoparticles (SPION samples) with the capability of loading PTX. We pursued this investigation to provide biologists and possibly clinics with new theranostic tools. We depicted SPION features and potentialities, starting with the design, passing from the synthesis to the structural and physicochemical characterization of both the final adducts and the intermediates, going on with TD-NMR investigation, and ending with the loading and release of PTX.

As anyone can recognize in current research, the nanomedicine field is becoming immeasurable. It could be compared to a dark forest where it is very difficult to find one's bearings. As an example, a scholar intending to update the enhanced permeability and retention (EPR) of nanoparticles in tumors could not avoid considering the paper of Nichols and Bae, published in 2014, where they presented a solid overview of EPR limits and perspectives [40]. We offer these remarks to clarify the thinking we followed to project Fe_3O_4·DA-BSA/HA. First, we judge that the theranostic approach is still valid to fight cancer, and that its rationale is the best to pursue, as far as we know. Additionally, we decided that, in this war, our chemical approach must be not too sophisticated, while structural and physicochemical characterization needed to be as in-depth as possible. The synthetic strategy for creating SPIONs was based on well-known reactions. Dopamine (DA) has been shown to easily bind to Fe_3O_4 as a bidentate enediol ligand [41] and to be a robust and stable anchor group to functionalize iron oxide nanoparticles with functional molecules [42]. In Fe_3O_4·DA-BSA/HA, dopamine (DA) is the spacer between BSA and HA and the iron core. Furthermore, DA is very convenient as a bifunctional molecule suitable to functionalize the terminal amino group, for example by condensation with the carboxylic group of glycosaminoglycans [43] and of proteins [44]. BSA and HA were separately cross-linked to DA by an amide bond, affording BSA-DA and HA-DA, as detailed in the result and experimental sections. Of note, a dialysis procedure was used to remove nonpolymeric materials and undesired byproducts from the BSA-DA and HA-DA crude reactions. The reagents ratio employed for HA/BSA and DA crosslinking was decided with the aim of not functionalizing all the carboxylic groups of DA and HA, because in our minds HA and BSA have to maintain their biological and physical properties to act by targeting glycosaminoglycan (HA) and biocompatible protein (SA). It is well known that charges are crucial for the electrostatic interaction so important in biological environments.

A significant effort was made to characterize both the dialyzed crude reactions, putting in evidence the amido linkage formation and estimating the substitution degree of the HA and BSA carboxylic groups with DA: see Sections 2.1.1 and 2.1.2 The medium average derivatization of BSA was estimated 20 molecules of DA for each molecule of BSA. The medium average derivatization of HA was estimated at two molecules of DA for each 10 disaccharide building blocks.

BSA-DA and HA-DA solutions were used in a one-pot reaction to perform ligand exchange on iron oleate (OA) nanoparticles, Fe_3O_4·OA, prepared in organic solvent [45,46]: see Sections 2.1.3 and 2.1.4. Oleic acid coating was used to stabilize and enhance the exchange with DA adducts. Fe_3O_4·OA ligand exchange with DA-BSA and DA-HA provided Fe_3O_4·DA-BSA/HA as a bioactive adduct suitable for suspensions in buffer solution [47]. As far as we know, Fe_3O_4·DA-BSA/HA is a new nanostructure, in terms of its covalent DA linkages and DA chelation of Fe. HA and BSA undergo strong interactions that could be associated with significative bioactivities and synergic effects in stabilizing SPION and targeting citotoxic drugs to tumor mass. Different Fe_3O_4·DA-BSA/HA (SPIONs) were prepared by changing the DA-HA:DA-BSA ratios: see Table 3 and Section 4.2.4. We assume that modified DA reactivity towards Fe does not depend on the cross-linked polymers. This assumption is justified by the high affinity between DA and Fe and by the fact that steric effects are, in our opinion, not very important because of the distance between the diol and the amino group. Therefore, the initial DA-HA:DA-BSA ratio affords Fe_3O_4·DA-BSA/HA composition. SPIONs were all characterized by IR spectroscopy that supports the Fe_3O_4·DA-BSA/HA structure and gives evidence of CTA as positive counter ions of the carboxylic groups not involved in the amidation. The relevant rule that CTAB plays in modulating the interactions of magnetic nanoparticles with biomolecules [34] is noteworthy.

For convenience, the SPION2 spectrum is shown and detailed: see Figure 8. TEM images were reported in Figures 9–11 and partly discussed in the results. Before further discussing SPION2-6 TEM and DLS results, let us have a look to SPION1, which is the precursor of Fe_3O_4·DA-BSA/HA. SPION1 could be described as a nanostructured organic salt or complex. Its morphology is shown in Figure 7. It shows iron cores surrounded by the organic layer of oleic acid. After the ligand exchange, the situation dramatically changes. The Fe_3O_4·DA-BSA/HA morphology resembles a pomegranate, with several iron cores covered by a single organic envelopment. The size of the iron cores does not seem to vary significantly in the different SPIONs. On the other hand, SPION size distribution depends on the different ratios between the inorganic and organic parts, as reported in Table 3. SPION2 was prepared starting from same amount of HA-DA and BSA-DA. In SPION3 preparation, the amount of HA-DA was strongly reduced, and this was even less for SPION4. SPION2 presents a much higher size distribution than SPION3; SPION4 shows the same trend. From TEM, it appears that SPION2 and SPION3 have quite the same morphology (see Figures 9 and 10). We can argue that SPION2 and SPION3 are representatives of the Fe_3O_4·DA-BSA/HA nanosystem, where both HA-DA and HA-BSA contributes to the morphology. This is not true for SPION4 (see Figure 11). In other words, SPION4 cannot be described as a Fe_3O_4·DA-BSA/HA nanosystem.

SPION DLS analysis was also provided and summarized in Table 2 and Figure 12. They confirm the difference between SPION1 and the other SPIONS. The DLS data correspond well to most of the engineered SPIONs proposed in the literature. After ligand exchange, the hydrodynamic radius of the newly formed HA/BSA SPIONs increases to 70 nm. Table 2 shows that all the different Fe_3O_4·DA-BSA/HA fall in the range of standard SPION (50–150 nm). Noteworthy SPION that are 10–100 nm in size are considered to be optimal for intravenous administration [15]. This observation makes Fe_3O_4·DA-BSA/HA promising for future biomedical applications. Since the iron cores are not modified, this confirms that the assembly of large particles, as seen in Figure 9, is modulated by the interaction between biomolecular coronas and water, resulting in complex hierarchical (pomegranate) structures. Looking to the SPIONs' morphology and size distribution, we argue that some Fe_3O_4·DA-BSA/HA properties could be modulated by changing the ratios between HA and DA and between them and Fe. Note especially the zeta potential (ξ) values reported in Table 4 for HA, BSA, BSA-DA, HA-DA, and SPION2, 3 and 6. The ξ values change from negative, for HA-DA and BSA-DA, to positive for SPION2 and SPION3, perfectly agreeing with surface charges due to the CTA cation [34]. The presence of CTA as counter ion can be correlated with a very good colloidal stability as observed in Ref. [34]. Furthermore, the magnetic properties of our SPIONs discussed on the base of their TD-NMR results support the biomedical diagnostic potentiality of the system Fe_3O_4·DA-BSA/HA plus CTA.

SPION2 and SPION3 were loaded with PTX to obtain SPION5 and SPION6, as explained in Section 2.2.1. PTX was easily dispersed by the SPION2 and SPION3 suspensions. Both of the SPION5 and SPION6 DLS and TEM measurements of the obtained drug vehicle did not highlight any significant morphological variation (see Table 2 and Figures S7 and S8). Zeta potential values were also not affected ($\xi = 17.5 \pm 2.21$ mV, Table 4). The maintenance of size, morphology and ξ support the PTX loading within SPION2 and SPION3 affording SPION5 and SPION6. In advance, the Fe_3O_4·DA-BSA/HA capability to load PTX can be correlated with the PTX hydrophobic interaction with BSA. Since the nanoparticle albumin-bound paclitaxel has been discovered, many approaches have been attempted to put it in more complex systems to avoid the undesired effects of PTX anticancer drug. As a matter of fact, unfortunately the nanoparticle albumin-bound paclitaxel alone cannot solve the PTX limits and drawback. Layer-by-layer assembly of hierarchical nanoarchitectures has been investigated to enhance the systemic performance of nanoparticle albumin-bound paclitaxel [48]. The biodegradability has been pursued in one-step fabrication of agent-loaded biodegradable microspheroids for drug delivery and imaging applications [49]. A quite similar approach has been the thermoreversible gelation of poly(ethylene glycol)/poly(ester anhydride) triblock copolymer nanoparticles for injectable drug delivery systems [50]. Nanoparticle albumin-bound paclitaxel has been loaded into a nanoporous solid multistage nanovector to enhance therapeutic efficacy [51]. Finally, drug-induced self-assembly of modified albumins has been proposed for tumor-targeted combination therapy [52]. The rational of our approach to load PTX within Fe_3O_4·DA-BSA/HA perfectly agrees with References [48–52] and enhances the BSA role in Fe_3O_4·DA-BSA/HA structures.

As shown in Figure 13, PTX was released by SPION6 at 90% in nine days: see Section 2.2.2. In about one day, 60% of PTX was released. Both the PTX loading and the preliminary release data associated with the physicochemical characterization of SPION5 and SPION6 are strongly encouraging for the development of Fe_3O_4·DA-BSA/HA as PTX delivery nanosystems, where loaded PTX was made bioavailable in buffer solution and matched with the Fe_3O_4·DA-BSA/HA targeting potentiality according to the hope of reducing the PTX administered dose.

Section 2.3 reports the results obtained by TD-NMR experiments and highlights useful comments. In particular, the SPIONs' magnetic properties appear crucial to recognition that Fe_3O_4·DA-BSA/HA can also be tested as an innovative contrast agent: see Table 5 and Figure 14. Figure 14b shows the very important result about the R_2 relaxation of SPION2 compared with SPION3: the same NP weight concentration, but different Fe contents (SPION3 > SPION2), corresponds to a higher R_2 relaxation for SPION3 than for SPION2.

SPIONs were reported to be excellent MRI T2 contrast agents. As excepted, in vitro T2w MRI scanning of SPION3 and SPION4 demonstrated significant dark signal having a great potential for targeted imaging. The approximate blood volume of a mouse is 77–80 μL/g weight. After IV injection (200 μL) to mice, the sample is diluted in the blood stream (1.9–2 mL) and concentrated in the tumor so the dilution of the sample is up to 10 fold. From the MRI in vitro result (Figure 15), even after 10-fold dilution the darkening effect of SPION3 and SPION4 is significant, thus we can deduct from this experiment that a sufficient signal will be presumably observed in mice. Moreover, at higher dilution, SPION4 has a better darkening signal due to its lower concentration of HA.

We can argue not only that SPION3 could be more suitable as contrast agent, but also that the synthetic strategy approached in this paper can modulate Fe_3O_4·DA-BSA/HA properties. The TD-NMR experiments also confirm Fe_3O_4·DA-BSA/HA stability, a feature that is essential for further developments. Finally, the fact that the inclusion of PTX did not at all modify the magnetic properties of Fe_3O_4·DA-BSA/HA strongly supports the achievement of using Fe_3O_4·DA-BSA/HA as theranostic agent.

4. Materials and Methods

4.1. General

Chemicals: Ferric chloride hexahydrate ($FeCl_3 \cdot 6H_2O$), ferrous chloride tetrahydrate ($FeCl_2 \cdot 4H_2O$), sodium chloride (NaCl), potassium chloride (KCl), sodium hydrogenphosphate (Na_2HPO_4), potassium dihydrogen phosphate (KH_2PO_4), dopamine hydrochloride (DA·HCl), bovine serum albumine (BSA), cetyl trimethylammonium bromide (CTAB), *N*-(3 dimethylaminopropyl)-*N′*-ethylcarbodiimide hydrochloride (EDC·HCl), hydrochloric acid (HCl, 37%), sodium hydroxide (NaOH), and paclitaxel (PTX) were purchased from Sigma Aldrich (St. Louis, MO, USA). Oleic acid ≥85% and sodium oleate were purchased from Tokyo Chemical Industry (TCI), Tokyo, Japan. Sodium hyaluronate (5400 Da) was purchased from Lifecore Biomedical, Inc., Chaska, MN, USA.

Materials: Dialysis sacks were purchased from Sigma Aldrich (MWCO: 12,000 Da) (St. Louis, MO, USA) and from SpectrumLabs (Spectra/Por 3 Dialysis Tubing, MWCO: 3500 Da). Syringe filters (25 mm, 0.22 μm) were purchased from VWR International, Milan, Italy.

4.2. Synthetic Procedures

4.2.1. Synthesis of BSA-DA Adduct

The reaction flask was obscured to prevent denaturation of the BSA protein. First, 250 mg of BSA were dissolved in 20 mL of PBS buffer solution (NaCl 137 mM, KCl 3 mM, Na_2HPO_4 10 mM and KH_2PO_4 2 mM. pH = 7.4). Then 527.5 mg of 1-ethyl-3-(3′-dimethyl-aminopropyl)-carbodiimide (EDC) were added, under magnetic stirring. After a few minutes, 500 mg of dopamine hydrochloride were added to the solution, which rapidly became darker. The reaction lasted 20 h. The final mixture was dialyzed against several changes (6 × 1 L) of PBS buffer solution (MWCO: 12,000 Da). The recovered mixture was analyzed by MALDI–TOF.

4.2.2. Synthesis of HA-DA Adduct

The first 250 mg of Sodium Hyaluronate (5400 Da) were dissolved with 20 mL of PBS solution (pH = 7.4). A few drops of aqueous solution of HCl (1M) were added to adjust the pH to the value of 5–5.5. Then, 120 mg of Dopamine hydrochloride and 100 mg of EDC were added. The pH of the solution rapidly increased up to 8.0, and several drops of HCl 1M were added to the solution over time in order to keep the pH values between 5.0 and 6.0 during the reaction time (3 h). After 3 h, the pH no longer increased and the reaction was considered finished. The final mixture was dialyzed against several changes (3 × 1 L) of PBS buffer solution (MWCO: 3500 Da).

4.2.3. Synthesis of Fe_3O_4·OA Nanoparticles (SPION1)

The magnetite gel was formulated by coprecipitation. First, 3.44 g of $FeCl_2·4H_2O$ and 9.40 g of $FeCl_3·6H_2O$ were dissolved in 160 mL of distilled water under nitrogen gas with vigorous stirring, at 80 °C for 30 min. Next a mixture composed of 24 mL of NH_4OH solution (25% NH_3 in H_2O), 4 mL of oleic acid, and 4 mL of acetone was slowly added to the solution. The color of the reaction mixture immediately turned to black. Stirring lasted 30 min and then the solution was heated again, to 80 °C, for 30 min. Fe_3O_4·OA nanoparticle precipitation was promoted by adding 200 mL of EtOH 99% and putting a magnet under the reaction flask. The transparent liquid phase was removed and the recovered black solid material was dissolved in hexane (150 mL) and reprecipitated with ethanol (200 mL), with the simultaneous promoted magnetic sedimentation. After the removal of liquid supernatant, a last washing of the nanoparticles was performed by using acetone in an ultrasonic bath for 10 min. The SPIONs were collected and dissolved in hexane, a solvent that allows their storage for a long time avoiding any aggregation phenomena. The chemical structure of dried Fe_3O_4·OA nanoparticles (SPION1) was investigated by FTIR analysis; TEM and DLS characterization was also performed.

4.2.4. Synthesis of Fe_3O_4·DA-BSA/HA Nanoparticles (SPION2, SPION3, SPION4)

Once DA-BSA and DA-HA adducts were prepared, the exchange reaction between them and the oleic acid coating of nanoparticles was performed in a one-step procedure. In addition, 100 mg Fe_3O_4·OA (SPION1) were dispersed in 7 mL of chloroform. These dispersed nanoparticles were added to a solution of 1.33 g of cetyl trimethylammonium bromide (CTAB) in 66.5 mL of PBS buffer. Chloroform was carefully removed under reduced pressure. Suspended Fe_3O_4·OA nanoparticles were added, drop by drop and under vigorous stirring, to different mixtures of dissolved DA-BSA and DA-HA adducts in PBS (50:50, 80:20 and 90:10, respectively) in order to perform the ligand exchange reaction, resulting in the samples SPION2, SPION3, and SPION4, respectively. The products were soluble in PBS and the solid CTAB and the oil had to be discarded through centrifugation (9000 rpm, 30 min, r.t.). The final mixtures were dialyzed against several changes (3 × 1 L) of PBS buffer solution (MWCO: 12,000 Da). The samples were characterized with FTIR, DLS, and TEM and then submitted to further evaluations by means of TD-NMR experiments.

4.2.5. Inclusion of PTX in Fe_3O_4·DA-BSA/HA Nanoparticles (SPION5, SPION6)

An aliquot of milky aqueous dispersion of paclitaxel (0.5 mg/mL) was added to Fe_3O_4·DA-BSA/HA NPs (SPION2 or SPION3) within a starting volumetric ratio of 1:1 (*v/v*). The preparation was sonicated for 10 min. Then, a further aliquot of NPs was added, with a final 1:3 (*v/v*) ratio (PTX:NPs). After a further sonication of 10 min, the system was maintained for approximately 48 h under constant stirring.

4.3. Characterization Methods

4.3.1. Fourier Transform Infrared Spectroscopy (FTIR)

The solid phase FTIR spectra of the powdered sample with infrared grade KBr were generated using an ALPHA spectrometer (Bruker, Bremen, Germany). Data were analyzed using OPUS software, version 7.0 (Bruker, Bremen, Germany).

4.3.2. Transmission Electron Microscopy (TEM)

TEM micrographs and selected area electron diffraction (SAED) patterns were acquired using a Philips CM200 Field emission gun transmission electron microscope (Koninklijke Philips N.V., Eindhoven NETHERLANDS) operating at 200 kV. The suspensions of iron oxide nanoparticles and supraparticles were deposited onto a 200 mesh holey carbon-coated copper grid and let dry a few hours before the analysis. Image analyses of TEM micrographs were performed using ImageJ software, Research Services Branch (RSB) of the National Institute of Mental Health (NIMH) [53], which is quite useful for estimating the dimension and shape of nanoparticles and supraparticles. In particular, the mean values and widths of the statistical asymmetric distribution ($\sigma-$, $\sigma+$) of particles were evaluated by fitting the experimental values with a log-normal function (Table S4).

4.3.3. Dynamic Light Scattering (DLS)

Hydrodynamic diameter (Z_{av}) and zeta potential (ξ) values of nanosystems were measured using the Zetasizer Nano ZS (Malvern, Worcestershire, UK) with a fixed 173° scattering angle and a 633-nm-helium-neon-laser. Data were analyzed using Zetasizer software, version 7.11 (Malvern, Worcestershire, UK). The temperature was set at 298 K. SPION1 was collected from the bulk mixture after the first dispersion with hexane and directly submitted to DLS measurement. SPION2 and SPION3 were passed through a 0.22 µm syringe filter, sonicated for 10 min, and then submitted to DLS measurements. SPION5 and SPION6 were directly collected and analyzed after 10 min of sonication.

4.3.4. MALDI–TOF Measurements

Measurements of BSA samples and their corresponding dopamine derivatives were performed using an UV-MALDI–TOF Autoflex mass spectrometer (Bruker, Bremen, Germany) equipped with an ultraviolet laser (λ = 232 nm) operating in linear and positive ion mode in the mass range from 10 to 150 kDa. Each spectrum was recorded by averaging about 300 shots after appropriate mass range calibration performed with commercial standard proteins mixture (trypsinogen, protein A, albumin-bovine). The matrix solution, used either for analytes or standard proteins solution, was freshly prepared as a saturated solution of sinapinic acid (SA) in water 0.1% TFA:acetonitrile 2:1 (*v*/*v*). The analyte solutions were prepared at a concentration of 5–7 mg/mL in water (corresponding to about 100 pmol/µL of BSA protein) and mixed with the matrix solution in a 1:1 (*v*/*v*) ratio; then, 1 µL of this matrix/analyte mixture was loaded on the stainless steel probe and left to dry at room temperature.

4.3.5. HPLC/Mass Spectrometry Measurements

Analyses of hyaluronic acid and its dopamine derivative were performed on an HPLC system (Platin Blue, Knauer, Berlin, Germany) coupled to ESI-Q-TOF mass spectrometer (impact II, Bruker). Because of the polyanionic nature of hyaluronic acid, chromatographic separation of the numerous components contained in extremely complex mixture of the hyaluronic acid sample was performed by ion pairing reversed-phase liquid chromatography (IP RP LC method) using alkylamine for ion pairing.

The sample solution was prepared at a concentration of 1 mg/mL. 2 µL were injected on a 2.1 × 100 mm Kinetex reversed-phase C18 column with 2.6 µm particles (Phenomenex, Aschaffenburg, Germany) hold at 35 °C and run at a flow rate of 0.15 mL/min, by the mobile phases A (dibutylamine 10 mM, acetic acid 10 mM in water) and B (dibutylamine 10 mM, acetic acid 10 mM in methanol) according to the following gradient: isocratic step at 10% B for 5 min, followed by a first linear gradient from 10% to 31% B in 30 min and a second slower gradient from 31% to 45% B in 30 min; then, column washing at 90% B for 5 min and reconditioning in the initial conditions were performed.

The mass spectrometry detector was set to negative polarity (capillary voltage: +3500 V) in the mass range from *m*/*z* 140 to *m*/*z* 2500; nitrogen gas used as nebulizer and heater gases was set at 1.8 bar and 7.0 L/min, respectively.

Mass calibration was performed by using sodium formate solution (water–isopropanol 1:1 *v*/*v* solution containing HCOOH 0.2% and NaOH 5×10^{-3} N).

4.3.6. NMR Experiments

NMR spectra were recorded at 30 °C using a Bruker Avance HD spectrometer (500 MHz) equipped with a high sensitivity 5 mm TCI cryoprobe. Samples were dissolved in ^2H_2O (99.996%) and in 0.5 M NaCl, pH 7.4 and placed in 5-mm NMR tubes. Proton spectra were recorded with presaturation of the residual water signal with a recycle delay of 12 s and 8–16 scans. Bidimensional double quantum filter-COSY and two-dimensional Total Correlation Spectroscopy (TOCSY) spectra were acquired using 16 scans per series of 2048_320 data points with zero filling in F1 and F2 (4096_2048), and a shifted ($\pi/2$) squared cosine function was applied prior to Fourier transformation.

Heteronuclear single quantum coherence (HSQC) spectra were obtained in phase sensitivity-enhanced pure absorption mode with decoupling in the acquisition period and 24 scans while heteronuclear multiple bond correlation spectra (HMBC) were obtained with 64 scans. The matrix size of both experiments was 1024_320 data points and was zero-filled to 4096_2048 by application of a shifted ($\pi/2$) squared cosine function prior to Fourier transformation. Diffusion-ordered spectroscopy (DOSY) spectra were acquired using 32 scans and a series of 16 spin echo spectra registered with a time domain of 16 K zero-filled to 64 K.

4.3.7. ICP Experiments

For the experiments, 14.4 mg of both SPION2 and SPION3 (obtained by lyofilization) were mineralized with nitric acid (HNO_3) and subsequently analyzed using inductively coupled plasma (ICP) spectrometry. The employed instrument was a Perkin Elmer Optica 2300 (Perkin Elmer, Milan, Italy).

4.3.8. Time-Domain (TD) NMR Experiments

A 0.5 T Bruker Minispec was used for relaxometry. This instrument is a low-resolution NMR spectrometer with proton larmor frequency of 19.65 MHz, equipped with static probe and a BVT3000 temperature control unit working with nitrogen gas. The temperature was calibrated using an external thermometer with an accuracy of ± 1 K. The precision was 0.1 K; in these conditions, the temperature is stable within that range during the measurement.

All of the experiments were performed at a temperature of 303 K (29.85 °C), obtained using a Eurotherm nitrogen gas thermal apparatus (Como, Italy). Samples were prepared outside the NMR tube, and then 150 µL of each solution was inserted in a 10 mm o.d. tube, positioned in the magnet with the sample in the volume of maximum homogeneity of the B_0 and B_1 fields. All of the samples were thermalized for 10 minutes before performing the experiments.

For the $\pi/2$ and π, the pulse lengths were set to 2.07 µs and 4.15 µs, respectively. A good signal-to-noise ratio was obtained within a few scans, but due to the analytical nature of this work, each sample was measured with 128 scans during Carr–Purcell–Meiboom–Gill (CPMG) experiments and 64 scans per point during saturation recovery experiments.

For T_2 measurements, we made use of CPMG pulse sequence with parameters optimized for analytical use at low field [54]. This sequence consisted of a first 90° pulse followed by a train of equally spaced 180° pulses. The signal is measured in the midpoint between each pair of 180° pulses and the obtained decaying curve is fitted against $A\ \exp(-t/T_2)$.

For T_1, we implemented a saturation recovery sequence [55], a sequence composed by a pulse train that is optimized for defocusing the magnetization of the sample. Longitudinal magnetization was then measured using a single $\pi/2$ pulse after a set waiting time. Signal recovery as a function of time was then interpreted using the following equation:

$$M_z = M_0\left[1 - exp\left(-\frac{t}{T_1}\right)\right]. \tag{1}$$

4.4. *PTX-Release Experiments*

SPION6 (4 mL) was placed in a dialysis sack (MWCO: 3500 Da) and dialyzed against 30 mL of mixture containing 70% PBS buffer and 30% methanol. The experiment was conducted in a shaking water bath (SW22, Julabo) at room temperature and with a shaking frequency of 100 rpm. The amount of released PTX over time was monitored through quantitative UV-Vis (UV-spectrophotometer JASCO v-650; Cremella LC, Italy), SpectraManager software (Cremella LC, Italy). Several aliquots of dialysate mixture were collected at different times and immediately submitted to UV acquisitions, and then replaced in the mixture of the dialysis experiment. The calibration curve employed for the quantitative conversion of data over time was taken from existing literature ($y = 0.04x - 0.0626$; $R^2 = 0.9931$) [56,57].

4.5. In Vitro MRI

SPION3, SPION 4 and dilutions of those samples were scanned using a 9.4 T preclinical MRI scanner (Bruker, Bremen, Germany). Echo Time (TE) and Repetition Time (TR): TR/TE = 3000/60.

5. Conclusions

Our work was successful in identifying the synthetic strategy to obtain Fe_3O_4·DA-BSA/HA of 70–90 nm size containing different iron cores of 5 nm, quite homogenous and capable to afford well-dispersed and stable colloidal system. The synthetic strategy is quite easy, reproducible and up-scalable. Huge efforts were successfully done to modulate Fe_3O_4·DA-BSA/HA both in terms of the ratio between the inorganic core and the bioorganic layer, and the ratio between bovine serum albumin (BSA) and hyaluronic acid (HA) content in the bioorganic layer. Great attention was dedicated to structural and morphological characterization aspects. Fe_3O_4·DA-BSA/HA was capable of entrapping paclitaxel (PTX). Its physical-chemical characterization and preliminary release tests open the way to use Fe_3O_4·DA-BSA/HA as PTX delivery system. Noteworthy, Fe_3O_4·DA-BSA/HA increased the PTX bioavailability. Fe_3O_4·DA-BSA/HA gave good results in TD-NMR experiments to demonstrating their suitability to be developed as contrast agents in MRI.

Acknowledgments: Blerina Gjocka (Politecnico) and Gabriele Colombo (Ronzoni) for experimental works; Cesare Cosentino for NMR experiments. Bioiberica S.A., Barcelona Spain, for the contribution to the publication costs. Edith Suss-Toby, Ortal Schwartz and or Perlman for the professional assistance with the MRI experiments. La presente pubblicazione è stata realizzata con il contributo del Ministero degli Affari Esteri (MAE), Italy. (MAE, partial funding QUADRUGNOSTIC Project, MAE02674642013-11-27, bilateral project with Technion Department of Biotechnology and Food Engineering, Technion-Israel Institute of Technology, Haifa, 32000, Israel).

Author Contributions: E.V. was the main researcher, scientifically responsible and the supervisor of the MAE project. C.B., A.C. were devoted to synthesis, characterisation aspects, results and discussion. A.S. conducted the TEM experiments and wrote the discussion. M.M.R.S. was an expert researcher for the TD-NMR experiments and the discussion. S.B. was an expert researcher for DLS, Zeta Potential analysis, NMR experiments and the discussion. E.U. was an expert researcher for NMR and MALDI-TOF experiments and the discussion. R.E. conducted the in vitro MRI experiments. Y.G.A. was the Israeli partner involved in project conception and biological aspect supervision. Y.D.L. was the Israeli principal investigator and a partner from project conception, who was also responsible for the scientific co-supervision of the project.

References

1. Pelaz, B.; Alexiou, C.; Alvarez-Puebla, R.A.; Alves, F.; Andrews, A.M.; Ashraf, S.; Balogh, L.P.; Ballerini, L.; Bestetti, A.; Brendel, C.; et al. Diverse applications of nanomedicine. *ACS Nano* **2017**, *11*, 2313–2381. [CrossRef] [PubMed]
2. Sapsford, K.E.; Algar, W.R.; Berti, L.; Gemmill, K.B.; Casey, B.J.; Oh, E.; Stewart, M.H.; Medintz, I.L. Functionalizing nanoparticles with biological molecules: Developing chemistries that facilitate nanotechnology. *Chem. Rev.* **2013**, *113*, 1904–2074. [CrossRef] [PubMed]
3. Laurent, S.; Forge, D.; Port, M.; Roch, A.; Robic, C.; Vander Elst, L.; Muller, R.N. Magnetic iron oxide nanoparticles: Synthesis, stabilization, vectorization, physicochemical characterizations, and biological applications. *Chem. Rev.* **2008**, *108*, 2064–2110. [CrossRef] [PubMed]
4. Tartaj, P.; Morales, M.P.; Veintemillas-Verdaguer, S.; Gonzalez-Carreno, T.; Serna, C.G. Synthesis, properties and biomedical applications of magnetic nanoparticles. *Handb. Magn. Mater.* **2006**, *16*, 403–482.
5. Ramimoghadam, D.; Bagheri, S.; Hamid, S.B.A. Stable monodisperse nanomagnetic colloidal suspensions: An overview. *Colloids Surf. B Biointerfaces* **2015**, *133*, 388–411. [CrossRef] [PubMed]

6. Iyer, S.R.; Xu, S.; Stains, J.P.; Bennett, C.H.; Lovering, R.M. Superparamagnetic iron oxide nanoparticles in musculoskeletal biology. *Tissue Eng. Part B Rev.* **2017**. [CrossRef] [PubMed]
7. Gupta, A.K.; Gupta, M. Synthesis and surface engineering of iron oxide nanoparticles for biomedical applications. *Biomaterials* **2005**, *26*, 3995–4021. [CrossRef] [PubMed]
8. Gupta, A.K.; Naregalkar, R.R.; Vaidya, V.D.; Gupta, M. Recent advances on surface engineering of magnetic iron oxide nanoparticles and their biomedical applications. *Nanomedcine* **2007**, *2*, 23–39. [CrossRef] [PubMed]
9. Bertini, S.; Ferro, M.; Pizzolato, D.; Torri, G.; Valerio, A.; Vismara, E. Low molecular weight heparin-vectorized beta-cyclodextrin nanostructures. In Proceedings of the NSTI Nanotech Nanotechnology Conference and Trade Show, Technical Proceedings, Boston, MA, USA, 1–5 June 2008; Laudon, M., Romanowicz, B., Eds.; CRC Press: Boca Raton, FL, USA, 2008; Volume 2, pp. 487–490.
10. Bava, A.; Cappellini, F.; Pedretti, E.; Rossi, F.; Caruso, E.; Vismara, E.; Chiriva-Internati, M.; Bernardini, G.; Gornati, R. Heparin and carboxymethylchitosan metal nanoparticles: An evaluation of their cytotoxicity. *Biomed. Res. Int.* **2013**, *2013*, 1–10. [CrossRef] [PubMed]
11. Vismara, E.; Valerio, A.; Coletti, A.; Torri, G.; Bertini, S.; Eisele, G.; Gornati, R.; Bernardini, G. Non-covalent synthesis of metal oxide nanoparticle–heparin hybrid systems: A new approach to bioactive nanoparticles. *Int. J. Mol. Sci.* **2013**, *14*, 13463–13481. [CrossRef] [PubMed]
12. Huber, D.L. Synthesis, properties, and applications of iron nanoparticles. *Small* **2005**, *1*, 482–501. [CrossRef] [PubMed]
13. Gossuin, Y.; Gillis, P.; Hocq, A.; Vuong, Q.L.; Roch, A. Magnetic resonance relaxation properties of superparamagnetic particles. *Wiley Interdiscip. Rev. Nanomed. Nanobiotechnol.* **2009**, *1*, 299–310. [CrossRef]
14. Wei, H.; Bruns, O.T.; Kaul, M.G.; Hansen, E.C.; Barch, M.; Wiśniowska, A.; Chen, O.; Chen, Y.; Li, N.; Okada, S.; et al. Exceedingly small iron oxide nanoparticles as positive MRI contrast agents. *Proc. Natl. Acad. Sci. USA* **2017**, *114*, 2325–2330. [CrossRef] [PubMed]
15. Singha, N.; Jenkins, G.J.S.; Asadib, R.; Doaka, S.H. Potential toxicity of superparamagnetic iron oxide nanoparticles (SPION). *Nano Rev.* **2010**, *1*, 5358. [CrossRef] [PubMed]
16. Zaloga, J.; Janko, C.; Nowak, J.; Matuszak, J.; Knaup, S.; Eberbeck, D.; Tietze, R.; Unterweger, H.; Friedrich, R.P.; Duerr, S. Development of a lauric acid/albumin hybrid iron oxide nanoparticle system with improved biocompatibility. *Int. J. Nanomed.* **2014**, *9*, 4847–4866. [CrossRef] [PubMed]
17. Poller, J.M.; Zaloga, J.; Schreiber, E.; Unterweger, H.; Janko, C.; Radon, P.; Eberbeck, D.; Trahms, L.; Alexiou, C.; Friedrich, R.P. Selection of potential iron oxide nanoparticles for breast cancer treatment based on in vitro cytotoxicity and cellular uptake. *Int. J. Nanomed.* **2017**, *12*, 3207–3220. [CrossRef] [PubMed]
18. Shapira, A.; Livney, Y.D.; Broxterman, H.J.; Assaraf, Y.G. Nanomedicine for targeted cancer therapy: Towards the overcoming of drug resistance. *Drug Resist. Updat.* **2011**, *14*, 150–163. [CrossRef] [PubMed]
19. Livney, Y.D.; Assaraf, Y.G. Rationally designed nanovehicles to overcome cancer chemoresistance. *Adv. Drug Deliv. Rev.* **2013**, *65*, 1716–1730. [CrossRef]
20. Wang, Y.X.J. Superparamagnetic iron oxide based MRI contrast agents: Current status of clinical application. *Quant. Imaging Med. Surg.* **2011**, *1*, 35–40. [PubMed]
21. Bakhtiary, Z.; Saei, A.A.; Hajipour, M.J.; Raoufi, M.; Vermesh, O.; Mahmoudi, M. Targeted superparamagnetic iron oxide nanoparticles for early detection of cancer: Possibilities and challenges. *Nanomedicine* **2016**, *12*, 287–307. [CrossRef] [PubMed]
22. Barua, S.; Mitragotri, S. Challenges associated with penetration of nanoparticles across cell and tissue barriers: A review of current status and future prospects. *Nano Today* **2014**, *9*, 223–243. [CrossRef] [PubMed]
23. Journo-Gershfeld, G.; Kapp, D.; Shamay, Y.; Kopecek, J.; David, A. Hyaluronan oligomers-HPMA copolymer conjugates for targeting paclitaxel to CD44-overexpressing ovarian carcinoma. *Pharm. Res.* **2012**, *29*, 1121–1133. [CrossRef] [PubMed]
24. Choi, K.Y.; Chung, H.; Min, K.H.; Yoon, H.Y.; Kim, K.; Park, J.H.; Kwon, I.C.; Jeong, S.Y. Self-assembled hyaluronic acid nanoparticles for active tumor targeting. *Biomaterials* **2010**, *1*, 106–114. [CrossRef] [PubMed]
25. Misra, S.; Heldin, P.; Hascall, V.C.; Karamanos, N.K.; Skandalis, S.S.; Markwald, R.R.; Ghatak, S. HA/CD44 interactions as potential targets for cancer therapy. *FEBS J.* **2011**, *278*, 1429–1443. [CrossRef] [PubMed]
26. Unterweger, H.; Tietze, R.; Janko, C.; Zaloga, J.; Lyer, S.; Dürr, S.; Taccardi, N.; Goudouri, O.M.; Hoppe, A.; Eberbeck, D.; et al. Development and characterization of magnetic iron oxide nanoparticles with a cisplatin-bearing polymer coating for targeted drug delivery. *Int. J. Nanomed.* **2014**, *9*, 3659–3676. [CrossRef] [PubMed]

27. Li, H.; Yan, K.; Shang, Y.; Shrestha, L.; Liao, R.; Liu, F.; Li, P.; Xu, H.; Xu, Z.; Chu, P.K. Folate-bovine serum albumin functionalized polymeric micelles loaded with superparamagnetic iron oxide nanoparticles for tumor targeting and magnetic resonance imaging. *Acta Biomater.* **2015**, *15*, 117–126. [CrossRef] [PubMed]
28. Zhang, B.; Li, Q.; Yin, P.; Rui, Y.; Qiu, Y.; Wang, Y.; Shi, D. Ultrasound-triggered BSA/SPION hybrid nanoclusters for liver-specific magnetic resonance imaging. *ACS Appl. Mater. Interfaces* **2012**, *4*, 6479–6486. [CrossRef] [PubMed]
29. Lv, W.; Cheng, L.; Li, B. Development and evaluation of a novel TPGS-mediated paclitaxel-loaded PLGA-mPEG nanoparticle for the treatment of ovarian cancer. *Chem. Pharm. Bull.* **2015**, *63*, 68–74. [CrossRef] [PubMed]
30. Wang, W.; Wang, M.; Zhang, J.; Liu, H.; Pan, H. Cloud point thermodynamics of paclitaxel-loaded microemulsion in the presence of glucose and NaCl. *Colloids Surf. A Physicochem. Eng. Asp.* **2016**, *507*, 76–82. [CrossRef]
31. Sharma, S.; Singh, J.; Verma, A.; Teja, B.V.; Shukla, R.P.; Singh, S.K.; Sharma, V.; Konwarb, R.; Mishra, P.R. Hyaluronic acid anchored paclitaxel nanocrystals improves chemotherapeutic efficacy and inhibits lung metastasis in tumor-bearing rat model. *RSC Adv.* **2016**, *6*, 73083–73095. [CrossRef]
32. Zaloga, J.; Pöttler, M.; Leitinger, G.; Friedrich, R.P.; Almer, G.; Lyer, S.; Baum, E.; Tietze, R.; Heimke-Brinck, R.; Mangge, H.; et al. Pharmaceutical formulation of HSA hybrid coated iron oxide nanoparticles for magnetic drug targeting. *Eur. J. Pharm. Biopharm.* **2016**, *101*, 152–162. [CrossRef] [PubMed]
33. McWhirter, M.J.; Bremer, P.J.; Lamont, I.L.; McQuillan, A.J. Siderophore-mediated covalent bonding to metal (oxide) surfaces during biofilm initiation by pseudomonas aeruginosa bacteria. *Langmuir* **2003**, *19*, 3575–3577. [CrossRef]
34. Delina, J.; Rodriguez, R.D.; Verma, A.; Pousaneh, E.; Zahn, D.R.T.; Lang, H.; Chandra, S. Electrochemistry and surface-enhanced Raman spectroscopy of CTAB modulated interactions of magnetic nanoparticles with biomolecules. *RSC Adv.* **2017**, *7*, 3628–3634.
35. Caillé, J.M.; Lemanceau, B.; Bonnemain, B. Gadolinium as a contrast agent for NMR. *AJNR Am. J. Neuroradiol.* **1983**, *4*, 1041–1042. [PubMed]
36. Choi, H.S.; Liu, W.; Misra, P.; Tanaka, E.; Zimmer, J.P.; Itty Ipe, B.; Bawendi, M.G.; Frangioni, J.V. Renal clearance of quantum dots. *Nat. Biotechnol.* **2007**, *25*, 1165–1170. [CrossRef] [PubMed]
37. Blanco, E.; Shen, H.; Ferrari, M. Principles of nanoparticle design for overcoming biological barriers to drug delivery. *Nat. Biotechnol.* **2015**, *33*, 941–951. [CrossRef] [PubMed]
38. Bianchi, A.; Mauri, M.; Bonetti, S.; Koynov, K.; Kappl, M.; Lieberwirth, I.; Butt, H.J.; Simonutti, R. Hierarchical self-assembly of PDMA-b-PS chains into granular nanoparticles: Genesis and fate. *Macromol. Rapid Commun.* **2014**, *35*, 1994–1999. [CrossRef] [PubMed]
39. Skouras, A.; Mourtas, S.; Markoutsa, E.; de Goltstein, M.C.; Wallon, C.; Catoen, S.; Antimisiaris, S.G. Magnetoliposomes with high USPIO entrapping efficiency, stability and magnetic properties. *Nanomedicine* **2011**, *7*, 572–579. [CrossRef] [PubMed]
40. Nichols, J.W.; Bae, Y.H. EPR: Evidence and fallacy. *J. Control. Release* **2014**, *190*, 451–464. [CrossRef] [PubMed]
41. Xie, J.; Chen, K.; Huang, J.; Lee, S.; Wang, J.; Gao, J.; Li, X.; Chen, X. PET/NIRF/MRI triple functional iron oxide nanoparticles. *Biomaterials* **2010**, *31*, 3016–3022. [CrossRef] [PubMed]
42. Xu, C.; Xu, K.; Gu, H.; Zheng, R.; Liu, H.; Zhang, X.; Gu, Z.; Xu, B. Dopamine as a robust anchor to immobilize functional molecules on the iron oxide shell of magnetic nanoparticles. *J. Am. Chem. Soc.* **2004**, *126*, 9938–9939. [CrossRef] [PubMed]
43. Lee, Y.; Lee, H.; Kim, Y.B.; Kim, J.; Hyeon, T.; Park, H.; Messersmith, P.B.; Park, T.G. Bioinspired surface immobilization of hyaluronic acid on monodisperse magnetite nanocrystals for targeted cancer imaging. *Adv. Mater.* **2008**, *20*, 4154–4157. [CrossRef] [PubMed]
44. Montalbetti, C.A.G.N.; Falque, V. Amide bond formation and peptide coupling. *Tetrahedron* **2005**, *61*, 10827–10852. [CrossRef]
45. Zhang, L.; He, R.; Gu, H.C. Oleic acid coating on the monodisperse magnetite nanoparticles. *Appl. Surf. Sci.* **2006**, *253*, 2611–2617. [CrossRef]
46. Liu, X.; Kaminski, M.D.; Guan, Y.; Chen, H.; Liu, H.; Rosengart, A.J. Preparation and characterization of hydrophobic superparamagnetic magnetite gel. *J. Magn. Magn. Mater.* **2006**, *306*, 248–253. [CrossRef]

47. Wang, X.; Tilley, R.D.; Watkins, J.J. Simple ligand exchange reactions enabling excellent dispersibility and stability of magnetic nanoparticles in polar organic, aromatic, and protic solvents. *Langmuir* **2014**, *30*, 1514–1521. [CrossRef] [PubMed]
48. Ruttala, H.B.; Ramasamy, T.; Shin, B.S.; Cho, H.-C.; Yong, C.S.; Kim, J.O. Layer-by-layer assembly of hierarchical nanoarchitectures to enhance the systemic performance of nanoparticle albumin-bound paclitaxel. *Int. J. Pharm.* **2017**, *519*, 11–21. [CrossRef] [PubMed]
49. Heslinga, M.J.; Willis, G.M.; Sobczynski, D.J.; Thompson, A.J.; Eniola-Adefeso, O. One-step fabrication of agent-loaded biodegradable microspheroids for drug delivery and imaging applications. *Colloids Surf. B Biointerfaces* **2014**, *116*, 55–62. [CrossRef] [PubMed]
50. Liang, Y.; Qiao, Y.; Guo, S.; Wang, L.; Xie, C.; Zhai, Y.; Deng, L.; Donga, A. Thermoreversible gelation of poly(ethylene glycol)/poly(ester anhydride) triblock copolymer nanoparticles for injectable drug delivery systems. *Soft Matter* **2010**, *6*, 1915–1922. [CrossRef]
51. Tanei, T.; Leonard, F.; Liu, X.; Alexander, J.F.; Saito, Y. Redirecting Transport of Nanoparticle Albumin-Bound Paclitaxel to Macrophages Enhances Therapeutic Efficacy against Liver Metastases. *Cancer Res.* **2016**, *76*, 429–439. [CrossRef] [PubMed]
52. Chen, Q.; Wang, X.; Wang, C.; Feng, L.; Li, Y.; Liu, Z. Drug-Induced Self-Assembly of Modified Albumins as Nano-Theranostics for Tumor-Targeted Combination Therapy. *ACS Nano* **2015**, *9*, 5223–5233. [CrossRef] [PubMed]
53. Schneider, C.A.; Rasband, W.S.; Eliceiri, K.W. NIH Image to ImageJ: 25 years of image analysis. *Nat. Methods* **2012**, *9*, 671–675. [CrossRef] [PubMed]
54. Mauri, M.; Mauri, L.; Causin, V.; Simonutti, R. A method based on time domain nuclear magnetic resonance for the forensic differentiation of latex gloves. *Anal. Methods* **2011**, *3*, 1802–1809. [CrossRef]
55. Braun, S.; Kalinowski, H.O.; Berger, S. *150 and More Basic NMR Experiments: A Practical Course*, 2nd ed.; Wiley-VCH: Weinheim, Germany, 1998; p. 295.
56. Zhang, M.; Yilmaz, T.; Boztas, A.O.; Karakuzu, O.; Bang, W.Y.; Yegin, Y.; Luo, Z.; Lenox, M.; Cisneros-Zevallos, L.; Akbulut, M. A multifunctional nanoparticulate theranostic system with simultaneous chemotherapeutic, photothermal therapeutic, and MRI contrast capabilities. *RSC Adv.* **2016**, *6*, 27798–27806. [CrossRef]
57. Kesharwani, P.; Jain, K.; Tekade, R.K.; Gajbhiye, V.; Jain, N.K. Spectrophotometric estimation of paclitaxel. *Int. J. Adv. Pharm. Sci.* **2011**, *2*, 29–32.

10

Extended Physicochemical Characterization of the Synthetic Anticoagulant Pentasaccharide Fondaparinux Sodium by Quantitative NMR and Single Crystal X-Ray Analysis

William de Wildt [1], Huub Kooijman [2], Carel Funke [1], Bülent Üstün [1], Afranina Leika [1], Maarten Lunenburg [1], Frans Kaspersen [1] and Edwin Kellenbach [1,*]

1 DTS Aspen Oss B.V., 5223BB Oss, The Netherlands; wdewildt@nl.aspenpharma.com (W.d.W.); i.funke@kpnplanet.nl (C.F.); bustun@nl.aspenpharma.com (B.Ü.); aleika@nl.aspenpharma.com (A.L.); mlunenburg@nl.aspenpharma.com (M.L.); fmkaspersen@hotmail.com (F.K.)

2 Bijvoet Center for Biomolecular Research, Crystal and Structural Chemistry, Faculty of Science, Utrecht University, Padualaan 8, 3584 CH Utrecht, The Netherlands; Huub.Kooijman@shell.com

* Correspondence: ekellenbach@nl.aspenpharma.com

Abstract: Fondaparinux sodium is a synthetic pentasaccharide representing the high affinity antithrombin III binding site in heparin. It is the active pharmaceutical ingredient of the anticoagulant drug Arixtra®. The single crystal X-ray structure of Fondaparinux sodium is reported, unequivocally confirming both structure and absolute configuration. The iduronic acid adopts a somewhat distorted chair conformation. Due to the presence of many sulfur atoms in the highly sulfated pentasaccharide, anomalous dispersion could be applied to determine the absolute configuration. A comparison with the conformation of Fondaparinux in solution, as well as complexed with proteins is presented. The content of the solution reference standard was determined by quantitative NMR using an internal standard both in 1999 and in 2016. A comparison of the results allows the conclusion that this method shows remarkable precision over time, instrumentation and analysts.

Keywords: Fondaparinux sodium; extended physicochemical characterization; qNMR; single crystal X-ray structure; reference standard; iduronic acid conformation; Arixtra®

1. Introduction

Fondaparinux sodium (referred to as 'Fondaparinux' in this article; Figure 1) is a synthetic pentasaccharide [1] derived from the high affinity antithrombin III binding site in heparin, modified by a methyl group at the reducing end. It is the active pharmaceutical ingredient of GSK's anticoagulant drug Arixtra® and a selective aXa inhibitor through antithrombin III [2] and lacks aIIa activity as a result of its low molecular weight. As part of the extended physical characterization of Fondaparinux, both structure (by X-ray) and standard content (by qNMR) are described in this paper. The X-ray structures of Fondaparinux have previously been limited to co-crystals in complex with a number of proteins [3–8]. Also, related synthetic (penta) saccharides complexed with protein have been reported [9,10]. Furthermore, uncomplexed Fondaparinux (solution) structures determined by (a combination of) theoretical calculations and NMR spectroscopy have been described [11–15]. In solution, $^3J(^1H, ^1H)$ coupling constants allow to determine the conformation of the pyranose residues in heparin. The glucosamine and glucuronic acids residues adopt a stable $^4C_1$-conformation. However, the iduronate ring adopts $^1C_4$ and $^2S_0$ conformations rapidly interconverting on the NMR time scale [11,12]. Complexation by proteins locks the iduronate residue in a single $^2S_0$ conformation both in the crystal [5,6,9,10] and in solution [16]. Also in the crystal of uncomplexed Fondaparinux, the occurrence of a single iduronate conformation is foreseen. Here we report the X-ray single crystal structure of uncomplexed Fondaparinux and compare it to the conformation of Fondaparinux in solution, as well as complexed with proteins.

The content of ampoules of the Fondaparinux solution reference standard was determined in both 1999 and 2016 by quantitative NMR (qNMR) using an internal standard. The results of both determinations are discussed here. The ampoules of this standard are used to determine the Fondaparinux content of Fondaparinux batches. For consistency, the ability to assure the long-term stability of the standard content is crucial.

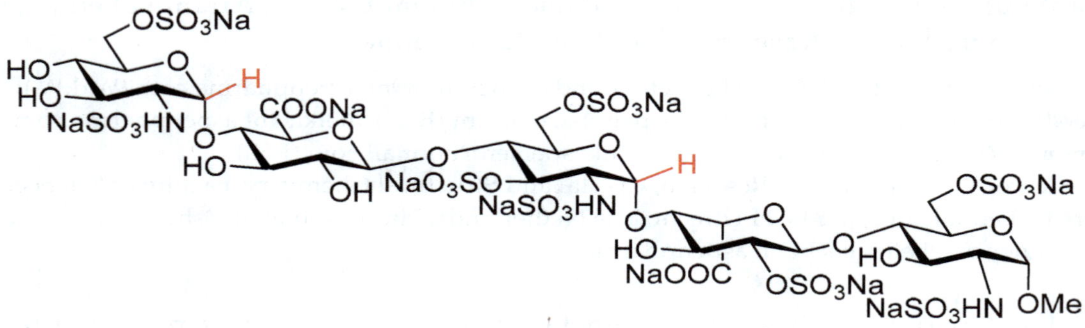

Figure 1. Structural formula of the synthetic anticoagulant pentasaccharide Fondaparinux sodium. The anomeric D1 and F1 protons used for qNMR integration have been indicated in red.

2. Results

qNMR is a well-established and accepted method for content determination [17–19] and is described in major pharmacopoeia [20–22]. The strength of qNMR lies in the fundamental property that, under the right conditions, the integrated response of a proton in ^{1}H-NMR will be identical in every molecule. This implies that a content determination can be carried out relative to a completely unrelated (but well-characterized) standard. We applied qNMR for the content determination of ampoules standard solution of the relatively complicated compound Fondaparinux using a maleic acid standard. Figure 2 shows an example of the 500 MHz ^{1}H-NMR spectrum of a mixture of the Fondaparinux standard and maleic acid in D_2O with the signals used for integration indicated. We performed these determinations on ampoules of the same standard both in 1999 and 2016 using an identical protocol which yields a unique opportunity to assess the long-term reproducibility of the qNMR method. The content determination in 1999 was performed at 400 MHz using a conventional probe whereas the content determination in 2016 was done at 500 MHz using a cryo probe. Different batches of maleic acid were used in 1996 and in 2017. For each experiment the tests were done by two different analysts and on two different days. The differences between the determinations are listed in the experimental section (Table 4).

The current analysis yields a content of 9.75 mg/mL with an SD of 0.06 mg/mL for the standard. The analysis performed in 1999 yielded a content of 9.64 mg/mL with an SD of 0.08 mg/mL. The two results are therefore not significantly different. The close correspondence between the two values obtained about 17 years apart demonstrates the intrinsic robustness of the qNMR content determination. Moreover, the differences between the two values is unlikely be due to degradation since the current content is slightly higher than the one determined 17 years ago and no signals pointing at degradation are currently detected in NMR.

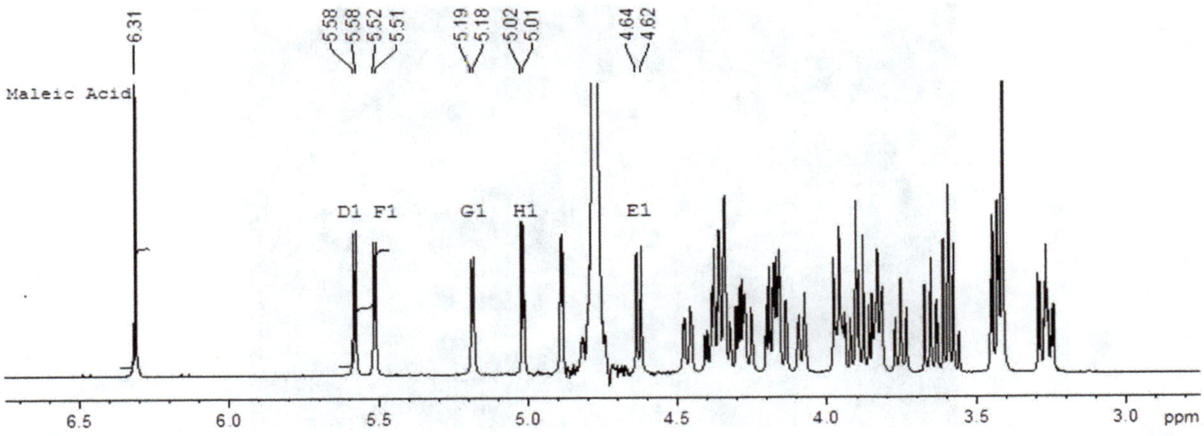

Figure 2. Example of the 500 MHz ^{1}H-NMR spectrum of a mixture of the Fondaparinux sodium standard and maleic acid in D_2O with the relevant integrated signals.

2.1. Fondaparinux Single Crystal X-ray Structure

Fondaparinux drug substance is industrially obtained as an amorphous powder as is evident from its X-ray powder diffractogram (XRPD; Figure 3; in green). Obtaining Fondaparinux single crystals was challenging, probably due to its inherent flexibility and linear structure. Ultimately, crystals were obtained as described in the Materials and Methods section. Several batches of crystals were produced. For a crystal from one batch, a full single-crystal structure determination was undertaken. A crystal from another batch was used for a unit-cell determination to ensure the similarity of these batches. Finally, an XRPD measurement was done for one batch of crystals see Table 7 for unit-cell comparison). In Figure 3, the blue trace shows the XRPD patterns of crystalline Fondaparinux. The XRPD pattern calculated from the crystal structure is shown as the red trace in Figure 3. A polarization microscopy image of representative crystals is displayed in Figure 4.

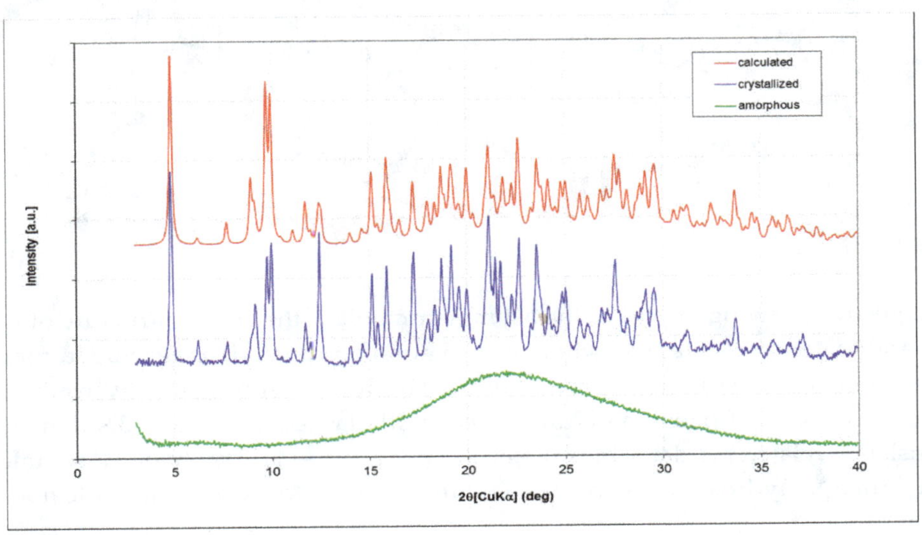

Figure 3. Comparison of the observed powder diffraction patterns of amorphous (green) and crystallized Fondaparinux (blue) with the pattern calculated from the single-crystal structure (red). The patterns are given an arbitrary displacement along the intensity axis to aid comparison. For the calculated pattern, the unit-cell parameters were refined using the Rietveld method to allow for the difference in data collection temperature. The reflection positions of observed and calculated patterns show a good correlation. The relative intensities show some differences, which are most likely due to the limited number of crystallites in the powder measurement, some preferred orientation effects and small changes in structure (especially in the water molecules) due to the temperature difference.

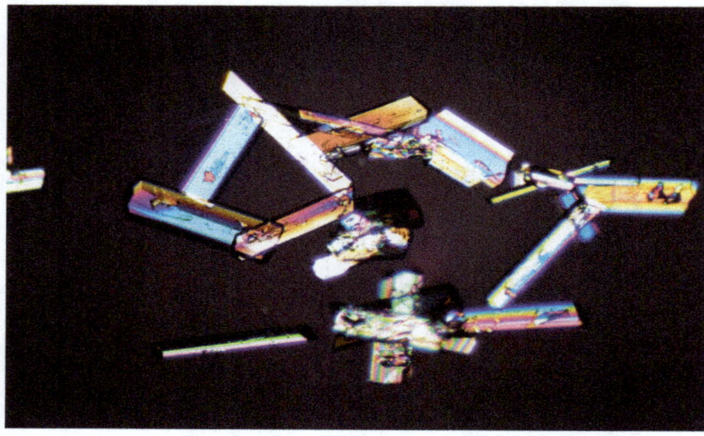

Figure 4. Polarized light microscopic picture at 40× magnification of Fondaparinux crystals formed from a water/ethanol solution.

2.2. Structural Features of the Crystal Structure

The asymmetric unit of the crystal structure of Fondaparinux contains a pentasaccharide anion, with one of the carboxylic groups protonated (vide infra), nine sodium cations, 17 water molecules coordinated to one or more sodium atoms and 15 non-coordinated water molecules. A perspective drawing of the molecular structure of the pentasaccharide Fondaparinux, along with the atomic labeling scheme of the non-hydrogen atoms and the labeling scheme of the rings is given in Figure 5.

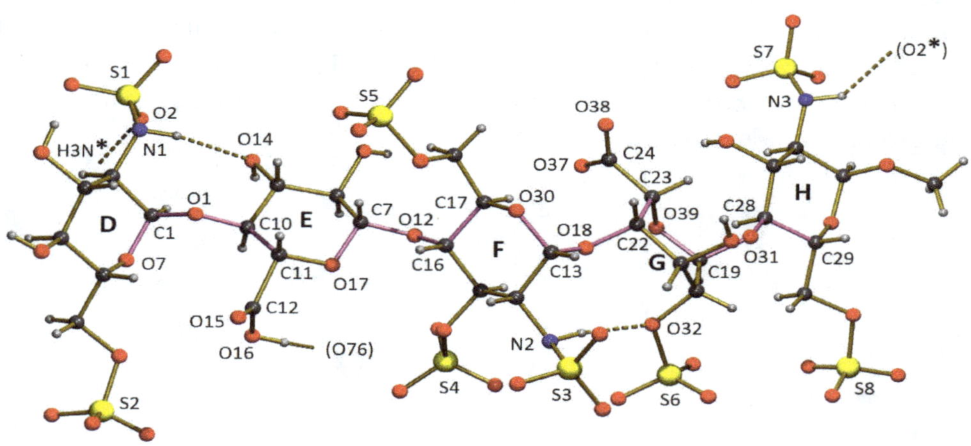

Figure 5. Perspective drawing of part of the asymmetric unit of the crystal structure of Fondaparinux. Sodium ions and water molecules (coordinated and non-coordinated) are excluded for clarity. Rings and atoms mentioned in the discussion are labelled. The bonds defining the glycosidic conformation are highlighted in pink. Hydrogen bonds are marked with dashed lines. N3-H3N donates a hydrogen bond to a translation related Fondaparinux molecule ($x-1, y, z-1$). The involved symmetry positions are indicated with a *. Hydroxyl O16 donates a hydrogen bond to a water molecule not shown.

The sodium ions are coordinated by numerous oxygen atoms from the pentasaccharide and extensively co-crystallized water molecules. The seven ordered sodium ions are coordinated by six oxygen atoms each. For the ordered ions, most Na...O distances fall in the range 2.3–2.7 Å. However, a small number of Na...O distances up to 2.9 Å are observed. The two disordered sodium ions are also surrounded by a total of six oxygen atoms that can be assigned to the coordination shell, but this shell is somewhat larger than that observed for the ordered sodium atoms. As a result of this, the sodium can take up several positions and some of the individual disorder components are only directly coordinated by five oxygen atoms. Full details of the observed coordination distances are given in the deposited Crystallographic Information File. Through these coordinative bonds an infinite three-dimensional structure is formed. A perspective drawing of the infinite substructure formed by sodium counter-ions, sulfate groups and coordinated water molecules is included in the Supporting Information. The final model contained no solvent accessible void. DFT calculations also indicated extensive coordination to both sodium ions and water (e.g., [13,15]).

3. Discussion

The individual glucosamine (D, F and H) rings have adopted the conventional stable $^4C_1$ chair conformation. The glucuronic acid ring (E) is in a slightly distorted $^4C_1$ chair-conformation. The iduronic acid G ring conformation has been the subject of intense debate [11–15,23–26]. Uncomplexed in solution, its structure cannot be described by a single conformer but is an equilibrium of $^1C_4$, chair and $^2S_0$. Skew-boat conformations with the equilibrium shifted to the $^2S_0$ conformation [11–15,23–26]. The conformation is $^2S_0$ in complex with antithrombin III [5,6,16].

In our crystal structure, the iduronic acid ring (G) is in a chair conformation, heavily distorted towards a half-chair conformation with the best-fitting local twofold rotation axis running through the midpoint of the bond ring O–C5 (crystal structure numbering O39–C23; see Table 1 for quantification using Cremer & Pople puckering parameters [27]). The iduronic ring conformation is therefore clearly different from the conformation reported by Johnson et al. [5], who found a skew-boat conformation (related Cremer & Pople puckering parameters are included in Table 1). A comparison of the conformations of the iduronic acid G ring in both structures is given in Figure 6. Interestingly, in the co-crystal of heparin and teichoic acid α-glycosyl transferase the iduronic acid adopts a chair conformation according to the coordinates reported by Sobhanifar et al. ([8], PDB entry 4X7R), related Cremer & Pople puckering parameters are also included in Table 1.

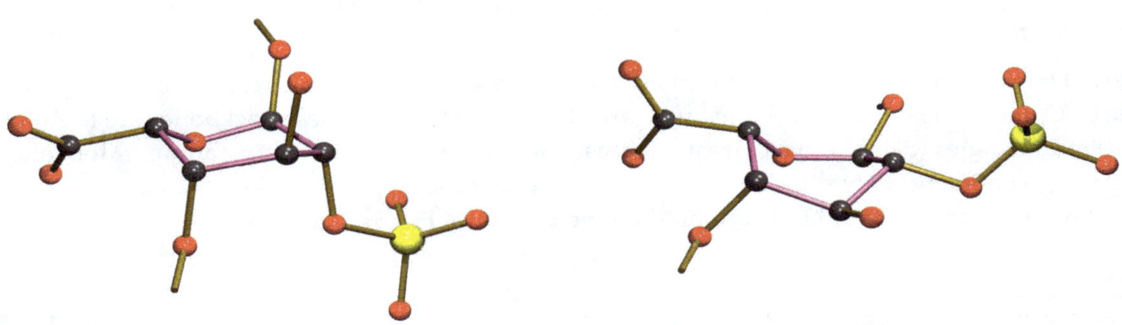

(a) (b)

Figure 6. A comparison of the conformations of the iduronic acid G ring structures in uncomplexed Fondaparinux (**a**) and Fondaparinux co-crystallized with antithrombin (**b**); from PDB entry 2GD4) [5].

The overall conformation of the pentasaccharide can be described in terms of the torsion angles of the glycosidic links between the carbohydrate rings. An alternative description uses the dihedral angles between least-squares planes fitted through the ring atoms. Numerical data for both descriptions are given in Table 2. Table 2 contains the same set of descriptors for the pentasaccharide molecules co-crystallized with antithrombin S195A, platelet factor 4 and a glycosyl transerase as well as for the structure in solution determined by NMR. A comparison of the free and co-crystallized pentasaccharide shows only relatively small differences when the glycosidic links between adjacent sugar rings are considered. In most cases the range of torsion angles observed is approximately 30 °C. However, in combination with the conformational change of the iduronic acid, these differences add up to a substantial difference for the overall conformation of the pentasaccharide. This can be convincingly illustrated by the angle between the least-squares planes fitted through rings D and H, which shows a difference of almost 60 °C. This difference in dihedral angles (which have a defined range of 0–90 °C) corresponds to the mean planes of rings D and H being almost parallel in the crystal structure of Fondaparinux while they are almost perpendicular in complex 2GD4.

Table 1. Cremer & Pople puckering parameters for the rings in the Fondaparinux structure published here (FP). Parameters for a selection of ideal conformations are included for comparison in a separate section; k is an integer number [27]. For comparison, the values calculated from the published coordinates of a selection of co-crystals of proteins and heparin. These are indicated with their PDB codes: 2GD4 is antithrombin S195A with heparin [5]; 4R9W is platelet factor 4 with heparin [7], 4X7R is wall teichoic acid glycosyl transferase [8]. The last column reports the values calculated from the coordinates of a solution NMR study [28]. 2GD4 and 4X7R contain two crystallographically independent heparin molecules; values for both are included.

Reference Values		
	θ	φ
Chair	0 or 180	(any value)
Half-chair	50.8 or 129.2	$k \times 60 + 30$
Boat	90	$k \times 60$
Skew-boat	90	$k \times 60 + 30$

Observed Values	**FP**		**2GD4 1**		**2GD4 2**		**4R9W**		**4X7R 1**		**4X7R 2**		**NMR Solution**	
	θ	φ	θ	φ	θ	φ	θ	φ	θ	φ	θ	φ	θ	φ
D	0	349	7	64	7	65	12	308	7	0	6	342	4	26
E	8	23	3	94	3	92	18	40	8	339	1	350	5	22
F	0	227	7	76	7	76	7	7	5	21	4	18	7	107
G	165	135	91	140	91	140	90	1	169	142	170	109	92	133
H	4	298	7	268	7	268	89	208	5	28	14	68	10	324

Table 2. Description of the overall conformation of the pentasaccharide in terms of torsion angles (deg.) of the C–O backbone in the glycosidic links (see also Figure 5 where these backbones are highlighted) and dihedral angles (deg.) between least-squares planes fitted through the ring atoms. Atom and ring labels are given in Figure 5; s.u.'s are included in parentheses. For comparison, the values for various other structures are included in the Table, see the legend of Figure 1 for details of the abbreviations used here.

Torsion Angles (deg)	**FP**	**2GD4 1**	**2GD4 2**	**4R9W**	**4X7R 1**	**4X7R 2**	**NMR Solution**
τ(O7–C1–O1–C10)	90.0(9)	101.4	101.4	69.5	96.4	95.5	76.9
τ(C1–O1–C10–C11)	−143.9(10)	−157.6	−158.0	−155.4	−128.2	−126.1	−151.4
τ(O17–C7–O12–C16)	−82.3(7)	−84.4	−84.3	−70.2	−94.6	−93.0	−55.2
τ(C7–O12–C16–C17)	−103.4(6)	−120.8	−121.0	−105.1	−100.5	−97.2	−111.0
τ(O30–C13–O18–C22)	88.5(7)	63.1	62.4	71.0	73.2	73.7	89.2
τ(C13–O18–C22–C23)	−145.9(6)	−157.0	−156.2	−132.0	−152.0	−146.2	−143.8
τ(O39–C19–O31–C28)	−72.0(7)	−67.8	−-67.5	−77.0	−65.2	−66.6	−73.0
τ(C19–O31–C28–C29)	−118.7(6)	−108.5	−108.7	−139.2	−106.8	−110.2	−134.0
Dihedral Angles (deg)	**FP**	**2GD4 1**	**2GD4 2**	**4R9W**	**4X7R 1**	**4X7R 2**	**NMR Solution**
χ (D,E)	57.4(5)	57.4	57.6	63.1	48.9	44.6	58.2
χ (D,H)	14.0(3)	71.3	71.4	31.7	13.6	12.7	30.3
χ (E,F)	57.3(5)	35.7	35.5	68.9	48.4	50.2	69.3
χ (F,G)	66.6(4)	78.8	78.8	89.7	69.7	72.2	84.0
χ (G,H)	39.3(4)	33.8	33.7	20.7	57.0	53.4	3.4

The intramolecular hydrogen bond between rings D and E, found in the Fondaparinux crystal structure, is also present in the co-crystal with antithrombin. In the latter, an even shorter donor-acceptor distance of 2.98 Å is found, suggesting a reasonably strong hydrogen bond. The intramolecular hydrogen bond between residues F and G (iduronic acid), found in the single-crystal structure of Fondaparinux, is not present in the pentasaccharide unit in the co-crystal. The conformational change of the iduronic acid to a twist-boat has moved the accepting sulfate out of reach of the sulfamido group. In the co-crystal, this sulfamido group rotated around the bond to which it is attached to the sugar ring so that an intramolecular hydrogen bond to the neighbouring sulfate group attached to the same sugar ring can be formed (donor-acceptor is 2.98 Å, also suggesting the presence of a reasonably strong intramolecular hydrogen bond).

The sulfamido groups play an important role in stabilizing the pentasaccharide molecule in a relatively linear conformation by forming two N-H...O intramolecular hydrogen bonds. The NH hydrogen of the sulfamido group in carbohydrate residue F is involved in an interresidue hydrogen bond to an oxygen of the 2-sulfate group residue G, as shown in Figure 5. This hydrogen bond is also found in solution [15]. Previously, in solution, an intraresidue hydrogen bond between the NH hydrogen of the sulfamido group in carbohydrate residue F and the adjacent 3-sulfo group [15,28] was found. This hydrogen bond is not observed in the crystal, possibly as a consequence of the different conformation of the iduronic acid G discussed above. Geometric details are given in Table 3.

Table 3. Geometric details of selected hydrogen bonds (Å, deg.). Standard uncertainties are given in parentheses (only available for *D*...*A* since H atoms were not freely refined). Hydrogen bond type refers to intramolecular or intermolecular hydrogen bonds. The listed hydrogen bonds are also indicated in Figure 5.

Involved Atoms	Type	*D*–H	H $\cdots$ *A*	*D* $\cdots$ *A*	*D*–H $\cdots$ *A*
N1–H1N $\cdots$ O14	intra	0.92	2.52	3.282(14)	141
N2–H2N $\cdots$ O32	intra	0.92	2.18	3.095(9)	172
N3–H3N $\cdots$ O2 $(x-1, y, z-1)$	inter	0.92	2.26	2.972(12)	134
O16–H16H $\cdots$ O76 (water)	inter	0.84	1.91	2.54(3)	131

Besides the items listed in Table 3, the crystal structure displays numerous hydrogen bonds, which further strengthen the infinite three-dimensional network formed by the pentasaccharide ions, sodium ions and water molecules. As can be expected in view of their acidic nature, all SO_3H groups are deprotonated, which is supported by the observed equality of the S–O bond lengths.

Interestingly, the geometry of the carboxylic acid group bonded to ring E strongly suggests a protonated, neutral acid group (d(C12–O15) = 1.09(2) Å, d(C12–O16) = 1.40(3) Å), in spite of the fact that the crystallization was carried out at neutral pH. Due to high anisotropic displacement parameters, the C–O distances appear shortened. The anisotropicity is also reflected by the accuracy of these bond lengths, which is significantly lower than that of similar bond lengths in other sections of the pentasaccharide anion. The presence of a hydrogen bond acceptor at hydrogen bonding distance from O16 (see Table 3) supports the model of a protonated acid group. However, the unfavorable value of the *D*–H $\cdots$ *A* angle (131 deg) does not suggest this is a particularly strong hydrogen bond.

The acid group bonded to ring G (iduronic acid) is deprotonated as expected, as is clearly shown by the similar lengths of the C–O bonds: d(C24–O37) = 1.242(11) Å and d(C24–O38) = 1.267(10) Å.

Based on the covalent angles between their substituents, the nitrogen atoms N1, N2 and N3 can be considered sp^3 hybridized, which is common for this type of group. The coordinates of the hydrogen atoms bonded to the nitrogen atoms were derived from the availability of hydrogen bond acceptors at reasonable distances from the nitrogen donor atoms (see "Crystal Structure Determination and Refinement").

Absolute Configuration

The Flack x-parameter and its standard uncertainty $u(x)$ can be used to assess absolute structure and absolute configuration [29,30]. A structure determination is considered to have strong inversion-distinguishing power if $u(x) < 0.04$. If the enantiopurity of a sample is certain, a less strict criterion is applied. When $u(x) < 0.08$, the experiment is considered to have enantiopure sufficient inversion-distinguishing power. If one of these criteria is met, a numerical value of x that lies within statistical fluctuation of zero, i.e., $|x| < 2\ u(x)$, assures a valid absolute structure (and absolute configuration) determination from a single crystal which is not twinned by inversion. The cited criteria are taken from Flack and Bernardinelli [31].

In this study, a value of −0.02(11) was found by classical fit to all intensities, which does not satisfy the criterion for enantiopure sufficient inversion-distinguishing power. However, as argued by Parsons et al. [32] anomalous dispersion differences can be obscured by other effects, such as absorption and extinction. If these effects are filtered out as proposed by these authors, and x-value of 0.017(14) is obtained, we can classify the current structure determination as having strong inversion-distinguishing power.

As a final alternative to assess the absolute configuration, the method of Hooft et al. [33] was considered. Using Bayesian statistics, these authors offer a method that gives reliable absolute structure determinations even in cases where only weak anomalous scatterers are present. According to this method, the probability that the absolute configuration was determined correctly is calculated to be 1.00, based on the assumption of an enantiopure sample. In case the measured crystal is a racemic twin, the twin ratio, expressed as the y-parameter, comparable to Flack's x-parameter, amounts to −0.002(14), further confirming the correct assignment of the absolute configuration of the enantiopure sample.

4. Materials and Methods

4.1. General Information

4.1.1. Materials

The Fondaparinux standard was prepared from a commercially manufactured Fondaparinux batch and underwent an additional ion exchange chromatography purification. Maleic acid batches were obtained from Acros (Geel, Belgium; in 1999) or Fluka (St. Louis, MO, USA; Lot BCBV2002V, in 2016) and used as such. The content of the maleic acid batches of 99.61 (1999) and 99. 99% (2016) was taken from the Certificate of Analysis from the supplier. D_2O was used as a solvent since both Fondaparinux and the standard maleic acid are charged molecules and well soluble in water. 0.01% w/v TSP-d_4 was used as a chemical shift reference at 0 ppm. The 500 MHz 1D ^{1}H spectrum of Fondaparinux and maleic acid is displayed in Figure 1 including the D1, F1 and maleic acid proton integrals used for content determination.

From an ampoule of Fondaparinux standard solution, 0.5 mL was transferred into an Eppendorf and 0.5 mL of a 0.67 mg/mL maleic acid standard solution was added. After stirring, the content of the Eppendorf was then frozen in a dry-ice ethanol mixture and subsequently lyophilized (>8 h, −50 °C, <300 mbar). After lyophilizing 0.7 mL D_2O was added to the freeze-dried material and subsequently stirred until complete dissolution. The solution was then transferred into a NMR tube. Five determinations were performed by two different analysts on two different days.

4.1.2. Fondaparinux Crystallization

Fondaparinux (100 mg) was dissolved in 2.5 mL of demineralized water in a flat-bottomed flask or bottle. The temperature was increased to 70 °C to dissolve the material. 5.5 mL of ethanol at room temperature was slowly added while maintaining the temperature at 70 °C to saturate the solution (the solution became slightly turbid). The solution (or even slightly turbid mixture) was then cooled to RT. No stirring was applied.

The turbidity of the mixture increased under cooling. Over time, the turbidity decreased, and in turn, an oily liquid (or drops) was formed on the bottom of the flask. After a while, the oily drops changed and crystallized (this procedure was not an optimized process and it took weeks before crystallization occurred). Various crystallization experiments of Fondaparinux (maximum concentration 16 mg/mL) were successful with an ethanol content between 70% and 90%. In addition, when available, seeding crystals were used to speed up the crystallization process.

4.2. Methods

4.2.1. qNMR

Spectrum Acquisition and Processing

^{1}H-NMR spectra were recorded on a Bruker NMR spectrometer (Bruker BioSpin, Billerica, MA, USA) according to the settings in Table 4.

Table 4. Acquisition and processing settings of the qNMR experiment.

Acquisition	1999	2016
Spectral frequency Probe	400 MHz 5 mm QNP probe	500 MHz TCI Cryo Probe
Temperature	25 °C/298 K	
Spinning	20 Hz	Off
Flip angle Relaxation delay	60° 30 s	
Dummy scans Number of scans	4 128	2 32
Number of data points	64 k	
Processing Exponential line-broadening Zero-Filling	 0.5 Hz 64 k	 0.3 Hz 132 k

The recorded spectra were manually phased and baseline corrected, and the signals of maleic acid and the anomeric protons D1 and F1 (indicated in red in Figure 1) were integrated as described in the protocol. The content of Fondaparinux in an ampoule was then calculated according to the formula: $C_{FP} = W_{MA}/V_{FP} \times I_{FP}/I_{MA} \times MW_{FP}/MW_{MA} \times P_{MA}/P_{FP}$ where C_{FP} = concentration of Fondaparinux in the ampoule, W_{MA} = weight of maleic acid (=concentration stock solution (mg/mL) × 0.5 mL); V_{FP} = volume of Fondaparinux taken from the ampoule (typically 0.5 mL); I_{FP} = integral of selected signals of Fondaparinux; I_{MA} = integral of maleic acid set at 2.0000 for each sample MW_{FP} = molecular weight of Fondaparinux (1728.088); MW_{MA} = molecular weight of maleic acid (116.07); P_{MA} = purity of maleic acid (99.99%); P_{FP} = purity of Fondaparinux (assumed to be 100%). The determination was performed in fivefold by two technicians on two different days and the average Fondaparinux content (mg/mL) was reported including the standard deviation and the relative standard deviation (RSD).

4.3. XRPD

X-ray powder diffractograms were obtained on a Miniflex600 diffractometer (Rikagu, Tokyo, Japan) using the settings listed in Table 5 below.

Table 5. XRPD settings.

XRPD Settings	
X-ray	40 kV, 15 mA
Goniometer	MiniFlex 600
Wavelength	Cu K_α (1.541 Å)
Filter	K_β(Ni)
Scan speed/Duration time	2.0000 deg/min
Step width	0.0200 deg
Scan axis	θ/2-θ
Scan range	3.0000–40.0000 °C ambient
Temperature	Ambient

4.4. Crystal Structure Determination and Refinement

A colorless, block-shaped crystal of approximate dimensions 0.10 × 0.20 × 0.20 cm was fixed to the tip of a glass capillary and transferred into the cold nitrogen stream on a kappa-CCD diffractometer (Bruker-Nonius, Billerica, MA, USA) on rotating anode. Raw data were reduced with DENZO [34]. Crystal data and details on data collection and refinement are presented in Table 6.

Table 6. Crystallographic data. Unit cell parameters are listed in Table 5.

Crystal Data	
Formula	$[C_{31}H_{44}N_3O_{49}S_8]^{9-}\cdot 9Na^+\cdot 32H_2O$
Molecular weight	2282.60
Crystal system	monoclinic
Space group	$P2_1$ (No.4)
D_{calc}, g cm^{-3}	1.784
Z	2
$F(000)$	2380
μ (Mo$K\alpha$), mm^{-1}	0.401
Crystal size	0.2 × 0.3 × 0.3
Data collection	
T, K	150
θ_{min}, θ_{max}, deg	1.00, 27.49
Wavelength (Mo$K\alpha$), Å	0.71073 (graphite monochromated)
Distance crystal to detector, mm	45
X-ray exposure time, h	7.0
Refined mosaicity, deg	0.914(1)
Data set (hkl-range)	−13:13, −29:29, −24:24
Completeness at $\sin\theta/\lambda = 0.6$ Å^{-1}	100.0% (no refl. missing)
Total data	81362 ($R_\sigma = 0.0498$)
Total unique data	19366 ($R_{int} = 0.0396$)
Refinement	
No. of refined parameters	1114
$wR2$	0.2211
R	0.0786 [for 16915 $F_o > 4\sigma(F_o)$]
S	1.041
w^{-1}	$\sigma^2(F^2) + (0.1328P)^2 + 11.21P$
$(\Delta/\sigma)_{av}$, $(\Delta/\sigma)_{max}$	<0.0001, 0.0002
$\Delta\rho_{min}$, $\Delta\rho_{max}$, e Å^{-3}	−0.84, 1.87 (near Na)

The unit-cell parameters were checked for the presence of higher lattice symmetry [35]. Data were not corrected for absorption. The structure was solved by automated direct methods (SHELXS86 [36]). Refinement on F^2 was carried out by full-matrix, least-squares techniques (SHELXL 2016-6 [37]); no observance criterion was applied during refinement. Two of the sodium ions and some of the water molecules coordinated with one of these sodium ions were found to be disordered. A disorder model with two positions for each of the atoms involved was introduced. The two sites for each sodium atom are close to each other. The site occupation factor of the major component refined to 0.502(11) for Na7 and 0.549(17) for Na9 and associated disordered water molecules. All hydrogen atoms were included in the refinement on calculated positions riding on their carrier atoms. The methyl hydrogen atoms and the hydroxyl hydrogen atoms were refined as rigid groups, allowing for rotation around the C–O bonds. Starting positions of the methyl hydrogen were derived from a difference Fourier map. The hydrogen atoms of the non-coordinated water solvent molecules could not be located on difference Fourier maps. Furthermore, the coordinates of these atoms could not be derived unambiguously from the distribution of potential hydrogen bond donors and acceptors. Most likely, there is extensive disorder in the hydrogen atoms of the non-coordinated water molecules. Displacement parameters of the oxygen atoms of the non-coordinated water molecules indicate that there is a slight disorder in their positions as well. Therefore, no further attempts were made to include these hydrogen atoms in the atomic model. All ordered non-hydrogen atoms were refined with anisotropic atomic displacement parameters. Atoms in the major disorder component were refined with isotropic displacement parameters, which were coupled to the isotropic displacement parameters of the related atoms in the minor component. Hydrogen atoms were refined with fixed isotropic displacement parameters related to the value of the equivalent isotropic displacement parameters of their carrier atoms by a factor of 1.5 for methyl, hydroxyl and water hydrogen atoms, and 1.2 for all other hydrogen atoms.

The Flack x-parameter [29], derived during the final structure-factor calculation, amounts to $-0.02(11)$ by classical fit to all intensities and 0.017(14) from 7033 selected quotients (Parsons' method, [32]). Refinement of the inverse absolute structure resulted in an x-parameter of 1.04(11) (value derived during final structure-factor calculation). Figures of merit for this inverted structure are $R1 = 0.0791$, $wR2 = 0.2223$ (weighting scheme not optimized) and $S = 1.0$. Refinement of a racemic twin model gave a twin ratio of reported versus inverted structure of 1.00(11):0.00; the twin model was therefore not used.

Neutral atom scattering factors and anomalous dispersion corrections were taken from the International Tables for Crystallography [38]. Geometrical calculations and illustration were performed with PLATON [39].

Unit Cell Determination

At $T = 150$ K, a data set was collected, consisting of a scan of 20 deg of φ divided into 20 image frames, using Mo$K\alpha$-radiation ($\lambda = 0.71073$ Å). The unit cell was determined using DENZO [28]. Results are summarized in Table 7.

Table 7. Unit cell parameters of Fondaparinux determined for the single-crystal study, the cell check of a second batch, and the powder diffraction study. In all cases systematic absences indicate the space group is $P2_1$. s.u.'s are included in parentheses.

	Single Crystal (DW1623B)	Cell Check (DW1637A)	Powder
a, Å	10.0296(2)	10.0132(18)	10.144(3)
b, Å	23.0353(6)	23.067(5)	22.992(5)
c, Å	18.9666(7)	18.820(3)	18.626(6)
β, deg	104.1420(14)	103.731(2)	102.65(2)
V, Å^3	4249.1(2)	4222.6(2)	4238.8(4)
Refined mosaicity, deg	0.914(1)	1.626(9)	-
T, K	150	150	ambient

5. Conclusions

Both Fondaparinux structure (X-ray) and content (qNMR) have been addressed in this paper. The content of ampoules of a Fondaparinux solution standard was determined using qNMR. For consistency, the ability to assess the long-term stability of the content of the standard is crucial since the standard content is used to determine the content of Fondaparinux batches. The 2016 analysis yielded a content of 9.75 mg/mL (SD 0.06 mg/mL) whereas the analysis performed in 1999 yielded a content of 9.64 mg/mL (SD of 0.08 mg/mL). qNMR shows remarkable precision over time, instrumentation and analysts, pivotal for consistent content determination.

The determination of the single crystal X-ray structure including the absolute configuration of Fondaparinux crystals allowed an unequivocal proof of structure. The iduronic acid residue in the uncomplexed Fondaparinux adopts a chair conformation heavily distorted towards a half chair. Interestingly, this iduronic acid conformation was also found in the complex of heparin with wall teichoic acid transferase according to the coordinates published [8]. The iduronic acid conformation also provides solid evidence of the thermodynamic accessibility of this chair conformation of iduronic acid within a pentasaccharide, (and thereby helps to extend our knowledge of the available conformational space).

Acknowledgments: The authors would like to thank Leendert van den Bos, Arno Bode and Marketta Uusi-Penttilä for carefully reading the manuscript and stimulating discussion. Judica Bootsma and Ineke Huiberts-Eeuwijk are thanked for their expert technical assistance and useful discussions. Anthony L. Spek is acknowledged for consultancy regarding the crystal structure determination. Cynthia Larive and Andrew Green made available the coordinates of their Fondaparinux solution structure [28] to us. The authors would also like to thank the referees for their critical comments and suggestions which helped us to considerably improve the original manuscript.

Author Contributions: C.F., F.K. and E.K. conceived and designed the experiments; W.d.W., M.L., A.L., H.K. and E.K. performed the experiments; H.K., B.Ü. and E.K. analyzed the data; E.K. and H.K. wrote the paper.

References

1. Petitou, M.; van Boeckel, C.A.A. A synthetic antithrombin III binding pentasaccharide is now a drug! What comes next? *Angew. Chem. Int. Ed.* **2004**, *43*, 3118–3133. [CrossRef] [PubMed]
2. Giangrande, P.L. Fondaparinux (Arixtra): A new anticoagulant. *Int. J. Clin. Pract.* **2002**, *56*, 615–617. [PubMed]
3. Tan, K.; Duquette, M.; Liu, J.H.; Zhang, R.; Joachimiak, A.; Wang, J.H.; Lawler, J. The structures of the thrombospondin-1 N-terminal domain and its complex with a synthetic pentameric heparin. *Structure* **2006**, *14*, 33–42. [CrossRef] [PubMed]
4. Tan, K.; Duquette, M.; Liu, J.-H.; Shanmugasundaram, K.; Joachimiak, A.; Gallagher, J.T.; Rigby, A.C.; Wang, J.H.; Lawler, J. Heparin-induced *cis*- and *trans*-dimerization modes of the thrombospondin-1 N-terminal domain. *J. Biol. Chem.* **2008**, *283*, 3932–3941. [CrossRef] [PubMed]
5. Johnson, D.J.; Li, W.; Adams, T.E.; Huntington, J.A. Antithrombin–S195A factor Xa-heparin structure reveals the allosteric mechanism of antithrombin activation. *EMBO J.* **2006**, *25*, 2029–2037. [CrossRef] [PubMed]
6. Langdown, J.; Belzar, K.J.; Savory, W.J.; Baglin, T.P.; Huntington, J.A. The critical role of hinge-region expulsion in the induced-fit heparin binding mechanism of antithrombin. *J. Mol. Biol.* **2009**, *386*, 1278–1289. [CrossRef] [PubMed]
7. Cai, Z.; Yarovoi, S.V.; Zhu, Z.; Rauova, L.; Hayes, V.; Lebedeva, T.; Greene, M.I. Atomic description of the immune complex involved in heparin-induced thrombocytopenia. *Nat. Commun.* **2015**, *6*, 8277. [CrossRef] [PubMed]
8. Sobhanifar, S.; Worrall, L.J.; Gruninger, R.J.; Wasney, G.A.; Blaukopf, M.; Baumann, M.; Lameignere, E.; Solomonson, M.; Brown, E.D.; Withers, S.G.; et al. Structure and mechanism of Staphylococcus aureus TarM, the wall teichoic acid α-glycosyltransferase. *Proc. Natl. Acad. Sci. USA* **2015**, *112*, E576–E585. [CrossRef] [PubMed]
9. Li, W.; Johnson, D.J.; Esmon, C.T.; Huntington, J.A. Structure of the antithrombin–thrombin–heparin ternary complex reveals the antithrombotic mechanism of heparin. *Nat. Struct. Mol. Boil.* **2004**, *11*, 857–862. [CrossRef] [PubMed]
10. Jin, L.; Abrahams, J.P.; Skinner, R.; Petitou, M.; Pike, R.N.; Carrell, R.W. The anticoagulant activation of antithrombin by heparin. *Proc. Natl. Acad. Sci. USA* **1997**, *94*, 14683–14688. [CrossRef] [PubMed]
11. Ferro, D.R.; Provasoli, A.; Ragazzi, M.; Torri, G.; Casu, B.; Gatti, G.; Jacquinet, J.C.; Sinay, P.; Petitou, M.; Choay, J. Evidence for conformational equilibrium of the sulfated L-iduronate residue in heparin and in synthetic heparin mono-and oligo-saccharides: NMR and force-field studies. *J. Am. Chem. Soc.* **1986**, *108*, 6773–6778. [CrossRef]
12. Ragazzi, M.; Ferro, D.R.; Perly, B.; Sinaÿ, P.; Petitou, M.; Choay, J. Conformation of the pentasaccharide corresponding to the binding site of heparin for antithrombin III. *Carbohydr. Res.* **1990**, *195*, 169–185. [CrossRef]
13. Remko, M.; von der Lieth, C.W. Conformational structure of some trimeric and pentameric structural units of heparin. *J. Phys. Chem. A* **2007**, *111*, 13484–13491. [CrossRef] [PubMed]
14. Remko, M.; Van Duijnen, P.T.; Broer, R. Molecular structure of basic oligomeric building units of heparan-sulfate glycosaminoglycans. *Struct. Chem.* **2010**, *21*, 965–976. [CrossRef]
15. Hricovíni, M. Solution structure of heparin pentasaccharide: NMR and DFT analysis. *J. Phys. Chem. B* **2015**, *119*, 12397–12409. [CrossRef] [PubMed]

16. Hricovíni, M.; Guerrini, M.; Bisio, A.; Torri, G.; Petitou, M.; Casu, B. Conformation of heparin pentasaccharide bound to antithrombin III. *Biochem. J.* **2001**, *359*, 265–272. [CrossRef] [PubMed]
17. Yang, Q.; Qiu, H.; Guo, W.; Wang, D.; Zhou, X.; Xue, D.; Zhang, J.; Wu, S.; Wang, Y. Quantitative ^{1}H-NMR method for the determination of Tadalafil in bulk drugs and its tablets. *Molecules* **2015**, *20*, 12114–12124. [CrossRef] [PubMed]
18. Holzgrabe, U. Quantitative NMR Spectroscopy in Pharmaceutical R & D. In *eMagRes*; Wiley: Hoboken, NJ, USA, 2015.
19. Holzgrabe, U. *NMR Spectroscopy in Pharmaceutical Analysis*; Iwona, W., Bernd, D., Eds.; Elsevier: Amsterdam, The Netherlands, 2011; Charter 5; pp. 131–137.
20. United States Pharmacopoeia. *General Chapter <761> Nuclear Magnetic Resonance*; United States Pharmacopoeia Convention Inc.: Rockville, USA, 2017.
21. European Pharmacopoeia. *General Chapter 2.2.33. Nuclear Magnetic Resonance Spectrometry*; Council of Europe: Strasbourg, France, 2017.
22. Goda, Y. Introduction of qNMR to the Japanese Pharmacopoeia (JP) for specification of marker compounds used for standardization of herbal medicines. *Planta Medica.* **2013**, *79*, SL79. [CrossRef]
23. Torri, G.; Casu, B.; Gatti, G.; Petitou, M.; Choay, J.; Jacquinet, J.C.; Sinay, P. Mono-and bidimensional 500 MHz ^{1}H-NMR spectra of a synthetic pentasaccharide corresponding to the binding sequence of heparin to antithrombin-III: Evidence for conformational peculiarity of the sulfated iduronate residue. *Biochem. Biophys. Res. Commun.* **1985**, *128*, 134–140. [CrossRef]
24. Casu, B.; Petitou, M.; Provasoli, M.; Sinay, P. Conformational flexibility: A new concept for explaining binding and biological properties of iduronic acid-containing glycosaminoglycans. *Trends Biochem. Sci.* **1988**, *13*, 221–225. [CrossRef]
25. Casu, B.; Guerrini, M.; Torri, G. Structural and conformational aspects of the anticoagulant and antithrombotic activity of heparin and dermatan sulfate. *Curr. Pharm. Des.* **2004**, *10*, 939–949. [CrossRef] [PubMed]
26. Rudd, T.R.; Skidmore, M.A.; Guerrini, M.; Hricovini, M.; Powell, A.K.; Siligardi, G.; Yates, E.A. The conformation and structure of GAGs: Recent progress and perspectives. *Curr. Opin. Struct. Biol.* **2010**, *20*, 567–574. [CrossRef] [PubMed]
27. Boeyens, J.C. The conformation of six-membered rings. *J. Cryst. Mol. Struct.* **1978**, *8*, 317–320. [CrossRef]
28. Langeslay, D.J.; Young, R.P.; Beni, S.; Beecher, C.N.; Mueller, L.J.; Larive, C.K. Sulfamate proton solvent exchange in heparin oligosaccharides: Evidence for a persistent hydrogen bond in the antithrombin-binding pentasaccharide Arixtra. *Glycobiology* **2012**, *22*, 1173–1182. [CrossRef] [PubMed]
29. Flack, H.D. On enantiomorph-polarity estimation. *Acta. Crystallogr. Sect. A* **1983**, *39*, 876–881. [CrossRef]
30. Flack, H.D.; Gérald, B. Absolute structure and absolute configuration. *Acta. Crystallogr. Sect. A* **1999**, *55*, 908–915. [CrossRef]
31. Flack, H.D.; Bernardinelli, G. Reporting and evaluating absolute-structure and absolute-configuration determinations. *J. Appl. Crystallogr.* **2000**, *33*, 1143–1148. [CrossRef]
32. Parsons, S.; Howard, D.F.; Trixie, W. Use of intensity quotients and differences in absolute structure refinement. *Acta. Crystallogr. Sect. B* **2013**, *69*, 249–259. [CrossRef] [PubMed]
33. Hooft, R.W.; Straver, L.H.; Spek, A.L. Determination of absolute structure using Bayesian statistics on Bijvoet differences. *J. Appl. Crystallogr.* **2008**, *41*, 96–103. [CrossRef] [PubMed]
34. Otwinowski, Z.; Minor, W. Processing of X-ray diffraction data collected in oscillation mode. *Methods Enzymol.* **1997**, *276*, 307–326. [PubMed]
35. Spek, A.L. LEPAGE—An MS-DOS program for the determination of the metrical symmetry of a translation lattice. *J. Appl. Crystallogr.* **1988**, *21*, 578–579. [CrossRef]
36. Sheldrick, G.M. *SHELXS86, Program for Crystal Structure Determination*; University of Gottingen: Gottingen, Germany, 1986.
37. Sheldrick, G.M. Crystal structure refinement with SHELXL. *Acta. Crystallogr. Sect. C* **2015**, *71*, 3–8. [CrossRef] [PubMed]

11

From Farm to Pharma: An Overview of Industrial Heparin Manufacturing Methods

Jan-Ytzen van der Meer *, Edwin Kellenbach and Leendert J. van den Bos

Development and Technical Support Aspen Oss, Kloosterstraat 6, P.O. Box 98, 5340 AB Oss, The Netherlands; ekellenbach@nl.aspenpharma.com (E.K.); lvandenbos@nl.aspenpharma.com (L.J.v.d.B.)
* Correspondence: jvandermeer@nl.aspenpharma.com

Academic Editors: Giangiacomo Torri and Jawed Fareed

Abstract: The purification of heparin from offal is an old industrial process for which commercial recipes date back to 1922. Although chemical, chemoenzymatic, and biotechnological alternatives for this production method have been published in the academic literature, animal-tissue is still the sole source for commercial heparin production in industry. Heparin purification methods are closely guarded industrial secrets which are not available to the general (scientific) public. However by reviewing the academic and patent literature, we aim to provide a comprehensive overview of the general methods used in industry for the extraction of heparin from animal tissue.

Keywords: heparin; heparin process; manufacturing methods; industrial

1. Introduction

Heparin is a strongly charged polysaccharide anticoagulant which has been used and produced for nearly a century [1,2]. The heparin manufacturing methods used rely strongly on the unique molecular properties of heparin, including its acidity, high charge density and stability. These characteristics enable the purification of heparin despite the low concentration present in the starting material (~160–260 mg/kg). Therefore a short summary of the old and current views on structure and biosynthesis of heparin is given below, for more elaborate reviews on these topics see references [2–5]. Discussions on the structure of heparin date back to the 1920s. By the 1940s it was concluded that heparin consisted of uronic acids and amino sugars with a high content of ester sulfates and that the amino groups were (partly) acetylated [6]. Further biochemical characterization studies indicated that desulphonation resulted in loss of heparin activity [7]. Additionally, fractional precipitation of active material suggested that heparin consisted of a mixture of closely related structures instead of a single structure. [6,8] More recent studies have shown that these observations and conclusions were correct. We now know that heparin is indeed a highly sulfated polysaccharide consisting of alternating glucosamine and uronic acid units. In the biosynthetic pathway towards heparin, these monosaccharides (i.e., *N*-acetyl-D-glucosamine (GlcNAc) and D-glucuronic acid (GlcA)) are added to a tetrasaccharide linkage region (GlcA-Gal-Gal-Xyl-) which is attached to proteins containing Ser-Gly repeats. After this elongation step, heparin chains of up to 100 kDa are generated. During and after the elongation, several modifications can occur which include: epimerization of GlcA leading to L-iduronic acid (IdoA), *N*-deacetylation, *N*-sulfation, 2-*O*-sulfation, 6-*O*-sulfation, and more rarely 3-*O*-sulfation of the glucosamine [4]. The most prevalent disaccharide present in heparin is depicted below in Figure 1.

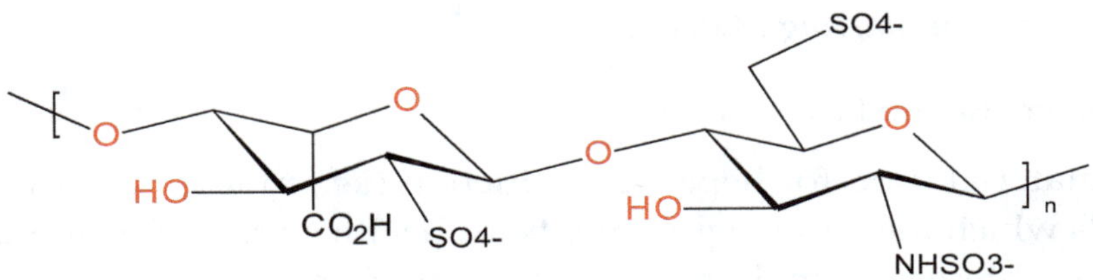

Figure 1. Major disaccharide found in heparin: (-4)-α-L-IdoA2S-(1-4)-α-D-GlcNS6S-(1-) [5].

The complete biosynthesis takes place in the Golgi compartment of mainly mast cells. These are a type of an immune cells containing heparin-rich granules. As a result of this biosynthesis and subsequent modifications, there are 32 theoretically possible disaccharides which make up heparin, making heparin more complex than other biopolymers such as proteins and nucleic acids [9]. Moreover, in contrast to proteins and nucleic acids, heparin is synthesized in a non-template directed fashion which results is a high degree of heterogeneity for all structural properties.

The anticoagulant activity of heparin is the result of its potentiating action on antithrombin (ATIII) which is an anti-coagulation factor. Potentiated ATIII, subsequently inhibits the action of pro-coagulation factors IIa (i.e., thrombin) and Xa by covalent binding, finally resulting in reduced coagulation. The molecular mechanism by which heparin potentiates ATIII differs for these two factors [5,10]. The potentiation of ATIII towards factor Xa mainly depends on an allosteric activation of ATIII by a specific pentasaccharide sequence in heparin. This pentasaccharide, which contains a unique 3-*O*-sulfate glucosamine triggers a conformational change in ATIII upon binding, which results in a ~1000-fold increasedaffinity of ATIII for Xa leading to increased inhibition of factor Xa [10]. The pentasaccharide sequence is sufficient for the Xa inhibition activity of heparin. For the inhibition of IIa, however, a heparin chain forms a bridge between ATIII and factor IIa by electrostatic interactions resulting in a stable ternary complex [10]. To enable this 'bridge' a heparin chain should be at least 15–16 saccharide units in length [11]. Besides chain length, also the overall charge (i.e., high sulfate to carboxylate ratio or S/C ratio) of a heparin chain is important for this mechanism since it enables strong interactions between heparin and ATIII and heparin and factor IIa.

The objective of the heparin manufacturing process is, therefore, to maximize the yield of highly charged, high molecular weight heparin chains present in the starting material without affecting the material by degradation (e.g., depolymerization and/or desulfation) caused by the applied process conditions. Typical industrial processes can be divided into five distinctive sections (Figure 2). Each of these section will be discussed in this review.

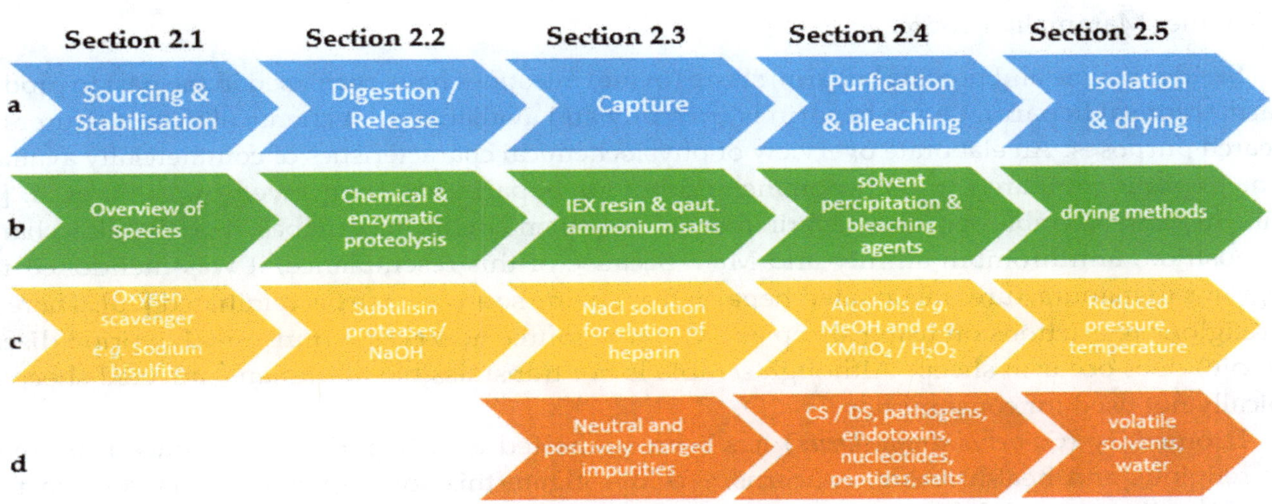

Figure 2. (**a**), Schematic representation of an industrial heparin purification process; (**b**) Discussed topics per section; (**c**) General process conditions and reagents; (**d**) Removed impurities per section.

1.1. Collection and Stabilization Starting Material

1.1.1. Regulatory Aspects Related to Sourcing

The biological material used for heparin production (i.e., mucosa or bovine lungs) should be derived from animals which meet the requirements for health suitable for human consumption [12]. This ensures the slaughtered animals are healthy and free of medication such as antibiotics. To guarantee this, several heparin producers provide full traceability of their starting material to the slaughterhouses and farms. Additionally, a polymerase chain reaction (PCR) or an immunochemical analysis is suggested by the FDA and European Pharmacopoeia to demonstrate the absence of any ruminant material in the starting material to mitigate the risk for contamination with BSE [12,13]. Moreover, from 2013 onwards, the complete supply chain of heparin, starting with the collection of the starting material, falls under EudraLex volume 4, annex 2 of the EU guidelines for "GMP for medicinal products for human and veterinary use" [14]. This indicates that the entire process falls under GMP control, albeit at different levels depending on the stage of the manufacturing process.

1.1.2. Sources: Porcine and Bovine

The first heparin production protocols used canine or bovine livers as a source. Later, mainly porcine mucosa and bovine lungs were used [15]. However, since porcine intestinal mucosa was found to be a much 'cleaner' source which required less degradation compared to bovine lungs and also as a result of the outbreak of bovine spongiform encephalopathy in the 1990s [3,16], heparin production from bovine material has decreased significantly. In fact, the only FDA-approved source of heparin is currently porcine mucosa [13,16]. However, several countries, including Brazil, Argentina and India, still allow bovine-derived heparin. Bovine heparin is preferred by some for religious reasons. Heparin is second only to insulin in application as a biological. To meet the annual heparin need, the offal of about 1.10^9 pigs are required, therefore there is a substantial risk for future heparin shortages. To prevent these potential shortages there is currently a strong debate ongoing to re-introduce bovine heparin in the USA [15]. Because strong drop of BSE prevalence in cows, the strongly increased knowledge on the disease and the prion reduction during the heparin purification process [17] the risks with respect to patient safety are now better understood [15]. This may facilitate the re-introduction of bovine heparin to the US market. There are however significant differences between porcine and bovine heparin. For instance, bovine heparin has substantially lower activity compared to porcine heparin [18] (see Table 1). A large amount of scientific literature is available describing structural differences between porcine and bovine derived heparin which might explain the difference in activity [15,17,19].

1.1.3. Other Mammalian Sources

Besides bovine and porcine heparin, sheep (ovine) intestines have been used in the past to produce pharmaceutical heparin. Ovine heparin is currently still available from chemical manufacturers for research purposes. An elaborate overview of physiochemical characteristics of commercially available ovine heparin compared to both porcine and bovine heparin has been given by Li Fu et al. [16]. Ovine heparin resembles porcine heparin more closely then bovine heparin based on the disaccharide composition, antithrombin affinity and M_W. Because of this resemblance, it was mentioned that programs to manufacture fractionated heparin from ovine sources have been initiated [20]. There are no religious restrictions on using sheep as a heparin-source however, a transmissible prion disease (scrapie) does occur in sheep. Although scrapie is not transmissible to humans, infected sheep are typically not used for consumption.

Dromedary (*Camelus dromedaries*) has been suggested as a heparin source since it is free of any religious and health reason concerns. To investigate this source heparin was isolated from dromedary intestines [21]. The disaccharide analysis in this study indicated that non- and monosulfated disaccharides were more abundant in dromedary heparin compared to porcine heparin. Consistent with this low degree of overall sulfation, dromedary raw heparin had a specific aXa activity of

~50–60 IU/mg which is approximately half of the activity of porcine heparin which was purified as a reference in that same study (see Table 1).

Table 1. Overview of characteristic of heparin derived from different sources.

Source	aXa Activity (IU/mg)	aPTT Activity	Average Mol. Weight (kDa)	S/C Ratio	Yield (mg/kg)	Refs
Porcine	148–219	168–277	15.0–19.0 [a]	2.31–2.57	160–260	[15,16,18,22]
Bovine [b]	123–156	103–181	16.2–16.5	2.29–2.40	n.d.	[16,18,19]
Ovine	142	150	22.9	3.66	n.d.	[16]
Dromedary	50–60	n.d.	24.0	2.0	400	[21]
Chicken	111	133	n.d.	2.26	n.d.	[18]
Turkey	16.6	n.d.	n.d.	n.d.	300	[23]
Salmon	110–137	n.d.	<8.0 [c]	2.20	n.d.	[24]
Shrimp	95–100	n.d.	8.5	n.d.	32	[25]
Clam	317	347	14.9	n.d.	2100	[26]

[a] Pharmacopoeial specification; [b] intestinal mucosa; [c] 96% was ≤8.0 Da.

1.1.4. Non-Mammalian Sources

By-products of the poultry industry might seem an obvious source for heparin production because of the high global chicken and turkey meat production. Active heparin can be derived from chicken intestines with a specific aXa activity of 111 IU/mg and slightly lower degree of sulfation compared to porcine heparin produced according to the same method (S/C ratio resp.: 2.26 and 2.40) [18]. In this study, however no yields have been reported. Heparin derived from chicken intestines appears to approach porcine-derived heparin based on disaccharide composition and aXa activity (111 IU/mg) [18]. The specific aXa activity of heparin derived from turkey intestines was extremely low (16.6 IU/mg) [23]. Although based on this information, chicken might be a potential source of biologically active heparin, to the best of our knowledge there is currently no heparin production on an (semi-) industrial scale using poultry-derived starting material. The obtained GAGs from turkey tissue mainly consisted of heparan sulfate. Differences between mammalian and avian immunological mechanisms might be an explanation for the absence of active heparin species in turkey [23].

A relatively recent report on heparin purification from salmon (*Salmo salar*) gills and intestines describes a partial purification where heparin was obtained with a low molecular weight (96% $\leq$ 8000 Da). The aXa activity of the salmon-derived heparin was in the range of clinically approved fractionated heparin (LMWH) [24].

Shrimp (*Penaeus brasiliensis*) heads can also be used as a source of natural LMWH with a yield of 32 mg/kg starting material [25]. This shrimp-derived heparin had a molecular weight of 8500 Da and an aXa activity of 95 IU/mg which is also comparable (on the low end) to LMWH. Nonetheless, in vivo experiments indicated that shrimp heparin had a slightly lower antithrombotic activity compared to pharmaceutical grade LMWH.

Heparin derived from clams (*Tapes phylippinarum*) was found to have substantially better aXa activity (317 IU/mg) compared to typical porcine heparin and an average molecular weight (Mw) of 14,900 Da, which is comparable to unfractionated heparin [26]. The yield of the clamp derived heparin was ~2.1 g/kg dry tissue which is a high yield. However, since the whole animal is used here, there is a strong competition with the food industry, which explains the high price of the starting material. To the best of our knowledge, there is currently no commercial heparin production from any of these sources.

1.1.5. Obtaining and Stabilizing Source Material

This section focusses on porcine intestinal mucosa, since this is the major source of the globally produced heparin. However, the processing steps also apply to bovine heparin. The mucosa production is highly linked to the production of casings for the sausage industry. A typical procedure starts with the removal of the content from the intestine and subsequent soaking of the intestine in a salt solution. After soaking, the mucosa is scraped from the intestines, yielding approximately 0.8 kg of mucosa per pig [22]. The emptied intestines are further processed as casings for the sausage industry and the mucosa is collected for further processing to heparin. Besides mucosa, whole porcine intestines can be used for heparin production and are referred to as "hashed porcine guts" [27,28]. It is known that chemical and/or enzymatic desulfation occurs after prolonged storage (mainly glucosamine 6-*O*-desulfation) resulting in decreased activity [18], therefore some sort of stabilization or preservation of the material is required. Typically, mucosa is preserved using an oxygen scavenger such as sodium bisulphite e.g., 1.5–2.5% *w*/*w* until further processing to limit microbiological growth [29]. Other preservatives which can be added to the mucosa include calcium propionate or phenol [22].

1.1.6. Heparin on Resin

To circumvent the transport of large volumes of mucosa and to reduce the risk of degradation during transport, a method was described [26] where the mucosa is hydrolyzed at the slaughterhouses and the resulting heparin subsequently loaded on an anion exchange resin. For this procedure, 3000–4000 L of intestinal mucosa (daily yield of a typical pig slaughterhouse) was enzymatically hydrolyzed using a subtilisin alkaline protease at 50–55 °C and at alkaline pH. After 3–4 h or when the viscosity was sufficiently reduced (threshold of 14.8 mPa·s) the enzyme was heat-inactivated and the hydrolysate was filtered. To this filtrate 24–30 kg of anion-exchange resin was added (examples described in the patent include Amberlite, Dowex, Duolite and Lewatit) and mixed for 10–13 h. The loaded resin was sieved off, dried and transferred to a container. As a preservative, 50 g/L of sodium bisulphite was added, and the container was shipped to a specialized chemical plant for further processing. Using this method the yield could be improved from 30,000 units per kg of mucosa to 48,000 units per kg mucosa, possibly because of the short processing times. Therefore, this approach can be highly advantageous, especially when sourcing mucosa at distant slaughterhouses. However, it does require more complex equipment, logistics and technical expertise at the slaughterhouses.

1.2. Digestion and Release of Heparin from Proteoglycans

The early heparin production procedures already included (e.g., [8]) a digestion step aiming to liberate the heparin from the (mast-) cells and proteoglycans. This digestion step can be done by autolysis, addition of pancreas extract, saliva, proteolytic enzymes or by chemical means. Chemical hydrolysis can be performed under acidic or alkaline conditions at high temperatures. This might affect the structure of the heparin. For instance, alkaline proteolysis at pH 11 leads to slight 2-*O*-desulfation of the uronic acids through base-catalyzed epoxide formation. [18] For an enzymatic digestion, a wide range of proteolytic enzymes (i.e., proteases) can be applied including trypsin, chymotrypsin [30], papaine [23] or subtilisin-type enzymes such as Alcalase® or Maxatase® [26,29,31]. For this enzymatic digestion, multiple tons of mucosa should be heated until the optimal temperature of the used enzyme (e.g., 50–60 °C for alcalase). Subsequently the pH should be set (e.g., 8.6 for subtilisins) [26,29] and the enzyme can be added at a typical enzyme:substrate ratio is 0.2–2 g/kg mucosa [31]. The reaction mixture is incubated for 4–16 h to ensure heparin is fully released from the proteoglycans.

1.3. Capture of the Heparin

Prior to the capture step, the heparin concentration in the digested starting material is extremely low (~0.01% *w*/*w*). Therefore, the aim of this step is to enrich the heparin content to enable further purification, at a higher concertation later in the process. Initial heparin extraction protocols describe the precipitation of heparin from autolyzed starting material by applying a low pH (2–2.5) and a high concentration of ammonium sulfate [7,8]. This step, most likely, precipitated mainly protein-bound heparins instead of free heparin, as the proteolytic (trypsin) digestion was conducted after this acid precipitation. The heparin crude obtained after this step still contained high amounts of protein [32]. Moreover, it was realized that this acid precipitation did not 'drop out all of the heparin' [33]. This is probably because heparin itself does not precipitate under these conditions. Therefore, in that latter patent a method was described using hydrophobic primary amines (such as hexylamine) which can form an insoluble complex with heparin under slightly acidic conditions due to their positive charge. This neutral heparin-amine complex was subsequently collected as a precipitate on the interface between the aqueous phase and an organic phase (e.g., methyl isobutyl ketone).

The principle of using ammonium cations such as in the example above is currently still the most widely used method for capturing heparin from digestion mixtures according to (patent-) literature. However, currently the quaternary ammonium cations are usually either immobilized on a resin (i.e., anion exchange resin) [29,31] or designed in such a way that they selectively form insoluble complexes with heparin (quaternary ammonium salts) [34,35]. Both methods exploit the polymeric nature and uniquely high charge density of heparin (~3.7 negative charges/disaccharide), distinguishing heparin from other biopolymers such as chondroitin sulfate (CS) (S/C ratio of ~1), dermatan sulfate (DS) (S/C ratio of ~1) or DNA/RNA (1 negative charge per disaccharide) present in the digestion mixture [36]. This allows a strong charge-based cooperative binding.

1.3.1. Precipitation with Quaternary Ammonium Salts

Several patents from the 1960s describe the precipitation of heparin with quaternary ammonium salts [34,35]. The general formula of such a salt is depicted below (Figure 3a) where the X represents any anion that does not render the salt water-insoluble, (e.g., chloride) and the ^{1}R and ^{2}R group represents an aliphatic hydrocarbon chain of at least eight carbons optionally interrupted by: aromatic rings, double bounds, oxygen- or nitrogen atoms and ^{2}R–^{4}R are groups consisting of 1–7 carbon atoms [35]. After incubation of the digestion mixture with such a salt, a water-insoluble complex is formed with the heparin chains. These insoluble complexes can be obtained as solids. One example of an applicable quaternary ammonium salt is Hyamine® 1622 (see Figure 3b) [34]. This patent describes a method were Hyamine 1622 is added to digested ground lungs, subsequently the precipitated Hyamine-heparin salt was filtered off and suspended in an organic solvent. This suspension was extracted with an aqueous solution, and from this solution the potassium salt of heparin precipitated by increasing the potassium acetate concentration to 30% (*w*/*v*). Approximately 0.6 g of crude material was obtained with an activity of 110 IU/mg from 2 kg of ground lungs using this method. Alternatively, the precipitated Hyamine-heparin complex can be extracted using a concentrated NaCl solution (i.e., 2M) to replace the heparin and subsequently precipitated with MeOH to obtain the heparin sodium salt [30]. Neither patents describe an extensive characterization on the obtained heparin, therefore there is no data on the amount of impurities such as nucleic acids and CS/DS.

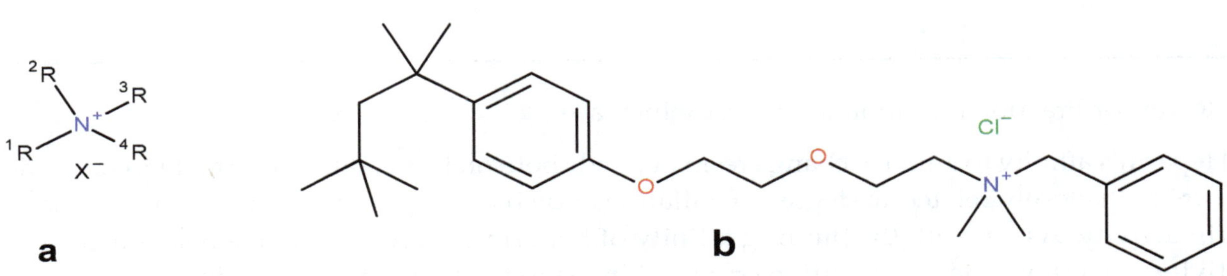

Figure 3. Structures of quaternary ammonium salts used for heparin capture by precipitation. (**a**) General structure of an applicable salt; (**b**) Structure of benzethonium chloride (Hyamine® 1622).

1.3.2. Ion Exchange Resins

Like Hyamine, the ion exchange resin can be added directly to the digestion mixture. Typical amounts of anion exchange resin include 2–4 L per 100 kg of mucosa [31]. Adsorption is typically done over several hours during which temperature, pH and salt concentration are critical parameters. Deviations on any of these parameters might result in increased binding of unwanted contaminants such as nucleic acids or other GAGs. After binding, the loaded resin has to be separated from the now heparin-free digestion mixture by sieving. To enable this sieving the anion exchanger (see Table 1, for functional groups) should be immobilized on a matrix which allows to be sieved. Examples thereof include crosslinked acrylic or polystyrene beads. After sieving the resulting waste stream (peptone) could be used as a fertilizer for farmlands, animal feed of for medical formulations for enteral or parental nutrition [37]. The loaded resin may be washed with water or a solution with a relatively low ionic strength (e.g., 5.8% NaCl m/v) to eliminate unbound material and to reduce less tightly bound compounds such as nucleic acids and other less charged GAGs [38]. This step can also be used to increase the activity of heparin (*vide infra*) by removing heparin with a low affinity to the resin. Subsequent elution with a high salt concentration (i.e., >14%) released the heparin from the column and enables further processing. There are several suitable anion exchange resins available on the market (Table 2). These resins might be the same type as the ones used for water treatment.

Table 2. Selected examples of functional groups used on anion exchange resins for heparin capture.

Resin Name	Functional Group	References
Amberlite IR-120, FPA98/, IRA900/CG-45	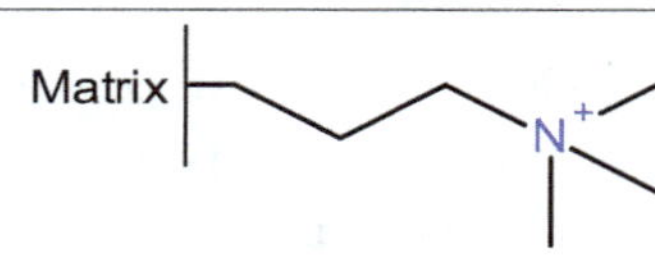	[24,29,31,36]
Dowex 22CL	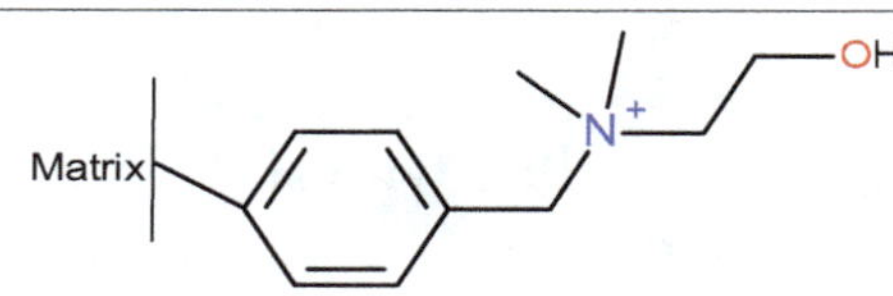	[23]
Lewatitt CA9249	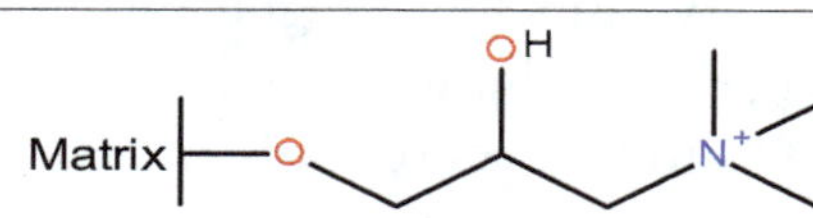	[26,31]
	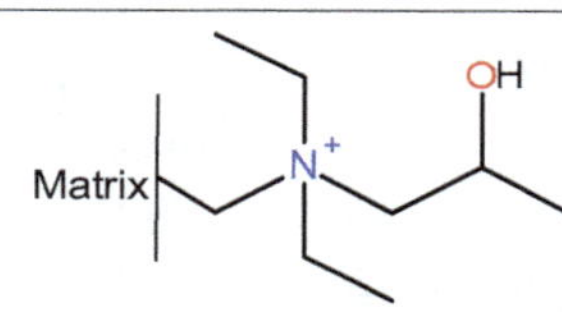	[39]
DEAE	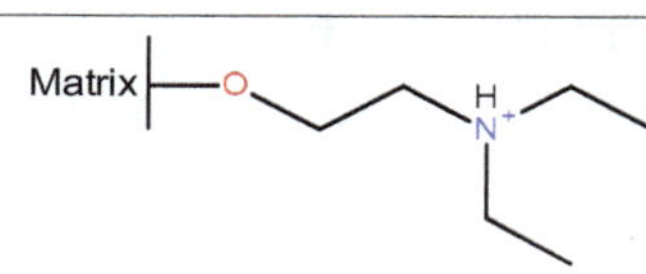	[39,40]

1.3.3. Resins or Fractional Elution for Activity Increase

Heparin's affinity to anion exchange resin depends both on its overall charge and its charge density. These are both closely related to degree of sulfation and chain length which are also important for its heparin activity. As a result, the binding affinity of heparin to anion exchange resin correlates with its activity. Therefore fractional elution or a washing step with a relatively low ionic strength (<3.5% NaCl) help to enrich highly active heparin chains [39–41]. Loaded resin (*N*-*N*-diethyl-2-hydroxypropyl ammonium functionalized cellulose) was washed with a ~2.3% NaCl solution. Subsequent fractional elution with a gradient from 2.3% to 8.2% NaCl enabled the inventors to obtain heparin fractions with a 2.5–5 fold increase of specific activity relative to the starting material yielding heparin with up to 500 IU/mg aXa activity and up to 400 IU/mg aIIa activity. Although for this invention purified heparin was fractionated instead of the more crude form of heparin which is bound to anion exchange resin, this patent illustrates the potential of applying the anion exchanger step to improve the activity, however at the expense of yield since low activity heparin still added to the initial yield. Other resin which can be used to improve heparin activity on lab scale include antihrombin-sepharose [42] and gel filtration columns. The first of these two selects heparin chains based on anti-thrombin affinity which is largely determined by the presence of the "high affinity pentasaccharide" and the second type separates heparin chains based on chain length. Both methods are highly useful analytical tools but due to scaling issues and considerable costs of the column material not practical for industrial scale heparin production.

1.4. *Purification and Bleaching*

At this stage of the production process, we have a heparin crude solution which is relatively pure. The main remaining contaminants at this stage are nucleic acids and non-heparin GAGs, such as chondroitin sulfate (CS) and dermatan sulfate (DS), which like heparin are biopolymers have a relatively high negative charge-density and therefore also adsorb to the anion exchange resin or precipitate with the quaternary ammonium salt. Moreover a variety of pathogens, including: viruses, bacteria and in the case of bovine starting material bovine spongiform encephalopathy (BSE) related prions may not have been adequately reduced to ensure patient safety. Therefore, the following steps are designed to reduce the inactive material such as DNA/RNA and to sufficiently reduce the infectious agents listed above.

1.4.1. (Fractional) Precipitation

Precipitation is both conducted to isolate the heparin or heparin crude from a solution and to remove impurities such as non-heparin GAGs and nucleic acids. It also serves to remove metal ions and small and/or less polar molecules such as peptide fragments generated during digestion and residues of chemicals used in processing: these will remain in the supernatant. For this step, different organic solvents such as methanol, ethanol, propanol, or acetone can be used [36,43]. As a result of decreasing polarity by addition of the antisolvent, the highly charged heparin chains precipitate. Most protocols in the literature apply either methanol or ethanol for this step with a percentage of ~50% (v/v). The concentration of the organic solvent is paramount at this stage as well as NaCl concentration and temperature. This was demonstrated by Volpi [36] who performed a fractional precipitation on a mixture of heparin, CS and DS with methanol, ethanol and propanol. Here it was observed that the order of precipitation of these compounds reflects their charge density (i.e., S/C ratios of resp. 2.4, 1.1 and 0.98). Using a relative volume of 1 methanol (i.e., ~50% v/v) precipitated nearly all the heparin from the mixture whereas a substantial concentration of CS and DS was still present in the supernatant (see Figure 4).

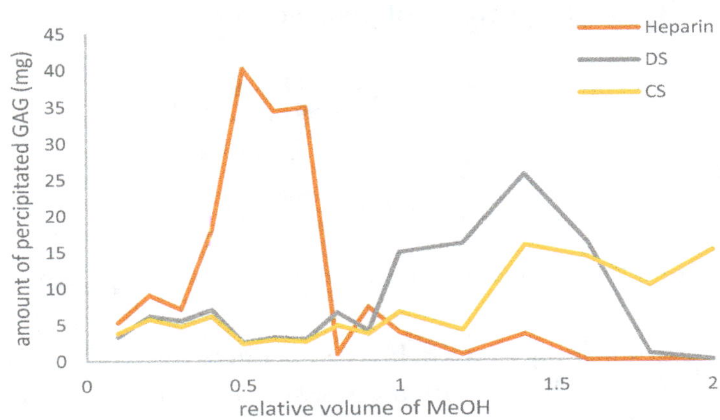

Figure 4. Fractional precipitation of heparin, DS and CS at different concentrations of methanol. Data derived from Volpi et al. [36].

1.4.2. Bleaching

The last step in most heparin processes usually includes an oxidation/bleaching step meant to remove/reduce color, endotoxins (depyrogenization), bacteria, mold, viruses and prions, followed by solvent precipitation sequence and a 0.22 μ sterile filtration to remove microbes and drying [43–47].

The oxidation is performed using e.g., potassium permanganate ($KMnO_4$) hydrogen peroxide (H_2O_2), peracetic acid (CH_3CO_3H), sodium hypochlorite (NaClO) or ozone (O_3) [48]. Prion reduction by hydrogen peroxide oxidation has been used by the FDA as a justification for the re-introduction of bovine heparin [15]. The term 'oxidation' is misleading here and 'bleaching' is more appropriate since the aim of the step is not to affect the heparin molecule by oxidation but rather to purify the heparin. However, this step can still result in the inadvertent modification of the heparin chains. This can result in damage to the heparin chain and/or a reduced biological activity [46,49,50]. In the wake of the 2008 contaminated heparin crisis, 1D ^{1}H-NMR was introduced as a pharmacopoeial release test. 1D ^{1}H-NMR had proved successful in detecting the contaminant oversulfated chondroitin sulfate which has a distinctive signal due to the glucosamine *N*-acetyl group [51–53]. This resulted in close inspection to heparin 1D ^{1}H-NMR spectra for unknown signals in specific spectral areas. Potassium permanganate oxidation has been shown to oxidize the reducing end hydroxyl of *N*-acetyl glucosamine to yield a carboxylate group resulting in a 2.10 ppm signal from the *N*-acetyl function in the NMR spectrum of potassium permanganate bleached heparin (see Figure 5, [54–57]).

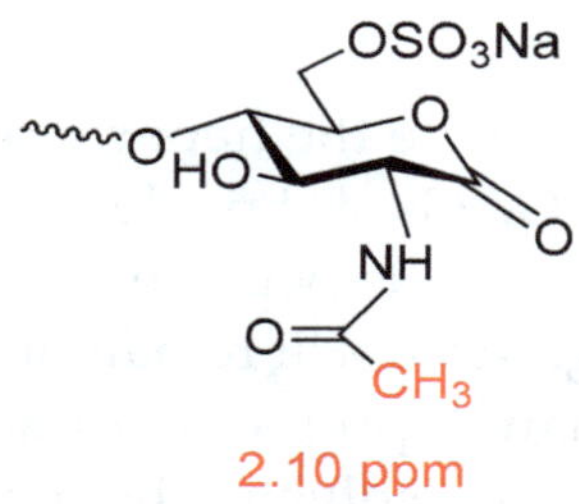

Figure 5. Reducing end oxidized *N*-acetylglucosamine heparin modification as a result of potassium permanganate bleaching.

Potassium permanganate oxidation also results in the reduction of the residual (glycol) serine at the reducing end of the heparin chain [50]. Oxidation by potassium permanganate results in an increase in carboxylate groups in heparin and concomitant chain breaks [50]. This should be taken into account when using the sulfate/carboxylate ratio which is commonly used as a measure for heparin sulfation [57]. Oxidation by peracetic acid results in the formation of 3-acetyluronic acid which displays a signal at 2.18 ppm in the ^{1}H-NMR spectrum of peracetic acid bleached heparin (Figure 6 [58]).

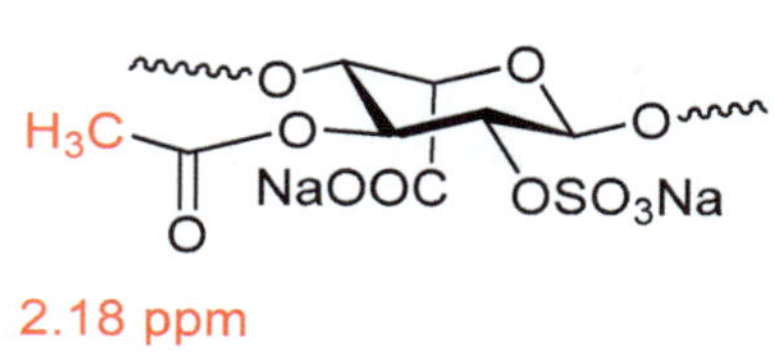

Figure 6. 3-Acetyluronic acid heparin modification as a result of peracetic acid bleaching.

Oxidation by other oxidation agents such as hydrogen peroxide and hypochlorite bleached heparin have not been reported to have a distinctive signals in its ^{1}H-NMR spectrum. Thus, these 'process signatures' allow to discriminate between oxidation methods used based on the ^{1}H-NMR spectroscopy [59]. Other products due to oxidation have been described in the literature [50]. Oxidation as purification step is only feasible because of the high intrinsic stability of the heparin molecule which is evident from a number of studies. [28,60,61] Less stable (bio-) molecules such as proteins would be degraded by these strongly oxidizing conditions, hence the strong virus/prion reductions achieved in this step [3,15]. The high stability of the heparin molecule together with its charged polymeric nature [60] enable it to be isolated in spite of being present at relatively low levels in the complex starting material [27].

1.5. Isolation and Drying

After this bleaching step, most properties of the heparin including: molecular composition, impurity profiles, microbial safety and color are determined. Therefore these steps are optimized to reach maximal yields and a minimum of residual solvents. There are several methods possible to isolate the heparin. Some of these methods include a precipitation step using a high percentage of methanol or ethanol ensuring that all heparin is precipitated. The precipitate is then collected and dried under vacuum at elevated temperatures (e.g., 40–75 °C) [62]. Alternatively, the heparin can be directly isolated from the solution by spray drying [63] or barrel drying [62].

2. Concluding Remark

Sourcing, isolation and purification of this 100 year old drug is still evolving for optimal efficacy and patient safety as well as production efficiency. The strict GMP regulations and pharmacopoeial criteria on the complete supply chain from farm to pharma will continue to assure the safety and efficacy of this WHO essential drug [64].

Acknowledgments: We thank Gijs van Dedem for critical reading of the paper and for his constructive comments.

Author Contributions: J.-Y.v.d.M., E.K. and L.J.v.d.B. constructed the idea for the manuscript, all authors contributed to the writing of the paper.

References

1. Torri, G.; Naggi, A. Heparin centenary—An ever-young life-saving drug. *Int. J. Cardiol.* **2016**, *212*, S1–S4. [CrossRef]
2. Yates, E.A; Rudd, T.R. Recent innovations in the structural analysis of heparin. *Int. J. Cardiol.* **2016**, *212*, S5–S9. [CrossRef]
3. Barrowcliffe, T.W. History of heparin. In *Heparin-A Century of Progress*; Lever, R., Mulloy, B., Page, C.P., Eds.; Springer: Berlin/Heidelberg, Germany, 2012; pp. 3–22.
4. Carlsson, P.; Kjellén, L. Heparin biosynthesis. In *Heparin—A Century of Progress*; Lever, R., Mulloy, B., Page, C.P., Eds.; Springer: Berlin/Heidelberg, Germany, 2012; pp. 23–41.
5. Mulloy, B.; Hogwood, J.; Gray, E.; Lever, R.; Page, C.P. Pharmacology of heparin and related drugs. *Pharmacol. Rev.* **2016**, *68*, 76–141. [CrossRef] [PubMed]
6. Jorpes, E. On the chemistry of heparin. *Biochem. J.* **1942**, *36*, 203–213. [CrossRef] [PubMed]
7. Charles, A.F.; Scott, D.A. Studies on heparin: Observations on the chemistry of heparin. *Biochem. J.* **1936**, *30*, 1927–1933. [CrossRef] [PubMed]
8. Kruizenga, M.H.; Spaulding, L.B. The preparation of highly active barium salt of heparin and its fractionation into two chemically and biologically different constituents. *J. Biol. Chem.* **1943**, *148*, 641–647.
9. Shriver, Z.; Raman, R.; Venkataraman, G.; Drummond, K.; Turnbull, J.; Toida, T.; Linhardt, R.; Biemann, K.; Sasisekharan, R. Sequencing of 3-*O* sulfate containing heparin decasaccharides with a partial antithrombin III binding site. *Proc. Natl. Acad. Sci. USA* **2000**, *97*, 10359–10364. [CrossRef] [PubMed]
10. Olson, S.T.; Richard, B.; Izaguirre, G.; Schedin-Weiss, S.; Gettins, P.G. Molecular mechanisms of antithrombin-heparin regulation of blood clotting proteinases. A paradigm for understanding proteinase regulation by serpin family protein proteinase inhibitors. *Biochimie* **2010**, *92*, 1587–1596. [CrossRef] [PubMed]
11. Petitou, M.; Hérault, J.P.; Bernat, A.; Driguez, P.A.; Duchaussoy, P.; Lormeau, J.C.; Herbert, J.M. Synthesis of thrombin-inhibiting heparin mimetics without side effects. *Nature* **1999**, *398*, 417–422. [CrossRef] [PubMed]
12. European Pharmacopeia. *Monograph for Heparin Sodium Heparinum Natricum*, 9th ed.; 01/2017:0333; Council of Europe: Strasbourg, France, 2017.
13. Guidance for Industry-Heparin for Drug and Medical Device Use: Monitoring Crude Heparin for Quality. Available online: https://www.fda.gov/downloads/Drugs/GuidanceComplianceRegulatoryInformation/Guidances/UCM291390.pdf (accessed on 19 April 2017).

14. EudraLex. The Rules Governing Medicinal Products in the European Union, Volume 4: EU Guidelines for Good Manufacturing Practice for Medicinal Products for Human Van Veterinary Use, Annex 2 Manufacture of Biological Active Substances and Medicinal Products for Human Use. Ref. Ares(2012)118531-28/06/2012. Available online: https://ec.europa.eu/health/sites/health/files/files/eudralex/vol-4/vol4-an2__2012-06_en.pdf (accessed on 16 June 2017).
15. Keire, D.; Mulloy, B.; Chase, C.; Al-Hakim, A.; Cairatti, D.; Gray, E.; Hogwood, J.; Morris, T.; Mourão, P.A.S.; da Luz Carvalho Soares, M.; et al. Diversifying the Global Heparin Supply Chain: Reintroduction of Bovine Heparin in the United States? *Pharm. Technol.* **2015**, *28*, 36.
16. Fu, L.; Li, G.; Yang, B.; Onishi, A.; Li, L.; Sun, P.; Zhang, F.; Linhardt, R.J. Structural Characterization of Pharmaceutical Heparins Prepared from Different Animal Tissues. *J. Pharm. Sci.* **2013**, *102*, 1447–1457. [CrossRef] [PubMed]
17. Bett, C.; Grgac, K.; Long, D.; Karfunkle, M.; Keire, D.A.; Asher, D.M.; Gregori, L. A Heparin Purification Process Removes Spiked Transmissible Spongiform Encephalopathy Agent. *AAPS J.* **2017**, 1–7. [CrossRef] [PubMed]
18. Bianchini, P.; Liverani, L.; Mascellani, G.; Parma, B. Heterogeneity of unfractionated heparins studied in connection with species, source, and production processes. *Semin. Thromb. Hemost.* **1997**, *23*, 3–10. [CrossRef] [PubMed]
19. St. Ange, K.; Onishi, A.; Fu, L.; Sun, X.; Lin, L.; Mori, D.; Zhang, F.; Dordick, J.S.; Fareed, J.; Hoppensteadt, D.; et al. Analysis of heparins derived from bovine tissues and comparison to porcine intestinal heparins. *Clin. Appl. Thromb. Hemost.* **2016**, *22*, 520–527. [CrossRef] [PubMed]
20. Hoppensteadt, D.; Maia, P.; Silva, A.; Kumar, E.; Guler, N.; Jeske, W.; Kahn, D.; Walenga, J.M.; Coyne, E.; Fareed, J. Resourcing of Heparin and Low Molecular Weight Heparins from Bovine, Ovine, and Porcine Origin. Studies to Demonstrate the Biosimilarities. *Blood* **2015**, *126*, 4733. [CrossRef]
21. Warda, M.; Gouda, E.M.; Toida, T.; Chi, L.; Linhardt, R.J. Isolation and characterization of raw heparin from dromedary intestine: Evaluation of a new source of pharmaceutical heparin. *Comp. Biochem. Physiol. C Toxicol. Pharmacol.* **2003**, *136*, 357–365. [CrossRef] [PubMed]
22. Vreeburg, J.W.; Baauw, A. Method for Preparation of Heparin from Mucosa. Patent No. WO2010/110654 A1, 24 March 2009.
23. Warda, M.; Mao, W.; Toida, T.; Linhardt, R.J. Turkey intestine as a commercial source of heparin? Comparative structural studies of intestinal avian and mammalian glycosaminoglycans. *Comp. Biochem. Physiol. B Biochem. Mol. Biol.* **2003**, *134*, 189–197. [CrossRef]
24. Flengsrud, R.; Larsen, M.L.; Ødegaard, O.R. Purification, characterization and in vivo studies of salmon heparin. *Thromb. Res.* **2010**, *126*, e409–e417. [CrossRef] [PubMed]
25. Dietrich, C.P.; Paiva, J.F.; Castro, R.A.; Chavante, S.F.; Jeske, W.; Fareed, J.; Gorin, P.A.; Mendes, A.; Nader, H.B. Structural features and anticoagulant activities of a novel natural low molecular weight heparin from the shrimp *Penaeus brasiliensis*. *Biochim. Biophys. Acta* **1999**, *1428*, 273–283. [CrossRef]
26. Cesaretti, M.; Luppi, E.; Maccari, F.; Volpi, N. Isolation and characterization of a heparin with high anticoagulant activity from the clam *Tapes phylippinarum*: Evidence for the presence of a high content of antithrombin III binding site. *Glycobiology* **2004**, *14*, 1275–1284. [CrossRef] [PubMed]
27. Liu, H.; Zhang, Z.; Linhardt, R.J. Lessons learned from the contamination of heparin. *Nat. Prod. Rep.* **2009**, *26*, 313–321. [CrossRef] [PubMed]
28. Linhardt, R.J.; Gunay, N.S. Production and chemical processing of low molecular weight heparins. *Semin. Thromb. Hemost.* **1999**, *25*, 3–10.
29. Griffin, C.C.; Linhardt, R.J.; van Gorp, C.L.; Toida, T.; Hileman, R.E.; Schubert, R.L.; Brown, S.E. Isolation and characterization of heparan sulfate from crude porcine intestinal mucosal peptidoglycan heparin. *Carbohydr. Res.* **1995**, *276*, 183–197. [CrossRef]
30. Vidic, H.J. Process for Preparation of Heparin. U.S. Patent 4,283,530 A, 12 November 1976.
31. Van Houdenhoven, F.A.E.; Sanders, A.L.M.; van zuthpen, P.J.J. Process for the Purification of Heparin. U.S. Patent 6,232,093, 3 January 2000.
32. Homan, J.D.H.; Lens, J. A simple method for the purification of heparin. *Biochim. Acta* **1948**, *2*, 333–337. [CrossRef]
33. Bush, J.A.; Freeman, S.; Hagerty, E.B. Process for Preparing Heparin. U.S. Patent 2,884,358, 22 April 1957.

34. Nomine, G.; Pierre, B. Process of Purifying Heparin, and Product Produced Therefrom. U.S. Patent 2,989,438, 20 June 1961.
35. Mozen, M.M.; Evans, T.D. Process for Purifying Heparin. U.S. Patent 3,058,884, 14 September 1959.
36. Volpi, N. Purification of heparin, dermatan sulfate and chondroitin sulfate from mixtures by sequential precipitation with various organic solvents. *J. Chromatogr. B Biomed. Sci. Appl.* **1996**, *685*, 27–34. [CrossRef]
37. Van Gorp, C.L.; Vosburgh, F.; Schubert, R.L. Protein Hydrolysate from Mucosal Tissue. U.S. Patent 5,607,840, 30 November 1992.
38. Yamamoto, R.; Bellomo, E.G.; Kim, Y.; Rachana, V.Y.A.S. Method for Enhanced Heparin Quality. Patent No. WO2016/137471 A1, 26 February 2015.
39. Sache, E.; Maman, M.; Bertrand, H. New Heparin fractions Having Increased Anticoagulant Activities. Patent No. GB 2,051,103 A, 10 April 1980.
40. Toccaceli, N. Chromatographic Purification of Heparin. U.S. Patent 3,099,600, 30 July 1963.
41. Green, J.P. Fractionation of heparin on an anion exchanger. *Nature* **1960**, *186*, 472. [CrossRef] [PubMed]
42. Höök, M.; Björk, I.; Hopwood, J.; Lindahl, U. anticoagulant activity of heparin: Separation of high-activity and low-activity heparin species by affinity chromatography on immobilized antithrombin. *FEBS Lett.* **1976**, *66*, 90–93. [CrossRef]
43. Volpi, N. Fractionation of heparin, dermatan sulfate, and chondroitin sulfate by sequential precipitation: A method to purify a single glycosaminoglycan species from a mixture. *Anal. Biochem.* **1994**, *218*, 382–391. [CrossRef] [PubMed]
44. Arthur, B.E.; Ernest, H.J.; William, R.L. Process of Removing Colored Impurities from Heparin. U.S. Patent 2,830,931, 28 June 1954.
45. Bush, J.A.; Freeman, L.D.; Hagerty, E.B. Method for Purifying Sulfated Carbohydrates with Oxidizing Agents. U.S. Patent 31,356,660 A, 9 November 1956.
46. Ewards, F.R.; Horner, A.A. Purification of Heparin. U.S. Patent 3,179,566 A, 16 May 1963.
47. Celsus Website. Available online: https://www.heparin.com/manufacture_controls.php (accessed on 14 April 2017).
48. Coyne, E. Heparin—Past, present and future. In *Chemistry and Biology of Heparin*; Lundblad, R.L., Virgil Brow, W., Mann, K.G., Roberts, H.R., Eds.; Elsevier/North-Holland: Amsterdam, The Netherlands, 1981; pp. 9–17.
49. Yongjun, G. Refining Optimization Technology for Crude Heparin Sodium. Patent No. CN105,001,353 A, 17 August 2015.
50. Mourier, P.; Viskov, C. Process for Oxidizing Unfractionated Heparins and Detecting Presence or Absence of Glycoserine in Heparin and Heparin Products. Patent No. WO2005090411 A1, 24 March 2004.
51. Guerrini, M.; Beccati, D.; Shriver, Z.; Naggi, A.; Viswanathan, K.; Bisio, A.; Capila, I.; Lansing, J.C.; Guglieri, S.; Fraser, B.; et al. Oversulfated chondroitin sulfate is a contaminant in heparin associated with adverse clinical events. *Nat. Biotechnol.* **2008**, *26*, 669–675. [CrossRef] [PubMed]
52. Szajek, A.Y.; Chess, E.; Johansen, K.; Gratzl, G.; Gray, E.; Keire, D.; Linhardt, R.J.; Liu, J.; Morris, T.; Mulloy, B.; et al. The US regulatory and pharmacopeia response to the global heparin contamination crisis. *Nat. Biotechnol.* **2016**, *34*, 625–630. [CrossRef] [PubMed]
53. Szajek, A.Y.; Morris, T.S.; Koch, W.F.; Abernethy, D.R.; Williams, R.L. Inside USP: Heparin Monographs Further Revised. *Pharm. Technol.* **2009**, *33*, 136–137.
54. Beccati, D.; Roy, S.; Yu, F.; Gunay, N.S.; Capila, I.; Lech, M.; Linhardt, R.J.; Venkataraman, G. Identification of a novel structure in heparin generated by potassium permanganate oxidation. *Carbohydr. Polym.* **2010**, *82*, 699–705. [CrossRef] [PubMed]
55. Kellenbach, E.; Sanders, K.; Michiels, P.J.A.; Girard, F.C. 1H NMR signal at 2.10 ppm in the spectrum of KMnO4-bleached heparin sodium: Identification of the chemical origin using an NMR-only approach. *Anal. Bioanal. Chem.* **2011**, *399*, 621–628. [CrossRef] [PubMed]
56. Mourier, P.A.; Guichard, O.Y.; Herman, F.; Viskov, C. Heparin sodium compliance to the new proposed USP monograph: Elucidation of a minor structural modification responsible for a process dependent 2.10 ppm NMR signal. *J. Pharm. Biomed. Anal.* **2011**, *54*, 337–344. [CrossRef] [PubMed]
57. Casu, B.; Gennaro, U. A conductimetric method for the determination of sulphate and carboxyl groups in heparin and other mucopolysaccharides. *Carbohydr. Res.* **1975**, *39*, 168–176. [CrossRef]

58. Mourier, P.A.; Guichard, O.Y.; Herman, F.; Viskov, C. Heparin sodium compliance to USP monograph: Structural elucidation of an atypical 2.18 ppm NMR signal. *J. Pharm. Biomed. Anal.* **2012**, *67*, 169–174. [CrossRef] [PubMed]
59. Lee, S.E.; Chess, E.K.; Rabinow, B.; Ray, G.J.; Szabo, C.M.; Melnick, B.; Miller, R.L.; Nair, L.M.; Moore, E.G. NMR of heparin API: Investigation of unidentified signals in the USP-specified range of 2.12–3.00 ppm. *Anal. Bioanal. Chem.* **2011**, *399*, 651–662. [CrossRef] [PubMed]
60. Jandik, K.A; Kruep, D.; Cartier, M.; Linhardt, R.J. Accelerated stability studies of heparin. *J. Pharm. Sci.* **1996**, *85*, 45–51. [CrossRef] [PubMed]
61. Liu, L.; Linhardt, R.J.; Zhang, Z. Quantitative analysis of anions in glycosaminoglycans and application in heparin stability studies. *Carbohydr. Polym.* **2014**, *106*, 343–350. [CrossRef] [PubMed]
62. Huang, L.; Tang, J.; Wang, Z.; Zhou, J.; Yan, H. Method for Drying Heparin by Atomization. Patent No. CN1,218,058, 26 November 1997.
63. Raghavan, R.; Jett, J.L. Method to Produce a Solid Form of Heparin, U.S. Patent 2004/0176581, 27 February 2004.
64. WHO Model Lists of Essential Medicines. Available online: http://www.who.int/medicines/publications/essentialmedicines/EML_2015_FINAL_amended_NOV2015.pdf?ua=1 (accessed on 8 May 2017).

12

Structural Characterization of the Low-Molecular-Weight Heparin Dalteparin by Combining Different Analytical Strategies

Antonella Bisio [1,*], Elena Urso [1], Marco Guerrini [1], Pauline de Wit [1,2,†], Giangiacomo Torri [1] and Annamaria Naggi [1]

1 Istituto di Ricerche Chimiche e Biochimiche G. Ronzoni, 20133 Milan, Italy; urso@ronzoni.it (E.U.); guerrini@ronzoni.it (M.G.); pdewit@nl.aspenpharma.com (P.d.W.); torri@ronzoni.it (G.T.); naggi@ronzoni.it (A.N.)

2 Department of Cell and Applied Biology, Faculty of Science, Radboud University Nijmegen, 6525 HP Nijmegen, The Netherlands

* Correspondence: bisio@ronzoni.it

† Current address: Aspen Oss B.V., Kloosterstraat 6, 5349 AB Oss, The Netherlands.

Abstract: A number of low molecular weight heparin (LMWH) products are available for clinical use and although all share a similar mechanism of action, they are classified as distinct drugs because of the different depolymerisation processes of the native heparin resulting in substantial pharmacokinetic and pharmacodynamics differences. While enoxaparin has been extensively investigated, little information is available regarding the LMWH dalteparin. The present study is focused on the detailed structural characterization of Fragmin® by LC-MS and NMR applied both to the whole drug and to its enzymatic products. For a more in-depth approach, size homogeneous octasaccharide and decasaccharide components together with their fractions endowed with high or no affinity toward antithrombin were also isolated and their structural profiles characterized. The combination of different analytical strategies here described represents a useful tool for the assessment of batch-to-batch structural variability and for comparative evaluation of structural features of biosimilar products.

Keywords: low-molecular-weight heparin; dalteparin; NMR; LC-MS; affinity chromatography

---

1. Introduction

Low molecular weight heparins (LMWHs) are heterogeneous mixtures of sulfated glycosaminoglycans with notable pharmacological activity. They were developed as alternative therapies to heparin in the prophylaxis and treatment of venous and arterial thrombotic disorders, to overcome its uncommon but potentially serious side effects, such as bleeding and thrombocytopenia, and relative unpredictability [1]. LMWHs are derived from unfractionated heparin (UFH) through controlled chemical or enzymatic depolymerization processes to yield fragments which are approximately one third the size of the original chains with Mws ranging from 1000 to 10,000 Da [2,3]. Owing to their lower molecular size they typically possess more predictable pharmacological action, better bioavailability and longer half-life [4,5]. Depending on manufacturing process, marketed LMWHs mainly differ in degree of depolymerisation, and in the chemical structure of their terminal units, as well as their therapeutic and pharmacological properties.

Apart from characteristic terminal residues [6], their linear internal sequences are primarily composed by 1,4-linked repeating trisulfated disaccharides units containing 2-*O*-sulfated iduronic acid (I_{2S}) and *N*-sulfated glucosamine 6-*O*-sulfated ($A_{NS,6S}$). These trisulfated regions alternate with undersulfated sequences containing non-sulfated uronic acids—iduronic (I) and in lower proportion glucuronic (G)—which are usually preceded by *N*-acetylated glucosamine units (A_{NAc}). The specific pentasaccharide sequence -$A_{NAc,6S}$-G-$A_{NS,3S,6S}$-I_{2S}-$A_{NS,6S}$-(AGA*IA), present only in some of the chains, constitutes the antithrombin binding site (AT-bs), essential for a high anticoagulant and antithrombotic activity of LMWHs, such as that of UFH. LMWH structures can also include traces of the linkage region (LR), the non-sulfated sequence G-Gal-Gal-Xyl which links the original heparin chain to the core protein of its natural proteoglycan precursor through a serine (Ser) residue [7].

Due to the structural diversity and heterogeneity arising from the different methods of preparation, the LMWHs available for clinical use are regarded as chemically and pharmacologically distinct entities, each one with its own unique efficacy and safety profile, and their therapeutic interchange is considered inappropriate. Correlating the biological properties with particular structural motifs has been the most important challenge in the design of new LMWHs as well as in the development of generic versions of these drugs [6].

For the LMWH dalteparin, approved indications include the prevention of venous thromboembolism (VTE) in patients undergoing hip replacement or abdominal surgery and in acutely ill medical patients with severely restricted mobility, in long term secondary prevention of VTE, in patients with VTE and cancer, and in acute coronary syndromes as unstable angina and non-Q wave myocardial infarction [8].

Dalteparin is produced from porcine intestinal mucosa through a relatively simple and low cost method based on a controlled deaminative cleavage with nitrous acid followed by reduction, resulting in the formation of an anhydromannitol (aM.ol) ring at the reducing end. The complete structural characterization of dalteparin, such as of all LMWHs, should supply information on the size of the chains, the monosaccharide composition in terms of iduronic/glucuronic acid, *N*-sulfated/*N*-acetylated glucosamine content and sulfation pattern and the sequence of these residues along the chains. No single technique is able to fulfil all these requirements and only a combination of orthogonal analytical approaches can provide a thorough characterization. Among the analytical approaches used for structure investigation of LMWHs, NMR spectroscopy and mass spectrometry (MS) represent the most effective techniques [3]. In particular, a growing interest has been registered in the last two decades in the application of MS, by increasingly sophisticated instruments with higher mass resolution and accuracy. A relevant contribution to the analysis of very complex mixtures such as LMWHs was provided by the direct connection of mass spectrometry to liquid chromatography systems (LC-MS) [9–11]. Among the most recent academic studies, fingerprint analysis by reversed-phase ion-pairing ultra-performance liquid chromatography coupled to high resolution mass spectrometry (RPIP-UHPLC–MS), has been proved to be a very important analytical method to ensure, in a very fast way, drug quality and collection of extremely interesting information about oligosaccharide structure, chain length and chemical modification [12,13]. Nevertheless, due to the extremely high complexity of samples exhibiting large polydispersity over a large molecular weight distribution together with several isomers, further approaches are necessary to obtain a detailed understanding of the samples and make ensure the comparability between different samples and lot-to-lot variability. Heparin/heparan sulfate fragment mapping by enzymatic digestion either with either heparinase I, II and III or using a mixture of them is a very common strategy reported in several studies and different analytical methods to run the depolymerized solutions and record interesting information in function to the technique used are often described [14–18]. Moreover, it was recently described that the quantitative NMR-HSQC analysis, applied to determine the mono- and disaccharide composition of heparin and LMWHs, can be used for detailed structural comparison studies between generic or biosimilar drugs with the reference product [19].

The present work describes the in-depth structural characterization of dalteparin by 2D-NMR and LC-MS techniques, applied both to intact chains and to their enzymatic products. The sample depolymerization by two strategies involving the exhaustive digestion with a cocktail of heparinases I, II and III and heparinase III bottom up fragment mapping, allows one to obtain samples of reduced complexity and at the same time point out eventual structural motifs. As a further level of detailed analysis, investigation of appropriate size-exclusion chromatography fractions, such as octa- and decasaccharides, and of their sub-fractions endowed of high affinity (HA) or no affinity (NA) for antithrombin was performed. The overall analytical approach here described represents an effective strategy for comparative purposes of structural features of different lots of dalteparin samples either concerning the appraisal of batch-to-batch variability or the evaluation of biosimilar products.

2. Results and Discussion

2.1. NMR Characterization

The mono/disaccharide percentage content of eleven different batches of Fragmin® was determined by applying a recently validated method [19]. The HSQC spectrum reported in Figure 1 shows all major and minor signals used for integration. Results are presented in Table 1.

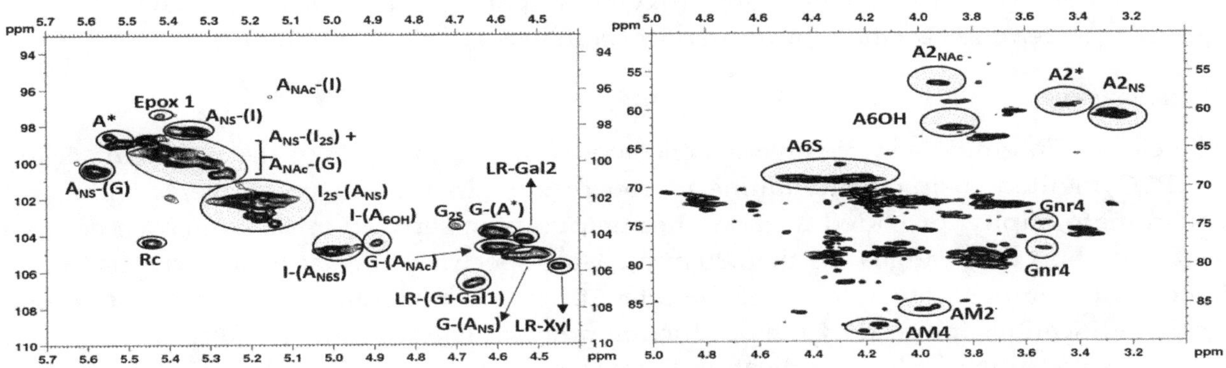

Figure 1. Anomeric (left) and ring (right) regions of $^{1}H/^{13}C$ HSQC NMR spectrum of Frag-5. AM corresponds to aM.ol.

Table 1. Percent content of variously substituted glucosamine and uronic acid residues in different disaccharide sequences of Fragmin® samples, together with typical linkage region residues.

	Frag-1	Frag-2	Frag-3	Frag-4	Frag-5	Frag-6	Frag-7	Frag-8	Frag-9	Frag-10	Frag-11
Amines											
A_{NS}-(I_{2S})	55.7	56.6	55.2	55.8	57.2	58.1	56.3	57.2	59.0	55.2	55.7
A_{NS}-I	7.6	5.9	7.0	7.6	6.6	6.8	6.9	7.1	6.5	7.5	8.1
A_{NS}-(G)	5.9	6.0	5.8	5.9	5.9	5.6	6.0	5.9	5.7	5.6	5.6
A*	5.9	5.5	6.1	5.3	5.6	4.9	5.5	5.2	4.7	5.5	5.1
A_{NAc}-(G)	9.4	9.5	9.0	9.5	9.3	9.2	9.2	9.3	8.9	9.7	9.7
A_{NAc}-(I)	nd	nd	nd	nd	nd	nd	nd	nd	nd	nd	nd
A_{NH2}	nd	nd	nd	nd	nd	nd	nd	nd	nd	nd	nd
A-epox	nd	nd	0.8 *	0.6 *	0.6 *	0.7 *	0.8 *	0.6 *	nd	1.1 *	nd
A-(GalA)	1.6	1.9	1.4 *	1.0 *	1.1 *	1.1 *	0.5 *	1.0 *	0.9 *	2.0	1.4
A_{6S}	90.7	90.5	90.6	90.4	89.9	90.3	90.6	89.8	90.2	91.0	90.8
aM.ol	12.9	13.3	13.5	13.3	12.9	12.6	13.9	12.7	13.2	12.7	13.3
Rc	1.0 *	1.2 *	1.0 *	0.9 *	0.8 *	1.0 *	1.0 *	0.9 *	1.1 *	0.7 *	1.2 *
Uronic acids											
I_{2S}	75.3	77.3	76.4	76.9	76.2	76.5	75.8	76.6	76.7	73.2	74.1
I-(A_{6S})	8.3	7.2	7.4	7.2	7.0	7.4	7.1	7.0	7.0	8.3	8.6
I-(A_{6OH})	0.6	0.7 *	0.8 *	1.0 *	0.7 *	0.7 *	0.9 *	0.9 *	0.7 *	0.8 *	0.9 *
G-(A*)	4.9	4.4	4.4	4.4	4.4	4.5	4.7	4.4	4.5	5.0	4.7
G-(A_{NS})	6.0	5.2	5.8	5.8	5.9	5.4	5.8	5.3	5.7	5.7	6.8
G-(A_{NAc})	3.9	4.6	3.9	4.1	4.5	4.7	4.9	4.5	5.3	4.1	3.8
Gnr	nd	nd	nd	nd	nd	nd	nd	nd	nd	nd	nd
epox	nd	nd	0.8 *	0.6 *	0.6 *	0.7 *	0.7 *	0.6 *	nd	1.0 *	nd
GalA	1.1	0.7 *	0.5 *	nd	0.5 *	nd	nd	0.7 *	nd	1.7	1.1 *
Linkage region											
Gal1+G	1.6 *	1.2 *	1.6	2.1	2.0	1.8	2.1	2.0	1.9	1.3 *	1.4
Gal2	1.3 *	1.0 *	1.3 *	1.6	1.5	1.4 *	1.6	1.4	1.6	1.2 *	1.0 *
Xyl-Ser-ox	0.8 *	0.6 *	0.8 *	0.9 *	0.9 *	1.0 *	1.0 *	0.9 *	1.1	0.6 *	0.7 *
Xyl-Ser	nd	nd	nd	nd	nd	nd	nd	nd	nd	nd	nd

nd indicates values under the limit of detection (LOD); * indicates values under the limit of quantification (LOQ); Gnr indicates glucuronic acid located at the non-reducing end.

The main structural features of dalteparin revealed by HSQC NMR analysis were the presence of an anhydromannitol ring as the only detectable residue at the reducing end, the relatively high content of sulfated monosaccharides and a substantial percentage of G-(A*) marker of the binding site for antithrombin, in agreement with previous results [20], the absence of N-acetylated glucosamine linked to non-sulfated iduronic acid [A_{NAc}-(I)] and a modest presence of linkage region. Moreover, traces of anomalous structures were also detected, such as epoxide and 2-deoxy-2-C-hydroxymethylpentafuranosidic residues. The former is the result of alkaline treatments possibly suffered by the parent heparin and are identified by typical H2/C2 and H3/C3 signals at 3.74/54.2 and 3.82/53.3 ppm, respectively. Such epoxides can convert to L-galacturonic acid (GalA) during the processes for preparation of both unfractionated heparin and LMWH and this structure was identified too. The latter structure is a side effect of nitrous acid treatment of heparin used to obtain dalteparin. Actually, some internal glucosamine residues can undergo a deamination to give, by ring contraction (Rc), a 2-deoxy-2-C-hydroxymethylpentafuranosidic residue, which hexocyclic CH_2 groups are identified by the typical chemical shift at 5.45/104.5 ppm [21].

2.2. Chain Mapping

The eleven Fragmin® samples were subjected to LC-MS analysis of the whole intact mixture. The UHPLC method, using pentylamine as ion reagent in the ion pair reversed phase (IPRP) liquid chromatography, provided a good chromatographic separation of numerous components in a relatively short time range (less than 30 min). Mass spectral information allowed us to calculate oligosaccharide composition, in terms of chain length, number of sulfate and/or acetyl groups, and chemical modifications induced by the production process. The structure hypothesis was expressed using a code consisting of a letter indicating the non-reducing residue, such as U (uronic acid) or A (glucosamine) followed by three numbers indicating monosaccharide residues, sulfate groups and *N*-acetyl groups, respectively, followed by the aM.ol symbol for the fragment residues terminating with 2,5-anhydro-D-mannitol. All samples displayed highly similar UHPLC/MS profiles in terms of number and shape of peaks; in Figure 2 a representative base peak chromatogram (BPC) is reported. Mass spectra details of the main signals detected in all dalteparin samples are reported in Table S1.

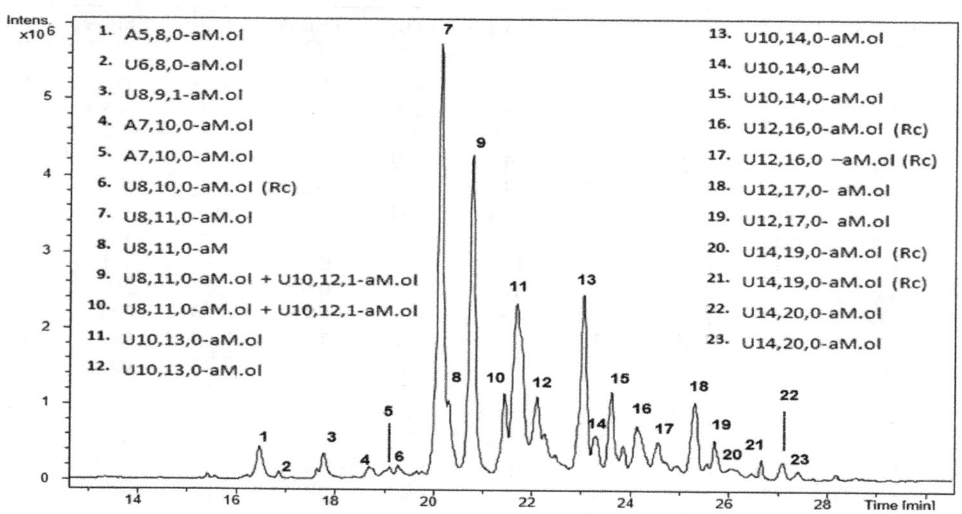

Figure 2. LC-MS profile (BPC) of a representative Fragmin® sample (Frag-5). Mass signals assignment of the main components is reported. LC conditions: isocratic step at 15% B for 1 min, followed by a linear gradient from 15% to 40% B in 31 min; then, column washing and reconditioning in the initial conditions were performed.

Twentythree main species ranging from pentamer to tetradecamer were detected. It is important to underline that the intensity of peaks observable in Figure 2 is not related to the content of oligomeric species. Actually, the ion desorption efficiency in mass spectrometry ionization source is strongly affected by structure and molecular weight of components. In general, the higher the molecular weight of a species the lower the MS response is. This explains the apparent discrepancy between the LC-MS profile displayed in Figure 2 and the oligomeric composition profiles obtained by size exclusion chromatography (Section 2.5, Figures S3–S5).

The main species detected are associated to anhydromannitol derivative structures, most of them having a high degree of sulfation and no acetyl group. Almost all the oligosaccharides have a high degree of sulfation, but a few monoacetylated species were also observed. Odd species (penta- and heptasaccharides) were detected as minor components. Since they have a glucosamine residue at the non-reducing end, they represent original terminal chains of the parent heparin which dalteparin was derived from.

Interestingly, a number of fully sulfated oligosaccharides were detected, such as U8,11,0-aM.ol, U10,14,0-aM.ol, U12,17,0-aM.ol and U14,20,0-aM.ol. They are expected to correspond to regular sequences made up of trisulfated disaccharides (I_{2S}-$Glc_{NS,6S}$) and terminating with the typical anhydromannitol moiety, i.e., (I_{2S}-$Glc_{NS,6S}$)$_n$-I_{2S}-aM.ol$_{6S}$, where n range from 3 to 6. Nevertheless, for each of the above oligomers at least two isomers were found: for U8,11,0-aM.ol in particular, two isomers were recorded as main components under the peaks 7 and 9, and a third one as minor species in the peak 10. Different isomers could contain a G-A* sequence in different positions (positional isomers).

The molecular mass of dalteparin oligosaccharides terminating with 2,5-anhydro-D-mannitol shows a loss of 15 Da with respect to the MW of unmodified heparin oligosaccharides, corresponding to the loss of an amino group produced by the depolymerization process.

Mass signals corresponding to a further loss of 15 Da can be often observed, suggesting an additional deamination, most probably occurred on glucosamine residues within the chain, with no subsequent depolymerization. In agreement with NMR data, such signals were associated to a ring contracted (Rc) unit, derived from a glucosamine residue [21]. Structures with the Rc unit were observed in nearly all peaks of the chromatogram. As reported in Figure 2, the presence of all these structures has been verified in peaks 6, 16, 17, 20 and 21. Minor mass signals corresponding to the expected molecular mass with 2 Daltons less were detected and identified as an aldehyde form (aM) produced by an incomplete reduction to the 2,5-anhydro-D-mannitol terminal residue.

2.3. Building Blocks Analysis by Heparinases I, II, III Digestion

Under exhaustive digestion conditions, 23 major entities were typically observed (Figure 3). Mass spectra details of the main signals detected in all dalteparin samples are reported in Table S2. Regular unsaturated disaccharides with different sulfation degree, but also monoacetylated and saturated disaccharides were observed. In particular, two isomers of the saturated disaccharide U2,3,0 were detected under the peak of the main trisulfated disaccharide ΔU2,3,0, suggesting the presence of the following isomers I_{2S}-$A_{NS,6S}$ and G-A* (Figure 3). Accordingly, a number of dalteparin chains starting with G-A* sequence at the non-reducing end are expected.

Several anhydromannitol residues were identified in different chains ranging from disaccharides to hexasaccharides. Minor signals were assigned to disaccharide ΔU2,1,0-aM.ol, ΔU2,2,0-aM.ol and to hexasaccharide ΔU6,6,1-aM.ol. The highest component in the tetrasaccharides region was attributed to ΔU4,5,0-aM.ol with five sulfate groups and the anhydro derivative at the reducing end glucosamine, followed by ΔU4,4,1 with four sulfates and an acetyl group. The former could be interpreted as ΔU_{2S}-$A_{NS,6S}$-I_{2S}-aM.ol$_{6S}$ and its survival can be explained by the presence of anhydromannitol derivative; the latter can be explained as ΔU-$A_{NAc,6S}$-G-A*. In fact, the presence of 3-*O*-sulfate glucosamine renders the glycosidic bond between *N*-acetylated, 6-*O*-sulfated glucosamine and the unsulfated glucuronic acid impervious to the action of heparinases [22]. This effect can be used to obtain interesting structural information, mainly in the tetra-hexasaccharides region. Actually, among the minor tetrasaccharide species, two interesting structures were detected such as ΔU4,5,0 and ΔU4,5,1, both deriving from the possible fragmentation of two structural variants of the binding site. Their most probable sequence interpretations are as follows: ΔU-$A_{NS,6S}$-G-A* and ΔU_{2S}-$A_{NAc,6S}$-G-A*, respectively.

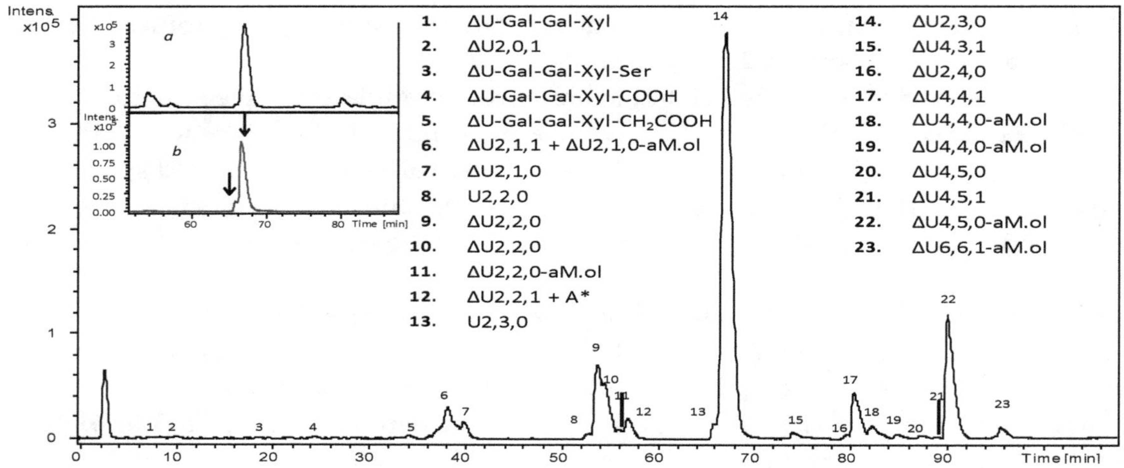

Figure 3. LC-MS profile (BPC) of a representative Fragmin® sample (Frag-5) depolymerized by a cocktail of Heparinase I, II, III. Mass signals assignment of the main components is reported. *Inset*: expansion of chromatogram portion with the main unsaturated trisulfated disaccharide (ΔU_{2S}-$A_{NS,6S}$) eluted (panel a); extracted ion chromatograms (EIC) of m/z 594.0 attributed to saturated trisulfated disaccharide (panel b): as indicated by arrows, two positional isomers were detected. LC elution conditions: isocratic step at 2% B for 10 min, followed by a linear gradient to 60% B in 90 min and final steps of column washing and reconditioning.

2.4. *Bottom up Analysis by Heparinases III Digestion*

Heparinase III cleaves the linkage between N-acetylated glucosamine A_{NAc}, with or without 6-O-sulfate, and glucuronic or iduronic acid, with preference for the former. As expected, all the fully sulfated oligosaccharides and their isomers, identified by the previous chain mapping analysis, were not recognized by this enzyme. The LC-MS profile and mass spectra assignment (Figure 4) show several oligosaccharides arising from the intact parent Fragmin® (with m/z values accounting for oligomers ranging from hexa- to hexadecasaccharides). Mass spectra details of the main signals detected in all dalteparin samples are reported in Table S3.

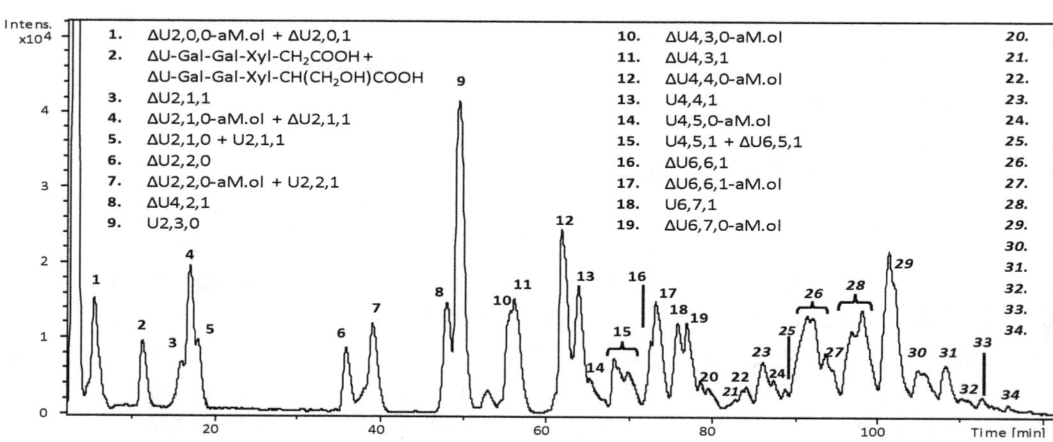

Figure 4. LC-MS profile (BPC) of a representative Fragmin® sample (Frag-5) following digestion with heparinase III. Mass signals assignment of the main components is reported. Components identified in the parent sample, before the enzymatic digestion, are indicated in italic font. LC elution conditions: isocratic at 10% B for 5 min, linear gradient from 10% to 50% B in 55 min, linear gradient from 50% B to 90% B in 80 min, followed by column washing and reconditioning.

Highly sulphated odd intact structures were also observed and identified as pentasaccharide A5,8,0-aM.ol and heptasaccharide A7,11,0-aM.ol. Confirmation of the sum formula of both oligosaccharides was provided by Ion Cyclotron Resonance-FT-MS (ICR-FT-MS) analysis (Figures S2 and S3, Supplementary Material). These unusual oligosaccharide composition can be explained by the presence of I_{2S}-A* sequence inside their chain, $(A_{NS,6S}$-$I_{2S})_{1or2}$-A*-I_{2S}-aM.ol_{6OS}. Such interpretation would be in agreement with the previous building blocks results where the disaccharide ΔU2,4,0, compatible with the structure ΔU_{2S}-A*, was detected.

2.5. Isolation of Octasaccharide and Decasaccharide Fractions

Fractionation of dalteparin by size exclusion chromatography into size homogeneous oligomeric fractions can be achieved both by Biogel P6 and Biogel P10 [20]. For the present work, all the analysed dalteparin samples underwent chromatographic fractionation on Biogel P6, to obtain a fingerprint of their overall oligomeric composition: their highly similar chromatographic profiles are compared in Figures S3–S5 (Supplementary Material). A series of peaks were resolved with each peak corresponding to a size-homogeneous oligomeric family. In particular, octa- and decasaccharide fractions were isolated from Frag-11 by implementing three chromatographic runs which yielded, after desalting, 27.6 mg of octasaccharides and 60.5 mg of decasaccharides, corresponding to 3.1% and 7.8%, respectively, of the whole sample.

2.6. Affinity Chromatography Separation of NA and HA Components

The isolated size-homogeneous oligosaccharide fractions were fractionated with regards to their ability to interact with AT-Sepharose column. Affinity chromatography of octa- and decasaccharides resulted in the separation of two components: the first one, considered devoid of affinity for AT as eluting at lower ionic strength (NA); the second one endowed of high affinity for AT as eluting at higher ionic strength (HA). The relative content of HA components for octa and decasaccharides with respect to the total fraction, were 5% and 6% respectively.

2.7. NMR Characterization of Octasaccharide and Decasaccharide Fractions and of their NA and HA Components

The isolated octa and decasaccharide fractions and their corresponding NA and HA components were studied through the quantitative compositional analysis method based on HSQC ^{1}H-^{13}C correlation measurement already applied for parent LMWH. The average monosaccharide content of all samples is presented in Table 2.

Table 2. Percent content of variously substituted glucosamine and uronic acid residues in octa and decasaccharide fractions, and in their corresponding HA and NA components. n.d. = not detected.

	Octa	HA-Octa	NA-Octa	Deca	HA-Deca	NA-Deca
Amines						
A_{NS}-(I_{2S})	56.6	34.5	58.6	58.1	27.0	59.8
A_{NS}-I	2.8	4.1	2.3	4.6	13.8	4.1
A_{NS}-(G)	4.4	10.3	2.8	5.3	9.0	5.1
A*	10.5	21.9	8.1	6.4	20.3	5.0
A_{NAc}-(G)	2.2	7.2	2.0	4.4	11.6	3.3
A_{NAc}-(I)	n.d.	n.d.	n.d.	n.d.	n.d.	n.d.
A_{NH2}	n.d.	n.d.	0.8	n.d.	n.d.	n.d.
A-epox	n.d.	n.d.	n.d.	n.d.	n.d.	n.d.
A-(GalA)	0.9	n.d.	0.8	0.9	n.d.	n.d.
A_{6S}	98.5	99.5	98.8	97.0	99.5	97.4
aM.ol	20.8	21.6	22.6	19.0	18.2	18.7
Rc	1.0	n.d.	1.0	1.3	n.d.	1.5

Table 2. *Cont.*

	Octa	HA-Octa	NA-Octa	Deca	HA-Deca	NA-Deca
Uronic acids						
I_{2S}	84.7	69.7	88.2	81.6	66.0	81.8
I-(A_{6S})	2.7	3.2	2.5	4.7	14.2	3.9
I-(A_{6OH})	n.d.	n.d.	n.d.	0.7	n.d.	0.6
G-(A*)	8.2	22.6	6.1	5.8	17.5	5.0
G-(A_{NS})	2.9	4.4	2.4	4.8	2.3	5.1
G-(A_{NAc})	0.6	n.d.	n.d.	1.5	n.d.	2.1
Gnr	4.6	traces	4.2	1.5	traces	2.9
G_{2S}	n.d.	traces	n.d.	n.d.	n.d.	n.d.
epox	n.d.	n.d.	n.d.	n.d.	n.d.	n.d.
GalA	0.9	n.d.	0.7	0.9	n.d.	1.4

Given the length of oligosaccharide sequences, additional structural information with respect to whole Fragmin® samples was determined (Table 1) such as the percent content of glucuronic acid located at the non-reducing end (Gnr). Whereas no significant differences were detected between octa- and decasaccharide composition, the most important diversities were displayed by each NA and HA components with respect to the parent oligosaccharides. Signals of residues associated with the AT-binding pentasaccharide sequence, e.g., A*, G-(A*) and A_{NAc}-(G), increased in HA components and their percentage content turned out to be about two-three times higher with respect to parent oligosaccharide fractions. Monodimensional ^{1}H-NMR spectra of HA and NA components of the two oligosaccharide fractions clearly revealed the main structural differences above mentioned (Figure 5). In both HA sub-fractions a substantial increase of the typical signals of AT-bs ($A_{NS,3S}$, GlcA and acetyl group) appeared accompanied by the expected decrease of N-sulfated glucosamine, A_{NS}. Additionally, in HA-deca, a significant increase of non-sulfated iduronic acid, which is expected to precede the AGA*IA sequence, was also observed and quantified. No trace of linkage region was detected in parent oligosaccharides or their derived components. Interestingly, despite a small amount of ring contracted unit (Rc) and galacturonic acid were detected in total octasaccharide and decasaccharide fractions, no traces of these structures appeared in both octa-HA and deca-HA components. The presence of anomalous monosaccharide units in so short sequences would impair definitely their interaction with AT.

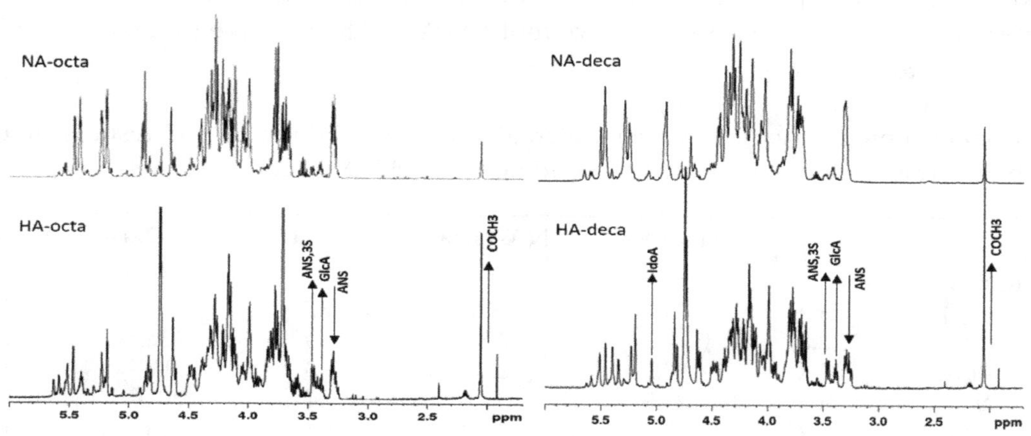

Figure 5. ^{1}H-NMR spectra of HA and NA components of octa and decasaccharide fractions. The direction of arrows, up or down, indicates the increase or decrease respectively of some characteristic signals in spectra of HA components.

2.8. LC-MS Analysis of Octasaccharide and Decasaccharide fractions

The compositional profiles of the isolated octa- and decasaccharide fractions are presented in Figure 6, together with the list of the main oligomeric species detected in BPCs. In the octasaccharide fraction, different octameric sequences were detected with a number of sulfate groups ranging from 9 to 11. In particular, nona- and decasulfated species, U8,9,1-aM.ol and U8,10,1-aM.ol respectively, contained also an acetyl group, whereas undecasulfated sequences, i.e., U8,11,0-aM.ol, accounted for a regular fully sulfated sequence. Two out of ten species are the most represented sequences, all accounting for the fully sulfated octasaccharide U8,11,0-aM.ol. A few species present in minor peaks, whose m/z ratio accounted for nona- and decasaccharides, coeluted with octasaccharides, including two isomers of a highly sulfated nonasaccharide sequence bearing 13 and 14 sulfate groups, respectively (A9,13,0-aM.ol and A9,14,0-aM.ol). As previously discussed, oligosaccharides with a glucosamine residue located at the non-reducing end represent the original terminal chains of the parent heparin.

The decasaccharide fraction turned out to be composed by eight main species bearing from 12 to 14 sulfate groups and including three monoacetylated dodecasulfated isomers. A sequence containing a ring contracted unit (Rc) was also detected. As for octasaccharide fraction, also in this case two isomers of the fully sulfated sequence U10,14,0-aM.ol were detected.

As already discussed in "Chain mapping" paragraph, together with octa and decasaccharides with regular structure $(I_{2S}\text{-}A_{NS,6S})_n\text{-}I_{2S}\text{-}aM.ol_{6S}$ ($n = 3$ or 4 respectively), isomers containing a G-A* in different positions are expected. Such oligosaccharides could either contain a fully sulfated AT-bs or a fragment if it. Actually, the presence of a G-A* located at the non-reducing terminal chain would be in agreement with the presence of Gnr detected by NMR in both oligosaccharide fractions.

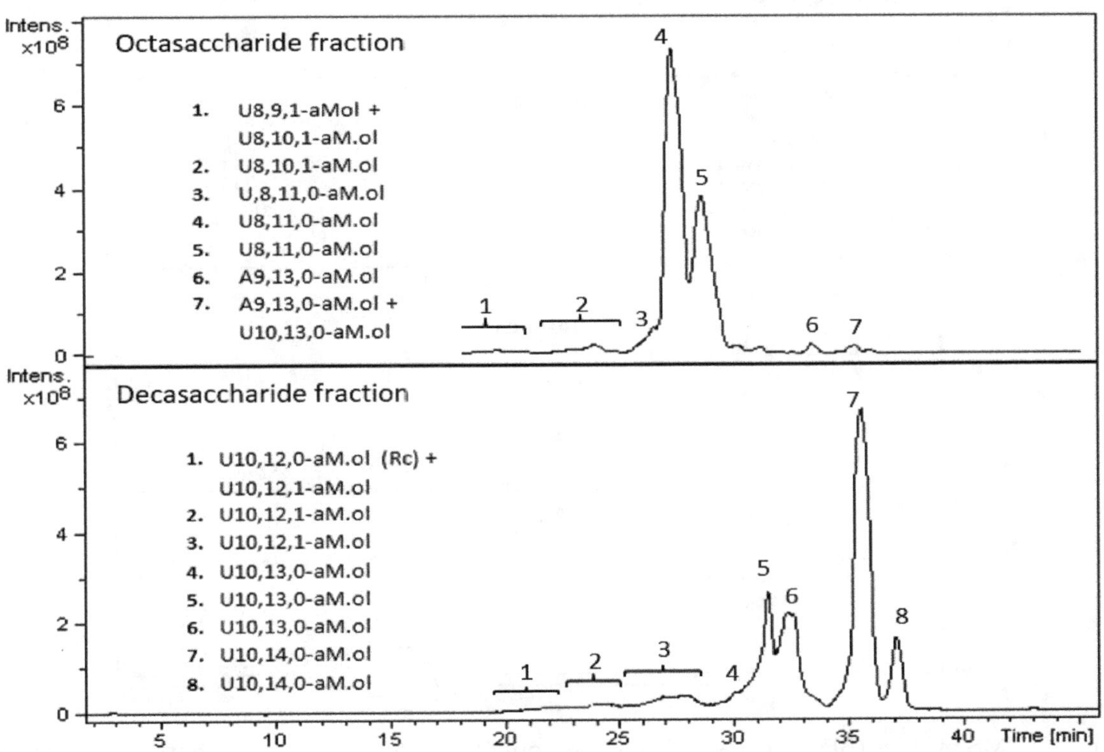

Figure 6. LC-MS profiles (BPC) of exemplary octasaccharide and decasaccharide fractions isolated from of Frag-5. Mass signals assignment of the main components is reported. LC elution conditions: linear gradients from 50% B to 57% B in 5 min and from 57% B to 80% B in 52 min, followed by column washing at 90% B and reconditioning in the initial conditions.

In principle, fully sulfated octa and decasaccharides could contain also G_{2S}–$A_{NS,6S}$ sequences in alternative to the prevailing trisulfated disaccharide. Nevertheless, the presence of G_{2S} residue was not detected by NMR spectra, possibly because under the sensitivity of the technique (Table 2). Further experiments are required to prove our hypothesis. Anyway, although such structural details were of great concern, their understanding did not meet the scope of the present paper.

2.9. LC-MS Analysis of NA and HA components of Octasaccharide and Decasaccharide fractions

It is important to underline that the sub-fractionation of oligosaccharide fractions based on their interaction with AT-Sepharose column, and then the composition of the resulting NA and HA components, greatly depend on the elution conditions applied (e.g., type of salt, salt concentration, type of gradient, etc.).

The compositional profiles of the obtained NA and HA components of both octa and decasaccharides greatly differed each other for the number and intensity of peaks (Figure 7). The reduced complexity of both sub-fractions allowed to detect also some species that were not observed in the whole corresponding oligosaccharide fractions, such as A7,9,1-aM.ol and A7,10,0-aM.ol in HA-octa, U8,8,1-aM.ol in NA-octa, and A11,15,0-aM.ol in HA-deca. In HA-octa sub-fraction five main octameric species were revealed including (i) two monoacetylated sequences (U8,9,1-aM.ol; U8,10,1-aM.ol), which are expected to contain the AGA*IA sequence; (ii) three fully sulfated octasaccharides, possibly containing an AT-bs with all N-sulfated glucosamines (U8,11,0-aM.ol) [23]; (iii) two coeluted heptasaccharides, a fully sulfated one, A7,10,0-aM.ol and the monoacetylated A7,9,1-aM.ol.

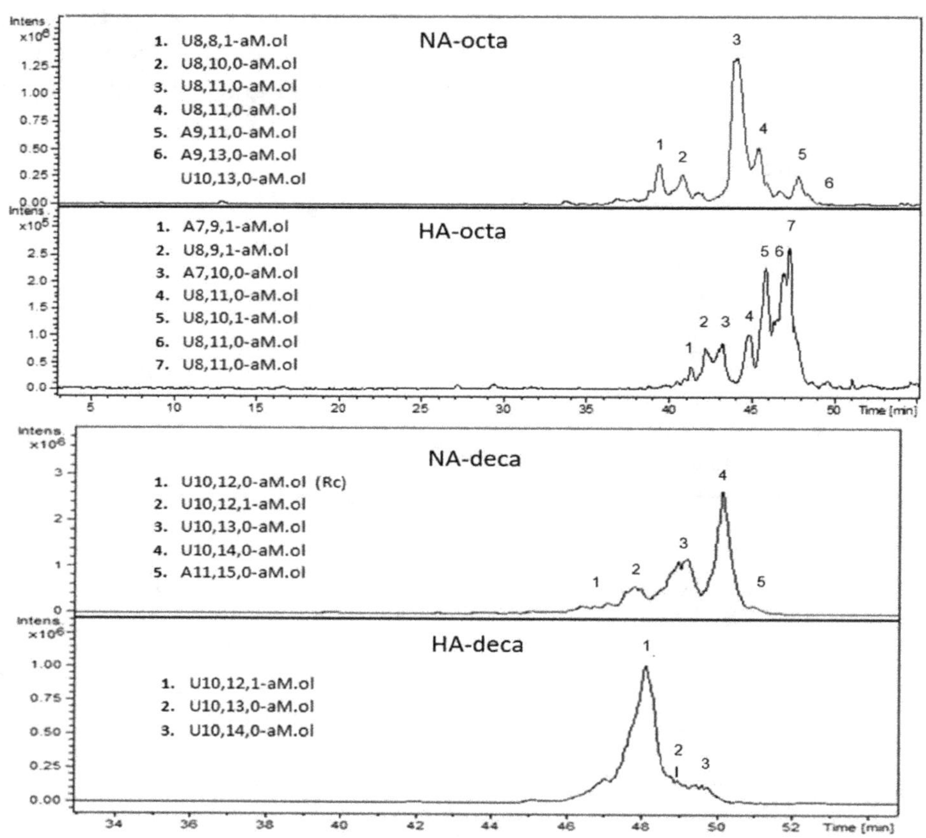

Figure 7. LC-MS profiles (BPC) of HA and NA components of octa- and decasaccharide fractions. Mass signals assignment of the main components is reported. LC elution conditions: isocratic at 20% Solvent B for 20 min, gradient elution from 20% B to 40% B for 10 min followed by a 20 min gradient from 40% B to 90% B; subsequently, 90% B was kept for 10 min.

In agreement with NMR data (Table 2) and building block analysis results (Figure 3), the structure of the main species detected in HA-octa fraction can be interpreted as shown in Table 3.

Heptasaccharides 1 and 3 are both compatible with the presence of AT-binding region, bearing an acetyl group or a sulfate group on the reducing glucosamine, respectively. Two possible interpretations have been reported for octasaccharide 2 (U8,9,1-aM.ol), both containing the AGA*IA pentasaccharide located in two different positions.

Table 3. Structure assignment of species detected in octa-HA sub-fraction.

Peak	Composition	Saccharide Sequence
1	A7,9,1-aM.ol	$A_{NAc,6S}$-G-A*-I_{2S}-$A_{NS,6S}$-I_{2S}-aM.ol_{6S}
2	U8,9,1-aM.ol	I-$A_{NAc,6S}$-G-A*-I_{2S}-$A_{NS,6S}$-I_{2S}-aM.ol_{6S} and/or I_{2S}-$A_{NS,6S}$-I-$A_{NAc,6S}$-G-A*-I_{2S}-aM.ol_{6S}
3	A7,10,0-aM.ol	$A_{NS,6S}$-G-A*-I_{2S}-$A_{NS,6S}$-I_{2S}-aM.ol_{6S}
5	U8,10,1-aM.ol	I_{2S}-$A_{NS,6S}$-I-$A_{NAc,6S}$-I_{2S}-A*-I_{2S}-aM.ol_{6S}
4, 6, 7	U8,11,0-aM.ol	I_{2S}-$A_{NS,6S}$-G-A*-I_{2S}-$A_{NS,6S}$-I_{2S}-aM.ol_{6S} I_{2S}-$A_{NS,6S}$-I_{2S}-$A_{NS,6S}$-G-A*-I_{2S}-aM.ol_{6S} G-A*-I_{2S}-$A_{NS,6S}$-I_{2S}-$A_{NS,6S}$-I_{2S}-aM.ol_{6S}

The octasaccharides U8,10,1-aM.ol, one of the most important peaks, could be explained by hypothesizing the presence of a I_{2S}-A* sequence instead of G-A*, in agreement with the previous detection of ΔU2,4,0 building block. Interestingly, a synthetic octasaccharide containing the sequence I_{2S}-A*-I_{2S} was found to be endowed of high binding affinity to AT [24]. As concerns the highly sulfated octasaccharide isomers U8,11,0-aM.ol two of the proposed structures contain the fully *N*-sulfated AT-binding region preceded by a 2-*O*-sulfated iduronic acid, and located in two different positions. Following cleavage with heparinase cocktail, these oligosaccharides are expected to generate the corresponding resistant tetrasaccharides U4,6,0 and ΔU4,6,0 respectively, which turned out to be almost undetectable in the whole dalteparin sample. Nevertheless, it is likely that the significant decreasing of structure polydispersity, such as in HA-Octa sub-fraction with respect to parent LMWH, allows the detection also of very minor sequences. The third undecasulfated isomer was interpreted as G-A*-I_{2S}-$A_{NS,6S}$-I_{2S}-$A_{NS,6S}$-I_{2S}-aM.ol_{6S}, which is in agreement with the finding of traces of non-reducing glucuronic acid in HA-Octa (Table 2). Despite such octasaccharide was expected to have a moderate AT-affinity, its presence in HA fraction is compatible with the elution conditions of AT-Sepharose column here applied, as the NA component was recovered at relatively very low salt concentration (50 mM NaCl). A possible additional or alternative interpretation of the third isomer U8,11,0-aM.ol, could be the presence of a G_{2S} instead of I_{2S}, taking into account that traces of 2-*O*-sulfated glucuronic acid were detected by NMR, but further investigation is required to confirm the exact structure. In the deca-HA subfraction three main decameric species were detected: U10,12,1-aM.ol, which is supposed to contain the I-$A_{NAc,6S}$-G-A*-I_{2S}-$A_{NS,6S}$ sequence; U10,13,0-aM.ol and U10,14,0-aM.ol, where both containing the fully N-sulfated AT-bs. As anticipated by the NMR results, the decasaccharide species containing a ring contracted unit (Rc) was recovered in the deca-NA fraction.

3. Materials and Methods

3.1. Materials

Dalteparin samples used in the present study were from different lots of injectable Fragmin® (Pfizer), named as follows: Frag-1 (lot 96223A51), Frag-2 (lot 96218B51), Frag-3 (lot 96231A51), Frag-4 (lot 96238A51), Frag-5 (lot 96240B51), Frag-6 (lot 96242A51), Frag-7 (lot 96228A51), Frag-8 (lot 96235A51), Frag-9 (lot 96225A51), Frag-10 (lot 96246A51) and Frag-11 (lot Z06358). Heparinases I (EC 4.2.2.7), II and III (EC 4.2.2.8) were purchased from Grampian Enzymes (Aberdeen, Scotland, UK). Dibutylamine (>99.5%), methanol (LC-MS grade), acetonitrile (LC-MS grade), acetic acid (glacial 99.9%), formic acid (98-100%), ammonium chloride (>99.5%), potassium phosphate monobasic were purchased from Sigma-Aldrich (Milan, Italy); sodium acetate was from Merck (Milan, Italy), and calcium acetate (>97%) from BDH (VWR Milan, Italy).

3.2. Fractionation by Size-Exclusion Chromatography

Fractionation by SEC to isolate octasaccharide and decasaccharide fractions was performed either on Biogel P10, as previously described [20] or Biogel P6. Briefly, on Biogel P6 column (5 × 190 cm) 300-350 mg sample dissolved in 5 mL purified water were loaded and eluted with 0.25 M NH_4Cl at a flow rate of 1.8 mL/min. The flow-through was collected in about 8 ml fractions and their UV absorbance was detected at 210 nm. Elution profile obtained by Biogel P6 is presented in additional material. Fractions of interest were collected and pooled. The pool volume was reduced to approximately 5 mL by evaporation under reduced pressure.

3.3. Desalting of Oligosaccharide Fractions

Desalting was performed using TSK-gel HW40S Toyopearl (Tosoh Bioscience, Yamaguchi, Japan) column 2.6 cm × 60 cm, particle size 20–40 μm. Samples were loaded onto the column and elution was performed in 10% EtOH in water at a flow rate of 1.4 mL/min. Two-point-one ml fractions were collected using a fraction collector. Absorbance at 210 nm was evaluated for each fraction. Fractions of interest were collected, pooled and lyophilized.

3.4. Affinity Chromatography on AT-Sepharose

Fifteen mg of octa and decasaccharide samples were dissolved in 5 mL equilibrium buffer (Tris-HCl 50 mM, pH 7.4, NaCl 50 mM), loaded onto a 30 mL of AT-Sepharose column (2 × 9.5 cm) and eluted first with 90 ml of equilibrium buffer to recover a fraction devoid of affinity for AT (NA), then with 90 mL of Tris-HCl 0.05M pH 7.4, 2.5 M NaCl, to recover a high affinity fraction (HA), at a flow rate of 0.5 mL/min. The flow-through was collected into 26 sub-fractions, 13 for NA and 13 for HA. Each sub-fraction was analysed for the uronic acid content [25]. HA and NA fractions were desalted as previously described [20].

3.5. NMR

Samples (8–20 mg) were dissolved in deuterium oxide containing 0.12 mM TSP (0.6 mL). NMR spectra were measured on a Bruker AVANCE III 600 MHz spectrometer or on a Bruker AVANCE IIIHD 500 MHz spectrometer (Bruker, Karlsruhe, Germany), both equipped with a 5 mm TCI cryo-genic probe. Proton spectra were measured with water suppression (decoupling power corresponding to 5 Hz linewidth). HSQC experiments (hsqcetgpsisp2.2 Bruker pulse sequence) were performed at 303 K, by using 32 dummy scans; from 60 to 48 scans; 2 s (500 MHz) or 2.5 s (600 MHz) relaxation delay; 8 ppm (F2) and 80 ppm (F1) spectral width; transmitter offset was set at 4.7 ppm(F2) and 80 ppm (F1); 1024 points were collected in F2 and 320 increments in F1. Zero filling was applied to 4k in F2 and, in F1, linear prediction to 640 points and zero filling to 1k; a 90 shifted squared sine bell-function was applied in both dimensions. Spectra were integrated by using the standard Topspin routine using rectangular integration domains with manual adjustment of regions according data published [19].

3.6. Exhaustive enzymatic Depolymerization with Heparin Lyases

Heparinase I, II, III. Each sample (20 μL of a 20 mg/mL solution in water) was incubated at 25 °C for 48 h in a total volume of 160 μL, containing 20 μL hep.ase I, II and III (0.4 IU/mL of each heparinase in 10 mM K_2HPO_4 buffer, pH 7.0) and 120 μL of 100 mM sodium acetate buffer pH 7.0, containing 2 mM of calcium acetate and 0.1 mg/mL bovine serum albumin (BSA).

Heparinase III. Each sample (20 μL of a 20 mg/mL solution in water) was incubated at 25 °C for 48h in a total volume of 160 μL, containing 20 μL hep.ase III (0.4 IU/mL 10 mM K_2HPO_4 buffer, pH 7.0) and 120 μL of 100 mM sodium acetate buffer pH 7.0, containing 2 mM of calcium acetate and 0.1 mg/mL BSA.

Enzyme inactivation. At the end of each incubation, enzymes were inactivated by a 2-min heating at 100 °C, and sample solutions were filtered onto 0.22 μm membrane.

3.7. LC-MS Analysis

Chain mapping analyses of intact samples were run on UHPLC system (Platin Blue, Knauer, Berlin, Germany) coupled to ESI-Ion Trap mass spectrometer (amaZon SL, Bruker Daltonics, Bremen, Germany). 5 μL of sample solution, prepared at the concentration of about 5 mg/mL, was injected on C_{18} Blue Orchid (150 mm × 2.0 mm i.d., 1.8 μm particle size, Knauer) column (maintained at 40 °C) and run at the flow rate of 0.3 mL/min, by the mobile phases A (10 mM pentylamine, 10 mM acetic acid in water/acetonitrile 95:5 *v*/*v*) and B (10 mM pentylamine, 10 mM acetic acid in acetonitrile) according to the following gradient: isocratic step at 15%B for 1 min, followed by a linear gradient from 15% to 40% B in 31 min; then, column washing by a gradient until 100% B kept for 5 min and reconditioning in the initial conditions were performed. The electrospray interface was set in negative ionization mode (Spray Voltage +4200 V), to record total ion current profiles in the m/z 300–2000 mass range. Nitrogen was used as a drying (9 L/min) and nebulizing gas (30 p.s.i.) and the ion transfer capillary was kept at 200 °C.

Building blocks composition and fragment mapping analyses were run on HPLC system (Ultimate 3000, Dionex, Sunnyvale, CA, USA) connected to ESI-Q-TOF mass spectrometer (micrOTOF$_Q$, Bruker Daltonics). Sample solutions at the concentration of 2 mg/mL in water were injected on C_{18} KINETEX column (100 mm × 2.1 mm i.d., with 2.6 μm particles, Phenomenex, Aschaffenburg, Germany) hold at room temperature and run by mobile phases A (10 mM dibutylamine and 10 mM acetic acid in water) and B (10 mM dibutylamine and 10 mM acetic acid in methanol) at 0.1 mL/min. Analyses of heparinases I, II, III digestion products were performed by injecting 5 μL of sample solution and eluting according to the following gradient: isocratic step at 2% B for 10 min, followed by a linear gradient to 60% B in 90 min and final steps of column washing and reconditioning. The separation method of heparinase III digestion products (injection volume of 10 μL) comprised an isocratic step of 5 min at 10% B, a linear gradient from 10% to 50% B in 55 min and a second linear gradient from 50% B to 90% B in 80 min, followed by column washing and reconditioning.

Mass spectrometry detector was set in negative polarity (Capillary voltage: +3200 V) in the mass range from m/z 200 to m/z 2000; nitrogen gas, used as nebulizer and heater gases, was set at 0.9 bar and 7.0 L/min, respectively; the ion transfer capillary was held at 180 °C.

Oligosaccharide fractions were run on Agilent 1100 HPLC system (Agilent Technologies, Santa Clara, CA, USA) coupled to ESI FT-ICR mass spectrometer (Solarix, Bruker Daltonics). Sample solutions at concentration of 10 mg/mL were injected (2 μL) on C_{18} KINETEX column (100 mm × 2.1 mm i.d., 2.6 μm partcles size, Phenomenex) held at room temperature and run by mobile phases containing 10 mM dibutylamine and 10 mM acetic acid (A: in water 100%, B: in methanol 100%) at 0.1 mL/min according to the following steps of linear gradient: from 50% B to 57% B in 5 min, from 57% B to 80% B in 52 min , from 80% B to 90% B in 16 min; then, 90% B was kept for 10 min and followed by column conditioning in the initial conditions. MS conditions were: capillary voltage at + 3200 V, nebulizer gas 1.0 bar, drying gas 3.7 liters/min, ion transfer capillary temperature 180 °C, mass range 200–3000 m/z.

Calibration of ESI-Q-TOF mass spectrometer was performed by using water -isopropanol 1:1 *v*/*v* solution containing HCOOH 0.2% and 5 mM NaOH; the ESI FT-ICR MS system was calibrated using sodium trifluoroacetate solution (0.05 mg/mL in water: acetonitrile 50:50 *v*/*v*), while low concentration tuning mix (Agilent Technologies) was employed for the mass range calibration of the ion trap detector. The LC-MS profiles and mass spectra were elaborated using the DataAnalysis software (Bruker Daltonics).

Octa-HA, octa-NA, deca-HA and deca-NA were run on an Agilent 1100 HPLC system (Agilent Technologies) coupled to an Esquire 3000 Plus (Bruker) as mass detector. Reversed-phase separation of LMWH fractions was carried out on a C_{18} KINETEX column (100 mm × 2.1 mm i.d., 2.6 μm partcles size, Phenomenex). Typically, 10 μg of each LMWH fraction was injected onto the column. The column was first eluted in isocratic conditions with 80% Solvent A (20 mM dibutylamine, 20 mM acetic acid in water) and 20% Solvent B (20 mM dibutylamine, 20 mM acetic acid in methanol) for 20 min. Then gradient elution gradient from 20% B to 40% B was applied followed for 10 min. The column was eluted at 40% B for 10 min. Subsequently, a 20 min gradient from 40% B to 90% B was applied and once 90% B was reached, this was kept for 10 min. Column conditioning for subsequent injections was established by a 5 min gradient from 90 % B to 20 % B and a 30 min equilibration at this solvent mixture. The flow rate and column temperature were maintained at 0.15 mL/min and 25 °C, respectively, throughout the run. The Chemstation software (Agilent Technologies) was used for instrument control.

Mass spectrometric analysis were performed on an Esquire 3000 Plus electrospray ion trap (Bruker Daltonics). Acquisition parameters for ESI-ion trap mass spectrometer were (set) negative polarity, mass range 300–1000 *m/z*, capillary +3166 V, nebulizer gas 60.0 psi, dry gas 12.0 L/min, dry temperature 350 °C.

4. Conclusions

In the present work, a combination of different methods for detailed structural investigation of dalteparin was proposed. The strategy involves a first analysis of the whole samples through a bi-dimensional NMR study, to determine the molar percentage of all differently substituted glucosamine and uronic acids. In parallel, high resolution LC-MS study was performed both on the whole samples and on their fragments obtained by digestion with a cocktail of heparinases I, II, III and heparinase III alone. For a more in-depth investigation, the same combined NMR and LC-MS approach was applied also to two size homogeneous oligosaccharide fractions, precisely octa and decasaccharides, and further on their sub-fractions endowed with and devoid of affinity toward AT. High resolution LC-MS approach applied provided information that was complementary to that produced by HSQC NMR, allowing to obtain an accurate and detailed picture of the oligomeric composition of dalteparin. The application of orthogonal analytical methods to the study of size homogeneous oligomeric families and of their HA and NA components permitted to identify a number of sequences, especially among the octasaccharide components endowed of affinity to AT.

The overall analytical approach here reported represents an effective strategy for comparative studies of dalteparin samples, either concerning the assessment of batch-to-batch variability or the appraisal of biosimilar drugs.

Supplementary Materials:
Figure S1: LC-MS analysis of dalteparin Frag-5 following heparinase III digestion: confirmation of A5,8,0-aM.ol composition by ICR-FT-MS. Figure S2: LC-MS analysis of dalteparin Frag-5 following heparinase III digestion: confirmation of A7,11,0-aM.ol composition by ICR-FT-MS. Figure S3: Elution profiles on Biogel P6 of dalteparin samples Frag-1–Frag-4. Figure S4: Elution profiles on Biogel P6 of dalteparin samples Frag-5–Frag-8. Figure S5: Elution profiles on Biogel P6 of dalteparin samples Frag-9–Frag-11. Table S1: Oligosaccharide family identified by LC-MS chain mapping in all the analysed dalteparin samples Frag-1–Frag-11: mass signal assignment. Table S2: Oligosaccharide fragments produced by heparinases I, II, III digestion observed in all the analysed dalteparin samples Frag-1–Frag-11: mass signal assignment. Table S3: Oligosaccharide fragments produced by heparinase III digestion observed in all the analysed dalteparin samples Frag-1–Frag-11: mass signal assignment. (*) In blue, species observed in the untreated sample too.

Acknowledgments: The authors thank Opocrin SpA for funding part of the work and Bioiberica for supporting the costs of publication.

Author Contributions: A.B. drew up the research plan and together with E.U., M.G., G.T. and A.N. discussed the experimental data; P.d.W. isolated oligosaccharide fractions, H.A. and N.A. sub-fractions; E.U. and M.G. performed LC-MS and NMR studies, respectively. A.B. and E.U. wrote the paper and together with M.G. edited and revised the manuscript. All the authors read and approved the final manuscript.

References

1. Fareed, J.; Jeske, W.; Hoppensteadt, D.; Clarizio, R.; Walenga, J.M. Low-molecular-weight heparins: Pharmacologic profile and product differentiation. *Am. J. Cardiol.* **1998**, *82*, 3L–10L. [CrossRef]
2. Bisio, A.; Mantegazza, A.; Vecchietti, D.; Bensi, D.; Coppa, A.; Torri, G.; Bertini, S. Determination of the molecular weight of low-molecular-weight heparins by using high-pressure size exclusion chromatography on line with a triple detector array and conventional methods. *Molecules* **2015**, *20*, 5085–5098. [CrossRef] [PubMed]

3. Guerrini, M.; Bisio, A. Low-molecular-weight heparins: Differential characterization/physical characterization. In *Heparin-A Century of Progress*; Lever, R., Mulloy, B., Page, C.P., Eds.; Springer: London, UK, 2012; pp. 127–157.
4. Hirsh, J.; Bauer, K.A.; Donati, M.B.; Samama, M.M.; Weitz, J.L. Parenteral anticoagulants: American college of chest physicians evidence-based clinical practice guidelines (8th edition). *Chest* **2008**, *133* (Suppl. 6), 141S–159S. [CrossRef] [PubMed]
5. Fareed, J.; Hoppensteadt, D.; Schultz, C.; Ma, Q.; Kujawski, M.F.; Neville, B.; Messmore, H. Biochemical and pharmacologic heterogeneity in low molecular weight heparins. Impact on the therapeutic profile. *Curr. Pharm. Des.* **2004**, *10*, 983–999. [CrossRef] [PubMed]
6. Guerrini, M.; Guglieri, S.; Naggi, A.; Sasisekharan, R.; Torri, G. Low molecular weight heparins: Structural differentiation by bidimensional nuclear magnetic resonance spectroscopy. *Semin. Thromb. Hemost.* **2007**, *33*, 478–487. [CrossRef] [PubMed]
7. Iacomini, M.; Casu, B.; Guerrini, M.; Naggi, A.; Pirola, A.; Torri, G. "Linkage region" sequence of heparin and heparan sulfate: Detection and quantification by nuclear magnetic resonance spectroscopy. *Anal. Biochem.* **1999**, *274*, 50–58. [CrossRef] [PubMed]
8. Fragmin (dalteparin sodium injection) Product Monograph, Pfizer Canada Inc, issued April 2016. Available online: www.pfizer.ca/sites/g/files/g10028126/f/201605/FRAGMIN_PM_193875_27April2016_E.pdf (accessed on 23 June 2017).
9. Henricksen, J.; Ringborg, L.H.; Roepstorff, P. On-line size-exclusion chromatography/mass spectrometry of low molecular mass heparin. *J. Mass Spectrom.* **2004**, *39*, 1305–1312. [CrossRef] [PubMed]
10. Korir, A.; Larive, C.K. Advances in the separation, sensitive detection, and characterization of heparin and heparan sulfate. *Anal. Bioanal. Chem.* **2009**, *393*, 155–169. [CrossRef] [PubMed]
11. Zaia, J. On-line separations combined with MS for analysis of glycosaminoglycans. *Mass Spectrom. Rev.* **2008**, *28*, 254–272. [CrossRef] [PubMed]
12. Langeslay, D.J.; Urso, E.; Gardini, C.; Naggi, A.; Torri, G.; Larive, C.K. Reversed-phase ion-pair ultra-high-performance-liquid chromatography-mass spectrometry for fingerprinting low-molecular-weight heparins. *J. Chromatogr. A* **2013**, *1292*, 201–210. [CrossRef] [PubMed]
13. Alekseeva, A.; Casu, B.; Torri, G.; Pierro, S.; Naggi, A. Profiling glycol-split heparins by high-performance liquid chromatography/mass spectrometry analysis of their heparinase-generated oligosaccharides. *Anal. Biochem.* **2013**, *434*, 112–122. [CrossRef] [PubMed]
14. Zhang, Q.; Chen, X.; Zhu, Z.; Zhan, X.; Wu, Y.; Song, L.; Kang, J. Structural analysis of low molecular weight heparin by ultraperformance size exclusion chromatography/time of flight mass spectrometry and capillary zone electrophoresis. *Anal. Chem.* **2012**, *85*, 1819–1827. [CrossRef] [PubMed]
15. Wang, B.; Buhse, L.F.; Al-Hakim, A.; Boyne li, M.T.; Keire, D.A. Characterization of currently marketed heparin products: Analysis of heparin digests by RPIP-UHPLC-QTOF-MS. *J. Pharm. Biomed. Anal.* **2012**, *67–68*, 42–50. [CrossRef] [PubMed]
16. Galeotti, F.; Volpi, N. Novel reverse-phase ion pair-high performance liquid chromatography separation of heparin, heparan sulfate and low molecular weight-heparins disaccharides and oligosaccharides. *J. Chromatogr. A* **2013**, *1284*, 141–147. [CrossRef] [PubMed]
17. Ouyang, Y.; Wu, C.; Sun, X.; Liu, J.; Linhardt, R.J.; Zhang, Z. Development of hydrophilic interaction chromatography with quadruple time-of-flight mass spectrometry for heparin and low molecular weight heparin disaccharide analysis. *Rapid Commun. Mass Spectrom.* **2016**, *30*, 277–284. [CrossRef] [PubMed]
18. Sun, X.; Guo, Z.; Yu, M.; Lin, C.; Sheng, A.; Wang, Z.; Linhardt, R.J.; Chi, L. Hydrophilic interaction chromatography-multiple reaction monitoring mass spectrometry method for basic building block analysis of low-molecular-weight heparins prepared through nitrous acid depolymerization. *J. Chromatogr. A* **2017**, *1479*, 121–128. [CrossRef] [PubMed]
19. Mauri, L.; Boccardi, G.; Torri, G.; Karfunkle, M.; Macchi, E.; Muzi, L.; Keire, D.; Guerrini, M. Qualification of HSQC methods for quantitative composition of heparin and low molecular weight heparins. *J. Pharm. Biomed. Anal.* **2017**, *136*, 92–105. [CrossRef] [PubMed]
20. Bisio, A.; Vecchietti, D.; Citterio, L.; Guerrini, M.; Raman, R.; Bertini, S.; Eisele, G.; Naggi, A.; Sasisekharan, R.; Torri, G. Structural features of low-molecular-weight heparins affecting their affinity to antithrombin. *Thromb. Haemost.* **2009**, *102*, 865–873. [CrossRef] [PubMed]

21. Alekseeva, A.; Casu, B.; Cassinelli, G.; Guerrini, M.; Torri, G.; Naggi, A. Structural features of glycol-split low-molecular-weight heparins and their heparin lyase generated fragments. *Anal. Bioanal. Chem.* **2014**, *406*, 249–265. [CrossRef] [PubMed]
22. Yamada, S.; Yoshida, K.; Sugiura, M.; Sugahara, K.; Khoo, K-H.; Morris, H.R.; Dell, A. Structural studies on the bacterial lyase-resistant tetrasaccharides derived from antithrombin III-binding site of porcine intestinal heparin. *J. Biol. Chem.* **1993**, *268*, 7, 4780–4787.
23. Loganathan, D.; Wang, H.M.; Mallis, L.M.; Linhardt, R.J. Structural variation in the antithrombin III binding region and its occurrence in heparin from different sources. *Biochemistry* **1990**, *29*, 4362–4368. [CrossRef] [PubMed]
24. Wang, Z.; Hsieh, P.-H.; Xu, Y.; Thieker, D.; En Chai, E.J.; Xie, S.; Cooley, B.; Woods, R.; Chi, L.; Liu, J. Synthesis of 3-*O*-sulfated oligosaccharides to understand the relationship between structures and functions of heparan sulfate. *J. Am. Chem. Soc.* **2017**, *139*, 5249–5256. [CrossRef] [PubMed]
25. Bitter, T.; Muir, H.M. A modified uronic acid carbazole reaction. *Anal. Biochem.* **1962**, *4*, 330–334. [CrossRef]

13

Sulfated Alginates as Heparin Analogues: A Review of Chemical and Functional Properties

Øystein Arlov [1] and Gudmund Skjåk-Bræk [2,*]

[1] Department of Biotechnology and Nanomedicine, SINTEF Materials and Chemistry, Richard Birkelands vei 3B, 7034 Trondheim, Norway; oystein.arlov@sintef.no

[2] Department of Biotechnology, Norwegian University of Science and Technology, Sem Sælands vei 6/8, 7034 Trondheim, Norway

* Correspondence: gudmund.skjak.brak@ntnu.no

Academic Editor: Giangiacomo Torri

Abstract: Heparin is widely recognized for its potent anticoagulating effects, but has an additional wide range of biological properties due to its high negative charge and heterogeneous molecular structure. This heterogeneity has been one of the factors in motivating the exploration of functional analogues with a more predictable modification pattern and monosaccharide sequence, that can aid in elucidating structure-function relationships and further be structurally customized to fine-tune physical and biological properties toward novel therapeutic applications and biomaterials. Alginates have been of great interest in biomedicine due to their inherent biocompatibility, gentle gelling conditions, and structural versatility from chemo-enzymatic engineering, but display limited interactions with cells and biomolecules that are characteristic of heparin and the other glycosaminoglycans (GAGs) of the extracellular environment. Here, we review the chemistry and physical and biological properties of sulfated alginates as structural and functional heparin analogues, and discuss how they may be utilized in applications where the use of heparin and other sulfated GAGs is challenging and limited.

Keywords: heparin; alginate; sulfated alginate; biomaterials

---

1. Introduction

Glycosaminoglycans (GAGs) are a group of negatively charged linear polysaccharides found in virtually all animal tissues. The majority of GAG subtypes are associated with the plasma membrane via a protein core, referred to as proteoglycans, and are key components of the extracellular matrix (ECM) in providing structural support and hydration. The sulfated GAGs have additional vital roles in the development, maintenance, and pathophysiology of mammalian tissues, and may serve as receptors, co-receptors, and reservoirs through electrostatic interaction with proteins. Heparin differs from other GAGs in that it is primarily produced by mast cells, and is released from storage granules into the extracellular space by exocytosis. Heparin is a potent anticoagulant, and is widely used in the clinic as an intravenously administered blood thinner and as a coating material for medical devices. While structurally related to heparan sulfate (HS), heparin undergoes a greater degree of enzymatic modification during synthesis, resulting in highly diverse biological activities. Heparin has the highest sulfation degree of the GAGs, and a higher charge density than any known biopolymer, thus associating with a plethora of proteins including coagulation factors, growth factors, cytokines, adhesion proteins, and pathogen-related proteins.

The use of heparin for other biomedical applications than anticoagulation is however limited, partly due to rapid turnover in biological systems and risks of excessive bleeding upon administration. Heparin has a high degree of heterogeneity in its monosaccharide sequence and modification pattern, depending on the source, and has few options for structural customizability. This complicates tuning of the drug's efficacy, as well as the characterization of biological activity and structure-function relationships required for exploring new potential applications. An additional aspect regarding widespread use of heparin is concerns regarding safety and sustainability in its production, as the most widely used derivatives of heparin are isolated from animal tissues [1]. For these reasons, over the last few decades numerous heparin derivatives and analogues from natural sources, chemical synthesis, and chemical and/or enzymatic functionalization of polysaccharides have been described [2–5]. Some of the heparin analogues described in the literature aim to emulate the anticoagulant properties of heparin, to provide more sustainable and safe drug manufacturing and/or allow greater control over pharmacokinetic and –dynamic properties. Others are directed toward novel pharmaceutical applications or as components in biomaterials, where the physicochemical properties and highly specific anticoagulating action of heparin pose limitations.

This review aims to present current knowledge and studies on sulfated alginates as novel heparin analogues, based on the authors' own work and the available recent literature. We further wish to discuss future directions of this research, as well as areas of application where sulfated alginates can potentially provide a viable alternative to heparin or other sulfated GAGs and derivatives.

1.1. Heparin Molecular Structure and Physical Properties

Heparin and heparan sulfate are synthesized as alternating copolymers of 1→4-linked *N*-acetylglucosamine (GlcNAc) and glucuronic acid (GlcA). During synthesis, the nascent chain is modified by a series of enzymes in the Golgi apparatus, namely N-deacetylase-N-sulfotransferases, C-5 epimerases, and 2-O, 3-O, and 6-O sulfotransferases [6]. Epimerization of GlcA into iduronic acid (IdoA) confers structural flexibility to the polysaccharide chains, in that IdoA can assume one of three stable conformations ($^4C_1$, $^1C_4$, or $^2S_0$) depending on the modification pattern and induced effects upon protein interaction [7]. The expression of tissue-specific isozymes [8,9] and varying combinations of modifications confer a high degree of structural complexity and variability to heparin and HS, requiring a great effort for their functional and structural characterization. Heparin has a higher degree of sulfation and epimerization compared to HS, where the trisulfated disaccharide IdoA2S-GlcNS6S (Figure 1) constitutes 60–85% of the heparin chain, depending on the source [10,11]. However, there are no repeating sequences in heparin as the trisulfated disaccharides are interspersed by undersulfated residues of varying lengths. Heparan sulfate exhibits long unmodified regions between heparin-like motifs with high sulfation and epimerization degrees [12]. Epimerization of GlcA to IdoA has been demonstrated in vitro, using Glucuronyl C5-epimerase isolated from bovine tissue and the K5 capsular polysaccharide (GlcA-GlcNAc) [13]. To the authors' knowledge, only one prokaryotic GlcA C5-epimerase has been identified and utilized for in vitro epimerization of K5. As the activity of the enzymes was relatively low, the results indicated that the native substrate differs from heparin and HS-like polysaccharides [14]. Of note, in vitro epimerization of GlcA is readily reversible, in contrast to the reaction in vivo due to subsequent O-sulfation following epimerization [13,15].

Commercial heparin is generally classified as unfractionated heparin (UFH, ~15 kDa), low molecular weight heparin (LMWH, ~6 kDa), or ultra-low molecular weight heparin (ULMWH, <2 kDa), where the most common ULMWHs are chemically synthesized oligosaccharides including the antithrombin (AT)-binding region [16]. Whereas chemical synthesis of heparin has had major limitations in terms of oligosaccharide length, recent advances have demonstrated production of up to 40-mers by iterative homologation of tetrasaccharides [17]. However, this approach generates repeating sequences, which are not found in native heparin.

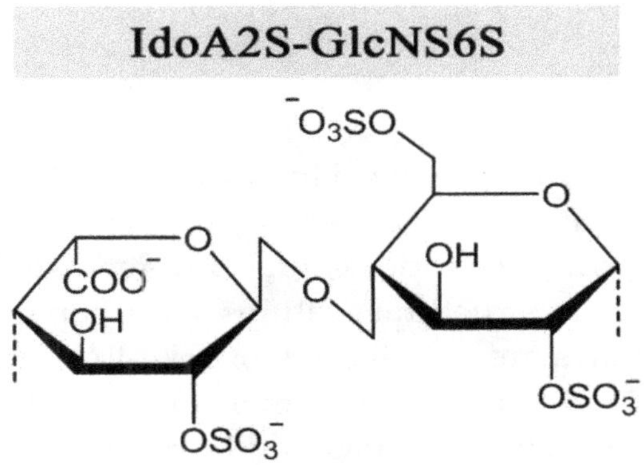

Figure 1. The prevalent disaccharide structure in heparin.

1.2. Biological Properties of Heparin and Structure-Function Relationships

Heparin has potent anticoagulating properties and has widespread use in the clinic as an intravenously administered drug and as a coating material on medical devices. Its anticoagulating effect is primarily mediated by highly specific binding and activation of antithrombin, which in turn inactivates several proteases of the coagulation cascade, namely thrombin and Factors X, IX, XI, and XII [18].

Furthermore, heparin has demonstrated anti-inflammatory effects, presumably by multiple functions due to its broad substrate affinity. For instance, heparin has long been known to bind complement factors, where its anti-coagulating effects can supplement this effect through cross talk between the complement and coagulation pathways [19,20], as well as pro-inflammatory cytokines [21]. Binding of heparin to these proteins can exert an inhibitory effect through preventing receptor interaction, conformational changes, or proteolytic cleavage. An additional postulated mechanism is the binding of heparin to P- and L-selectins, inhibiting interaction with endothelial proteoglycans and thus adhesion and extravasation of leukocytes [22]. Heparin has also been evaluated as a potential antiviral drug due to association with viral capsule proteins [23]. Heparan sulfate and other GAGs on the cell surface can be utilized as a receptor for pathogens initiating adhesion and eventual cell entry, where soluble heparin can serve as an antagonist [24].

Heparin has been demonstrated to bind a plethora of proteins with varying interaction strengths. Asides from the well characterized AT interaction, the selectivity of heparin-protein interactions, and whether specific sequences are "programmed" into the heparin chains, remains a controversial subject. For a more comprehensive discussion of the topic, the reader is referred to the works of Lindahl and associates [25,26]. As a relevant point to the present review, it is evident that variance in monosaccharide sequences and modification patterns can have a large impact on protein interaction strength, tied to optimal alignment for ionic interactions and van der Waals forces [7]. For example, Hu and co-workers generated a HS disaccharide library, demonstrating that only 4 out of 48 disaccharides bind fibroblast growth factor-1 (FGF-1) with high affinity [27]. The presence of IdoA has been demonstrated to be critical for the interaction strength to specific proteins, where a large degree of chain flexibility can contribute to improved alignment between heparin and the protein surface, compared to a more rigid polysaccharide with equivalent charge. For example, the $^1C_4$ conformation forms a kink in the heparin/HS chain which greatly enhances FGF interaction, but is not present in IdoA-containing dermatan sulfate due to the different interspersed monosaccharides and linkage patterns [28]. Studies have also shown the effect of various sulfation patterns in heparin on binding to P and L-selectins, revealing that 6-O-sulfation is critical for interaction with both selectins [29]. Furthermore, LMWH interacts less strongly with selectins compared with UFH, indicating an additional dependence of chain length, or that critical structural patterns are disrupted during fragmentation [30]. These examples emphasize that there are additional aspects beyond charge density that influence the biological activity of sulfated GAGs, which must be addressed in the design of functional analogues.

2. Sulfated Alginates

2.1. Properties of Alginate

Alginates, in contrast to GAGs, are produced in brown algae *(Pheaophyceae)*, where they serve as structural polysaccharides, or in certain genera of gram-negative bacteria (*Azotobacter* and *Pseudomonas* sp.) where alginates as exocellular polysaccharides confer different protective functions and virulence factors [31]. Still, they share some structural features with heparin and heparin sulfate besides all being linear uronans. Alginates are copolymers of 1➔4-linked β-D-mannuronic acid (M) and α-L-guluronic acid (G) (Figure 2), which are C-5 epimers of each other, analogous to GlcA and IdoA in heparin/HS. Moreover, they are arranged in G-and M-blocks of various length interspaced with regions of alternating sequences (MG-block) akin to the sulfate-, IdoA-rich and undersulfated GlcA-rich regions(NS and NA domains, respectively) found in heparan sulfate [32]. Alginates form hydrogels through ionic cross-linking with divalent cations such as calcium, where the gel properties are largely influenced by the content and length of the G-blocks [33]. Alginate is synthetized as homopolymeric mannuronan, which in a post-polymerization step is converted into alginate by C-5 epimerization, similar to the GlcA→IdoA conversion in the biosynthesis of heparin and heparan sulfate. Due to the action of these post-polymerization epimerases, both GAGs and alginate possess non-random block sequential structures. Whereas the introduction of IdoA in heparin/HS provides conformational flexibility significant for protein interactions, the main effect of epimerization in alginates is the introduction of calcium binding G-blocks responsible for gel formation. The alginate-producing bacterium *Azotobacter vinelandii* expresses seven exocellular epimerases (AlgE1-7), which have been cloned and can be used to engineer alginates with compositionally homogeneous structures not found in nature [34].

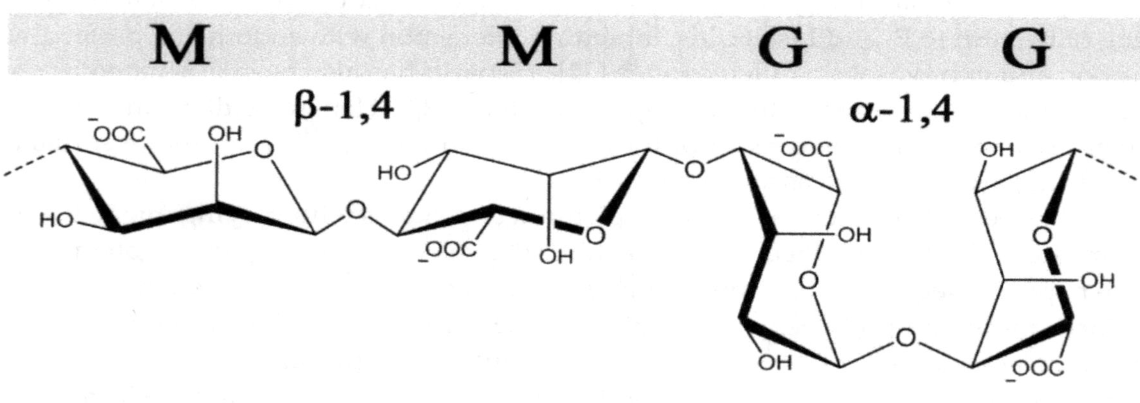

Figure 2. The structures and glycosidic bond conformations of β-D-mannuronic acid and α-L-guluronic acid in alginates.

Of note, the AlgE4 enzyme can be used to introduce an alternating sequence (poly-MG), similar to the basic backbone structure of heparin [35]. Enzymatic and chemical modifications of alginates have been extensively described in previous reviews, illustrating a great structural and functional versatility [36,37]. Alginate has been evaluated for numerous biomedical applications, primarily due to their gentle gelling conditions, including immunoisolation of cell transplants [38], slow-release systems [39], in vitro tissue engineering [40], and 3D-bioprinting [41]. Purified alginates are relatively inert toward cells and biomolecules, providing good biocompatibility but simultaneously discouraging favourable interactions with cell receptors and vital soluble factors that are characteristic of glycosaminoglycans in the extracellular matrix. Thus, great efforts have been made to functionalize alginates to provide a biomimetic environment, while maintaining their biocompatibility and gelling properties. One such strategy is by chemical sulfation, to emulate the structure of sulfated GAGs.

2.2. Synthesis and Characterization of Sulfated Alginates

Multiple strategies have been described for chemical sulfation of alginates (Figure 3). Huang and co-workers first employed chlorosulfonic acid ($HClSO_3$) in formamide, resulting in a reported degree of sulfation (DS) of approximately 1.2 sulfate groups per monosaccharide. As a means to reduce the adverse effects from over-sulfation, the sulfated alginates were conjugated with quaternary amine groups, allowing a controlled reduction of anti-coagulating properties [42]. We found that the sulfation degree could be reproducibly tuned by varying the chlorosulfonic acid concentration, but the DS was found to reach a plateau around DS = 1.0–1.2, depending on the monosaccharide sequence and their relative solubility in acid [43,44]. Sulfation of dextran has been performed using sulfur trioxide (SO_3) in pyridine, which was reported to result in a more homogeneous substitution compared with the $HClSO_3$/formamide method [45]. This approach was used for alginate by Mhanna and coworkers, using a tetrabutylammonium (TBA) salt of alginate to increase solubility in pyridine [46], but was found to have challenges related to reproducibility of the sulfation degree in following studies. An alternative strategy employs a carbodiimide-H_2SO_4 intermediate reacting directly with alginate [47], or via the TBA salt of alginate in DMF [48]. One challenge with the described methods is the strong acidic conditions used to obtain a high sulfation degree, resulting in partial depolymerization of high-molecular weight alginates [47], whereas the relatively low solubility of alginate in acid can reduce reaction reproducibility and throughput. Fan and co-workers reported a novel strategy for the sulfation of polysaccharides under non-acidic conditions, obtaining a DS of approximately 2 sulfates/monosaccharide at optimal conditions [49]. Although the authors of this review were not able to sulfate alginates using the method as described, the procedure could have a large potential for preventing depolymerization and allowing a DS approaching that of heparin, if successfully established.

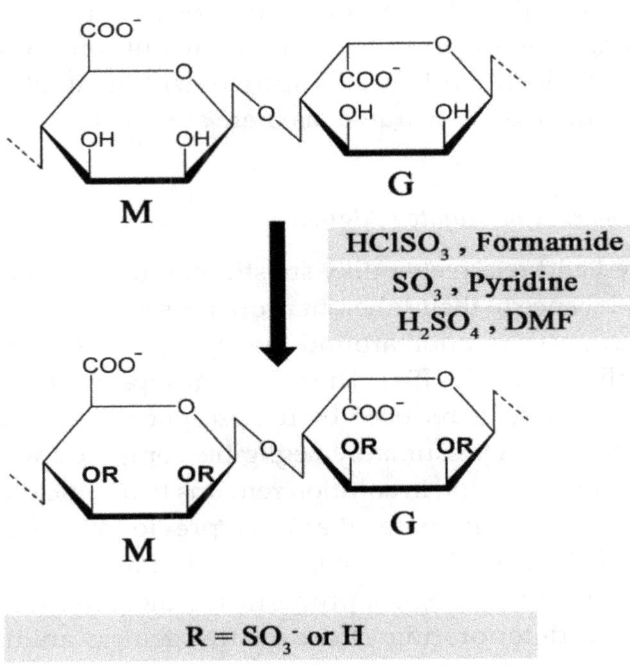

Figure 3. Published methods for chemical sulfation of alginate using different reagents [9,42,46,48].

The molecular structure of sulfated alginates has been characterized primarily by utilizing Fourier-transform infrared (FTIR) spectroscopy, Nuclear magnetic resonance (NMR), and Mass spectrometry (MS)-based methods. In the FTIR spectrum, sulfation of the hydroxyl groups in alginate results in the appearance of a distinct peak corresponding to the symmetric stretching of the S=O bond [42,48]. However, this method provides little qualitative data and cannot clearly distinguish substitution at C-2 from C-3, nor the M from G in alginate. NMR can provide detailed structural data, but generates highly complicated spectra due to the heterogeneity in the substitution patterns and monosaccharide sequences of sulfated alginates. We generated alginates with homogeneous sequences (poly-M, poly-G, and poly-MG) with three specific degrees of sulfation using $HClSO_3$, and employed various 2D NMR techniques to assign the 1D ^{13}C spectrum and identify the substitution pattern for the distinct alginate sequences [43,44]. Consistent with previous studies, the sulfation followed a random substitution pattern, indicated by the increase in spectrum heterogeneity at low sulfation degrees [43]. Based on the NMR data, no apparent selectivity was found for the substitution of M/G, or C-2/C-3. This was also found by Zhao and co-workers in an early study on low-molecular weight sulfated guluronate, by NMR characterization [50]. Following this presumption, the sulfate groups are evenly distributed along the polysaccharide chains and not organized in domains of varying density (e.g., following alginate block sequences), in contrast with heparan sulfate [51]. The degree of sulfation (DS) can thus be expressed as the average number of sulfates per monosaccharide, and determined by biochemical methods or mass spectrometry-based elemental analysis [44,52].

Chemical sulfation of alginates results in a less heterogeneous substitution pattern compared with natural heparin and heparan sulfate, as the sulfate groups are presumably equally distributed between C-2 and C-3 of the mannuronic acid and guluronic acid moieties. This provides as mentioned a relatively homogeneous charge distribution along the polysaccharide chain, which can contribute to the study of structure-function relationships while reducing batch-to-batch variability. The published methods demonstrate limitations in terms of sulfation degree, as the substitution is restricted to the free hydroxyl group, while di-sulfated monosaccharides are presumably discouraged from steric effects. The different substitution pattern and lower charge density of sulfated alginates can in turn lead to more transient protein interactions, or the utilization of alternative interaction sites compared with heparin/HS. Additional strategies for C-6 sulfation can therefore be explored to emulate highly sulfated moieties [53]. Furthermore, monosaccharide-specific sulfation of alginate would carry a substantial benefit, as sulfation of primarily mannuronic acid would allow unimpaired cross-linking of guluronic acid blocks and a vast improvement in sulfated alginate gel strength and stability. This is, however, yet to be demonstrated, as there are great challenges in discerning between the monosaccharides chemically.

2.3. *Chemical and Physical Properties of Sulfated Alginates*

Introduction of a charged and relatively bulky substituent notably alters the chemical structure of alginates, which is of great relevance to their inherent properties in solution and in ionically-crosslinked hydrogels. Steric hindrance reduces rotation around the glycosidic bond, conferring a more extended and rigid conformation in polysaccharides [54]. The sulfate groups can further promote intramolecular charge repulsion, although this effect is reduced by the presence of sodium counter ions similarly to the carboxyl groups of alginate and is presumably negligible compared with steric effects. The precise effect of sulfation on alginate conformation in solution remains to be elucidated, and can be approached utilizing homogeneous sequences of alginates that have previously been studied in terms of chain extension and bond rotation [55]. The stiffness of the polysaccharide chain can influence interaction strengths with proteins, and thus the biological properties of the polysaccharides.

Sulfation generally has a deteriorating effect on the gelling ability of alginates, where the resulting gels have a lower stiffness and increased rate of swelling and destabilization compared with unmodified alginate [46,56]. Negatively charged sulfate groups associate with divalent cations, but disrupt the long G-blocks that are responsible for the cooperative binding of ions and forming of cross-linking junction zones in the gel network, as described in the "egg-box" model [57]. In a recent study, we characterized gels made exclusively from sulfated alginates with varying sulfation degrees, as well as the effect of combining highly sulfated alginate (DS = 1) in unmodified alginate gels at various proportions. Sulfated alginate alone (150 kDa) was found to form stabile gels with calcium up to a sulfation degree of approximately 0.4, whereas increasing the sulfation level required either the inclusion of unmodified alginate or utilization of gelling ions with a higher affinity for alginate (e.g., barium, strontium) [58]. An alternative strategy that has not yet been explored to the authors' knowledge is covalent cross-linking between sulfated alginates, or to unmodified alginates, which can be a feasible approach where a higher gel stiffness is required. As highly sulfated alginates presumably only form transient cross-links within the hydrogel matrix, they diffuse out in the surrounding medium upon swelling of the gels at a higher rate than unmodified alginate, particularly at low molecular weight. Interestingly, a low amount (20%) of S-Alg mixed with unmodified alginate consistently demonstrated decreased stiffness but a lower swelling potential in saline than the alginate control, potentially due to a higher charge density, retention of gelling ions slowing the exchange with Na^+, and osmotic influx of water [58].

The use of heparin analogues in hydrogels are of great interest for encapsulation of cells and proteins (e.g., in tissue engineering). Sulfated alginates demonstrate great potential with its inherent gelling capability and has, similarly to native alginate, a great versatility in properties and gelling conditions to allow the tuning of hydrogel characteristics toward specific applications. These include enzymatic engineering to increase gel strength [34], and the utilization of alternative cross-linking ions [59] and gelling techniques, for example, $CaCl_2$ for immediate gelling versus $CaCO_3$ and glucono-δ-lactone GDL for a gradual release of calcium in injectable solutions and in situ gelation [60].

2.4. *Effects of Sulfated Alginates on the Coagulation Cascade*

As heparin is most widely known and used due to its potent anticoagulating properties, it is of great interest to investigate whether similar effects can be achieved utilizing the structurally analogous sulfated alginates. Huang and co-workers studied the activated partial thrombosis time (APTT), thrombin time (TT), and prothrombin time (PT) in plasma, using sulfated algal alginates with an approximate DS of 1.0 sulfate per monosaccharide. Although heparin was not included as a control in the present study, sulfated alginates prolonged the APTT with increasing treatment concentrations while showing no significant effects on the TT and PT [42]. Conversely, Ma and co-workers showed a pronounced elevation of the TT increasing with the sulfation degree and concentration of sulfated alginate, whereas no comparison with heparin was made. The authors further demonstrated a procedure for coating a polyethersulfone membrane with sulfated alginate, resulting in prolonged coagulation compared with the non-coated membrane [47]. By hydrolysis and separation, Li and co-workers prepared low-molecular weight (6–7 kDa) alginates enriched in mannuronic acid or guluronic acid, and studied the anticoagulating effects of their sulfated derivatives. Similarly to the study by Huang, SA was found to increase the APTT compared to the saline control and the non-sulfated alginates, whereas a two- and eight-fold greater effect was observed for LMWH and heparin, respectively, at similar concentrations [61]. The results indicate that sulfated alginates may inhibit the extrinsic coagulation pathway through binding and sequestration and/or prevention of protease activity of upstream factors, but are unable to bind antithrombin selectively to inhibit tissue factor (TF)-mediated activation of Factor X, and thrombin. Lacking AT activation was also evident from the TT test where sulfated alginate was unable to prolong coagulation time in the presence of excess thrombin. Heparin does not deactivate TF directly in vivo, but induces secretion of an inhibitor (TFPI) from endothelial cells, resulting in a less pronounced effect on the PT in vitro [62]. To the authors' knowledge, the release of TF has not been demonstrated for sulfated alginates or similar heparin analogues in in vivo models.

The mechanism behind the observed anticoagulating effects of sulfated alginates are still not clear, whereas the presented research does not strongly support the specific antithrombin activation that is characteristic of heparin. Presumably, the sulfated alginates non-specifically bind multiple coagulation factors, having a partial antagonizing or deactivating effect on the proteases or indirectly through other regulatory proteins (Figure 4). Alternatively, interaction outside the active sites may lead to aggregation and sequestration of precursors such as fibrinogen, as proposed for other heparin mimetics [63]. As the sulfated alginates were postulated to have a greater influence on the intrinsic coagulation pathway [42], interaction studies with individual coagulation factors can help further elucidate their effect on the coagulation cascade, by indicating whether the interactions are largely non-specific or if there is a selectivity for certain factors. Furthermore, platelet aggregation and activation are vital steps within the coagulation cascade, and should be studied for hydrogels or surface coatings of sulfated alginates to evaluate if they exhibit effects similar to heparin and other well-characterized heparin analogues [5,64].

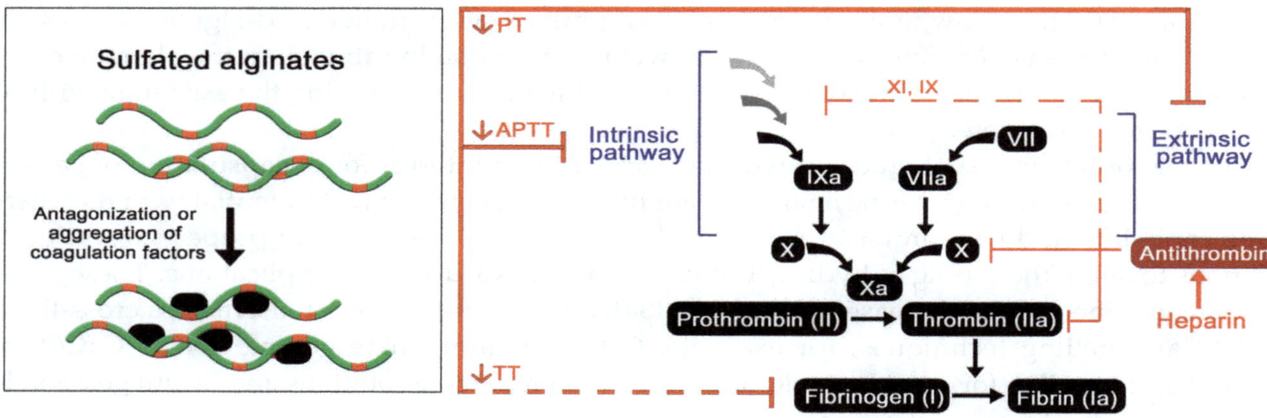

Figure 4. Postulated effect of sulfated alginates on the coagulation cascade resulting in prolonged coagulation time [42,47,49,50,61].

2.5. *Immunological Effects of Sulfated Alginates*

The mechanisms behind the anti-inflammatory properties of heparin and similar sulfated polysaccharides are still not fully understood. Several studies demonstrate interactions with cytokines, chemokines, growth factors, and signalling cascade factors, potentially resulting in altered protein half-life, sequestration of ligands from their receptors, and/or prevention of proteolytic cleavage or conformational changes in proteins. The cellular response to inflammation can also be affected more directly by heparin, through association with adhesion proteins that mediate extravasation of leukocytes across the endothelium [29].

To study the anti-inflammatory properties of sulfated alginates, we employed two different model systems, where multiple anti-inflammatory effects were observed (Figure 5). In the first study, sulfated alginates were incorporated in alginate microspheres either as a secondary coat on polycation-coated microcapsules or mixed with non-sulfated alginate in uncoated microspheres, followed by incubation in whole human blood anti-coagulated with lepirudin [65]. Microspheres with sulfated alginates were found to attenuate the inflammatory response, by lowering the expression of several inflammatory cytokines, including interleukin (IL)-1β, TNF, and IL-8. The sulfated alginate gels were found to inhibit the complement cascade in blood, as well as in plasma in soluble form [44], indicating direct interaction with complement factors as previously demonstrated for heparin [19,66]. Sequestration of complement factors prevents assembly of the convertases and terminal complement complex, whereas we additionally demonstrated interaction between sulfated alginates and complement inhibitory Factor H, which can contribute to suppression of the complement cascade on microsphere surfaces [65]. Lastly, there is significant cross talk between the coagulation and complement cascades [20,67], where the previously described anticoagulating activities of sulfated alginates can have an indirect influence on the inflammatory response. Sulfated alginates were further found to reduce integrin alpha M (ITGAM/CD11b) expression on leukocytes, which can be attributed to indirect effects from sequestration of cytokines and complement factors. In the second study, human chondrocytes were encapsulated in alginate or sulfated alginate gels, prior to inflammatory induction with IL-1β. Chondrocytes in sulfated alginate gels demonstrated lowered expression of inflammatory and catabolic markers, as well as reduced nuclear factor-kappa b NF-κB and p38-mitogen activated protein kinase (MAPK)-mediated signaling compared with the alginate controls. Sulfated alginate was found to bind IL-1β, presumably sequestering the cytokines in the gel matrix and preventing induction of the encapsulated cells [58]. Similarly, Freeman and co-workers demonstrated binding to IL-6, further indicating that sulfated alginates can regulate cytokine activity as well as their expression [48]. Inhibition of cytokine activity through binding can appear to contradict with the potentiating effect of binding growth factors, and will depend on whether the interaction sites between sulfated alginates and proteins interfere with receptor binding, or if there is a co-receptor functionality as previously established for heparan sulfate and FGF [68]. Heparin has previously been demonstrated to inhibit leukocyte activity through associating with L- and P-selectins [22], which has not yet been demonstrated for sulfated alginates, but can potentially reveal additional anti-inflammatory effects in alternative model systems. As a model for chronic inflammation, Zhao and co-workers studied granuloma formation in rats, and found that ingested sulfated guluronate reduced the size of the granuloma [50]. The mechanisms behind this effect are still unclear, and sulfated alginates may act on multiple levels such as inflammation and coagulation pathways, and adhesion molecules [69,70].

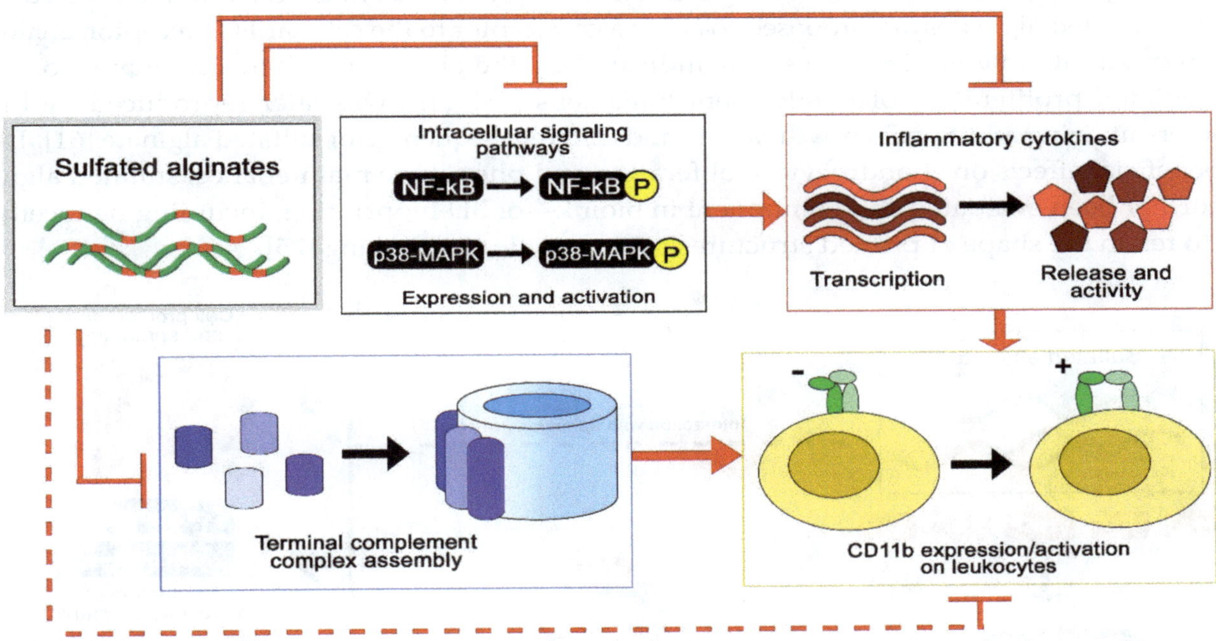

Figure 5. Anti-inflammatory effects of sulfated alginates from whole blood and cell culture models [58,65].

2.6. Sulfated Alginates in Tissue Engineering and Drug Delivery

The use of heparin and other GAGs in biomaterials intended for long-term implantation is limited partly due to their rapid turnover in vivo. The exploration of more stable analogues has therefore been encouraged for a range of applications in tissue engineering and encapsulation of therapeutics. Cohen and co-workers initially reported sulfated alginates to associate with multiple heparin-binding growth factors, highlighting their potential to serve as a reservoir and a slow-release system for growth factors toward tissue cultivation and drug delivery [48]. Sulfated alginate hydrogels loaded with growth factors were further found to promote angiogenesis and blood perfusion in animal tissues, and have been formulated as injectable solutions for gelation in situ [71,72]. In a separate study, heterogeneous hydrogels with layered organization of specific growth factors were found to support compartmentalized differentiation of mesenchymal stem cells into osteoblasts and chondrocytes [73]. In a recent study, Ruvinov and colleagues proposed a model where the multiple heparin-binding proteins and sulfated alginate chains spontaneously assemble into nanoparticles with a fiber-like structure and a net negative surface charge, which can subsequently be immobilized in injectable hydrogels such as unmodified alginates or various nanoparticle formulations [74]. This demonstrates a great potential and versatility for formulating hydrogel- and nanoparticle-based delivery of heparin-binding proteins, whereas modifications to the structure and sequence of the sulfated alginates can additionally contribute to the release rate by tuning the interaction strength with various proteins [43,44]. In addition to providing prolonged delivery of growth factors through their associative retention, the binding of sulfated alginate has been demonstrated to protect the proteins from proteolytic cleavage by trypsin [74], which is one of the postulated effects of heparin and other sulfated glycosaminoglycans in regulating cell signaling.

Zenobi-Wong and colleagues initially employed sulfated alginate hydrogels for the cultivation of cartilage, and found that the gels promoted proliferation and prolonged viability of the chondrocytes (Figure 6). Furthermore, the sulfated alginates were able to sustain the cartilaginous phenotype over long culture times, demonstrated by a high degree of collagen 2 expression and repressed collagen 1 expression [46]. The inductive effect on chondrocyte proliferation was attenuated by blocking beta1 integrins, indicating that the sulfated alginates interact (presumably indirectly) with integrins and potentially other adhesion proteins on the cell surface to support anchorage and migration. The chondrogenic effects were additionally related to a high degree of FGF retention in the hydrogels, where the sulfated alginates are proposed to act as a co-receptor to the cellular FGF receptor, analogous to heparan sulfate in vivo [56]. This was indicated by the ability of sulfated alginates to restore FGF-mediated proliferation of HS-deficient BaF3 cells [56], and was later reproduced by Li and co-workers utilizing additional growth factors and different sequences of sulfated alginate [61]. Due to their beneficial effects on chondrocyte proliferation and phenotype maintenance, sulfated alginates have further been evaluated as a component in bioinks for 3D-bioprinting, including nanocellulose fibers to retain the shape of printed structures prior to ionic crosslinking [75].

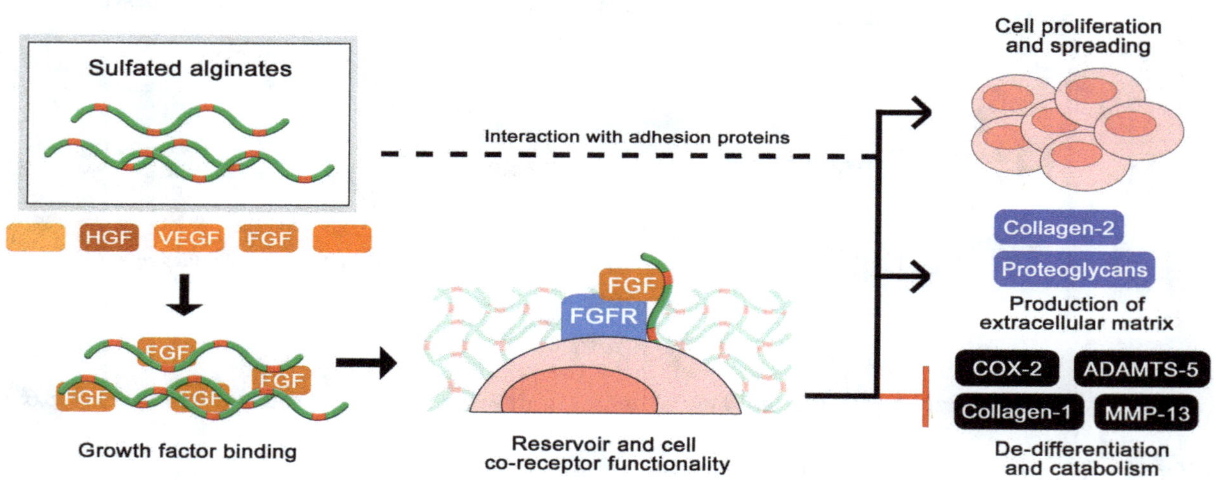

Figure 6. Sulfated alginates bind multiple growth factors [48], and have an inductive effect in chondrocyte cultivation [46,56,58].

Whereas the degradation of sulfated alginates has not yet been studied in vivo, alginates are not depolymerized by any known enzyme in mammals. Sulfated alginates may thus provide more stable hydrogels for long-term implants, where alteration of the sulfation degree, monosaccharide sequence, and gelling conditions can tune properties such as swelling and porosity, degradability, and retention of matrix-binding proteins. Despite a low inflammatory response from the innate immune system, in vivo experiments in certain rat models and primates have uncovered a fibrotic reaction to pure alginate implants, which will presumably occur in human subjects as well and impair the function of the hydrogels and encapsulated cells. As elaborated in the previous section, sulfated alginates show potent anti-inflammatory properties, which can reduce immunological rejection and fibrosis toward long-term implants and potentially overcome these challenges with alginate-based biomaterials. The encapsulation of cells in biomimetic matrices is a highly relevant approach for generating more advanced in vitro tissue models, and for clinical tissue engineering including matrix-assisted cell implantation and injectable matrices such as supporting scaffolds for tissue repair [76,77].

2.7. Structure-Function Relationships in Sulfated Alginates

The conformations of M and G are $^4C_1$ and $^1C_4$, respectively, with glycosidic bonds that are di-equatorial, di-axial, or equatorial-axial for MM, GG, and MG, resulting in varying orientations of the sulfated C2 and C3 hydroxyl groups (Figure 2). The sequences vary in their extension and rigidity, where the GG sequences have a more compact conformation with higher charge density per unit length compared with MM. The MG sequence was initially demonstrated by Smidsrød and colleagues to have a more flexible backbone compared with MM and GG [55], which is also supported by its higher solubility in water at low pH [78]. Similar to heparin, structural and conformational properties, alongside the negative charge density, can influence the interaction strength between sulfated alginates and proteins, emphasizing the importance of characterizing structure-function relationships.

Oligosaccharides of sulfated alginates have been utilized to study the minimal degree of polymerization (DP) required for binding to proteins. In one of our studies using a sulfated alternating alginate sequence (S-MG, DS~0.9), a minimum length of 8-mer was required for significant interaction with HGF, whereas 14-mers approached the interaction strength of poly-S-MG (DP = 80) and LMWH. For FGF-2, a low degree of interaction was observed for 6-mers of S-MG, whereas the 14-mers did not show the efficacy of poly-SMG. Overall, the S-MG samples showed a lower degree of interaction with FGF-2 compared with HGF, and did not approach the efficacy of heparin. Liu and co-workers prepared and sulfated (DS~1.5) M-rich oligosaccharides obtained from hydrolysis and separation of algal alginate, and studied the binding interaction to HIV envelope protein gp120, as a potential anti-HIV therapy. It was demonstrated that a minimal length of an 8-mer was required for interaction, whereas multivalent interactions were observed for >15–16 mers as well as a higher binding affinity compared with heparin [79]. As alginates can be reproducibly hydrolysed and separated into low-disperse fractions based on size and monosaccharide composition, optimizing the molecular weight of samples can potentially contribute to reducing adverse effects in therapeutic applications, similarly to the use of UFH/LMWH/ULMWH.

To assess the impact of the alginate monosaccharide sequence, we initially utilized homogeneous sequences (poly-M, poly-G, and poly-MG) of sulfated alginates with similar sulfation degrees and analysed the interaction with HGF [44]. Here, it was found that at high sulfation degrees (DS~1) the efficacy of the varying sequences was similar, whereas at intermediate sulfation degrees (DS~0.5) the interaction strength increased in the order of poly-M < poly-G < poly-MG. This points towards an influence of chain flexibility as the highly sulfated alginates are presumed to display a more rigid conformation, thus reducing the effect of backbone flexibility in the unmodified alginate sequences. To further investigate the effect of chain flexibility, we performed a periodate oxidation of sulfated poly-M alginates, causing hexuronic ring opening in non-sulfated monosaccharides and an introduction of flexible junction zones [43]. This resulted in increased interaction strength with HGF and FGF-2, correlated with the oxidation degree of the sulfated alginates. The importance of chain flexibility is expected to vary between proteins of different sizes and surface patterns of basic amino acid residues. It was discovered that sulfated poly-M alginates interacted more strongly to FGF-2 than the sulfated poly-MG alginates, while periodate oxidation had a smaller impact on interaction strength compared with that for HGF, indicating that the monosaccharide structure and charge orientation contributes to interaction strength alongside chain flexibility. This was again demonstrated by Li and co-workers, who found that sulfated G-rich oligosaccharides were more effective that M-rich oligosaccharides at prolonging coagulation time, and at mediating FGF-8 signalling in BaF3 cell cultures [61]. As over-sulfated alginates may exert a high degree of non-specific and potential adverse effects, chemo-enzymatic engineering of the backbone may provide a versatile tool to improve interaction strengths and potentially confer increased ligand selectivity compared to sulfation alone, similarly to the role of IdoA in heparin and heparan sulfate.

3. Conclusions and Future Directions

From the present status of knowledge, sulfated alginates show in particular promise for cell immobilization and tissue engineering applications, as presented through the works of Zenobi-Wong and Cohen with their respective groups. The sulfated alginates act as analogues of cell surface GAGs in mediating growth factor signalling, while creating a biomimetic physical environment for the proliferation and migration of cells, extracellular matrix deposition, and tissue maturation. Similarly, the sulfated alginate matrix may provide a reservoir for growth factors, where the affinity toward specific growth factors may be altered through chemo-enzymatic engineering of the alginate, for a tuned and sustained delivery to tissues. There have further been demonstrated anti-inflammatory properties in sulfated alginates, which can aid in matrix-assisted cell- and tissue transplantations by suppressing pro-catabolic and inflammatory responses from surrounding tissues and in encapsulated cells. However, additional in vivo studies to assess gel stability, immunological and fibrotic responses, and implant survival are required. Non-coagulating heparins have previously been evaluated for anti-inflammatory and anti-cancer therapeutics, highlighting an additional potential application for heparin analogues with customizable pharmacokinetic and -dynamic properties in treating acute and chronic inflammatory conditions.

Several studies on sulfated alginates have focused on their anti-coagulant properties. However, there are no clear indications of specific antithrombin activation, where substantially higher concentrations of sulfated alginates are required to approach the efficacy of heparin. While sequences of sulfated alginate with a higher affinity for antithrombin can potentially be generated through chemo-enzymatic engineering, emulation of the specific heparin pentasaccharide may prove challenging. As an intravenously administered drug with rapid onset, heparin benefits from a short half-life. Sulfated alginates are presumably eliminated through renal excretion alone, which is a slower mechanism compared to depolymerization, where extended activity may lead to a severe drop in blood pressure and additional adverse effects. The use of sulfated alginates as anticoagulants can therefore show greater promise as a coating for medical devices and biomaterials, where a high surface stability is desirable and the additional anti-inflammatory effects can potentially reduce fibrosis or immunological rejection of implanted devices or materials.

Chemical sulfation of alginates allows for the simple and reproducible synthesis of heparin-like molecules in large batches and at low cost. However, much work remains to explore novel strategies for milder and more selective syntheses, to further characterize and understand their interaction with heparin-binding proteins, and to evaluate the potential of sulfated alginates toward novel biomedical applications. Compared to GAGs and other heparin analogues, the utility of sulfated alginates is tied to their gelling capability and their structural customizability, allowing tuning of physical and biological properties, and bioavailability. The majority of studies have employed commercial algal alginates and have performed sulfation of C2 and C3, whereas exploring non-conventional sequence patterns (alternative sources, enzymatic engineering), novel sulfation strategies (M/G preference, C6-sulfation), and conjugation to other functional groups can provide new properties and potentially improved selectivity of protein interactions. Ideally, a sulfated alginate oligosaccharide library with defined modification patterns can be established and applied to gain a deeper understanding of their structure-function relationships. In conclusion, sulfated alginates have unique characteristics as heparin analogues, and while they are relatively unstudied, they demonstrate a wide range of biological properties and a structural versatility that can provide novel biomedical applications and a deeper understanding of the biological functions of sulfated glycosaminoglycans.

Acknowledgments: This work was supported by the Norwegian Research Council through the MARPOL project (grant no. 221576), and by SINTEF Materials and Chemistry, Trondheim, Norway.

Author Contributions: Ø.A. and G.S.-B. reviewed the literature and wrote the paper.

References

1. Liu, H.Y.; Zhang, Z.Q.; Linhardt, R.J. Lessons Learned from the Contamination of Heparin. *Nat. Prod. Rep.* **2009**, *26*, 313–321. [CrossRef] [PubMed]
2. Lindahl, U.; Li, J.P.; Kusche-Gullberg, M.; Salmivirta, M.; Alaranta, S.; Veromaa, T.; Emeis, J.; Roberts, I.; Taylor, C.; Oreste, P.; et al. Generation of "Neoheparin" from E Coli K5 Capsular Polysaccharide. *J. Med. Chem.* **2005**, *48*, 349–352. [CrossRef] [PubMed]
3. Codee, J.D.C.; Stubba, B.; Schiattarella, M.; Overkleeft, H.S.; van Boeckel, C.A.A.; van Boom, J.H.; van der Marel, G.A. A Modular Strategy toward the Synthesis of Heparin-Like Oligosaccharides Using Monomeric Building Blocks in a Sequential Glycosylation Strategy. *J. Am. Chem. Soc.* **2005**, *127*, 3767–3773. [CrossRef] [PubMed]
4. Jiao, G.L.; Yu, G.L.; Zhang, J.Z.; Ewart, H.S. Chemical Structures and Bioactivities of Sulfated Polysaccharides from Marine Algae. *Mar. Drugs* **2011**, *9*, 196–223. [CrossRef] [PubMed]
5. Deng, J.; Liu, X.Y.; Ma, L.; Cheng, C.; Shi, W.B.; Nie, C.X.; Zhao, C.S. Heparin-Mimicking Multilayer Coating on Polymeric Membrane Via Lbl Assembly of Cyclodextrin-Based Supramolecules. *ACS Appl. Mater. Interfaces* **2014**, *6*, 21603–21614. [CrossRef] [PubMed]
6. Sasisekharan, R.; Venkataraman, G. Heparin and Heparan Sulfate: Biosynthesis, Structure and Function. *Curr. Opin. Chem. Biol.* **2000**, *4*, 626–631. [CrossRef]
7. Raman, R.; Venkataraman, G.; Ernst, S.; Sasisekharan, V.; Sasisekharan, R. Structural Specificity of Heparin Binding in the Fibroblast Growth Factor Family of Proteins. *Proc. Natl. Acad. Sci. USA* **2003**, *100*, 2357–2362. [CrossRef] [PubMed]
8. Habuchi, H.; Tanaka, M.; Habuchi, O.; Yoshida, K.; Suzuki, H.; Ban, K.; Kimata, K. The Occurrence of Three Isoforms of Heparan Sulfate 6-*O*-Sulfotransferase Having Different Specificities for Hexuronic Acid Adjacent to the Targeted *N*-Sulfoglucosamine. *J. Biol. Chem.* **2000**, *275*, 2859–2868. [CrossRef] [PubMed]
9. Aikawa, J.; Grobe, K.; Tsujimoto, M.; Esko, J.D. Multiple Isozymes of Heparan Sulfate/Heparin Glcnac *N*-Deacetylase/Glcn *N*-Sulfotransferase-Structure and Activity of the Fourth Member, Ndst4. *J. Biol. Chem.* **2001**, *276*, 5876–5882. [CrossRef] [PubMed]
10. Sudo, M.; Sato, K.; Chaidedgumjorn, A.; Toyoda, H.; Toida, T.; Imanari, T. H-1 Nuclear Magnetic Resonance Spectroscopic Analysis for Determination of Glucuronic and Iduronic Acids in Dermatan Sulfate, Heparin, and Heparan Sulfate. *Anal. Biochem.* **2001**, *297*, 42–51. [CrossRef] [PubMed]
11. Guerrini, M.; Bisio, A.; Torri, G. Combined Quantitative H-1 and C-13 Nuclear Magnetic Resonance Spectroscopy for Characterization of Heparin Preparations. *Semin. Thromb. Hemost.* **2001**, *27*, 473–482. [CrossRef] [PubMed]
12. Maccarana, M.; Sakura, Y.; Tawada, A.; Yoshida, K.; Lindahl, U. Domain Structure of Heparan Sulfates from Bovine Organs. *J. Biol. Chem.* **1996**, *271*, 17804–17810. [CrossRef] [PubMed]
13. Hagner-McWhirter, A.; Lindahl, U.; Li, J.P. Biosynthesis of Heparin/Heparan Sulphate: Mechanism of Epimerization of Glucuronyl C-5. *Biochem. J.* **2000**, *347*, 69–75. [CrossRef] [PubMed]
14. Raedts, J.M.; Lundgren, M.; Kengen, S.W.M.; Li, J.P.; van der Oost, J. A Novel Bacterial Enzyme with D-Glucuronyl C5-Epimerase Activity. *J. Biol. Chem.* **2013**, *288*, 24332–24339. [CrossRef] [PubMed]
15. Lidholt, K.; Fjelstad, M.; Jann, K.; Lindahl, U. Biosynthesis of Heparin 25. Substrate Specificities of Glycosyltransferases Involved in Formation of Heparin Precursor and Escherichia-Coli K5 Capsular Polysaccharides. *Carbohydr. Res.* **1994**, *255*, 87–101. [CrossRef]
16. Lindahl, U.; Backstrom, G.; Hook, M.; Thunberg, L.; Fransson, L.A.; Linker, A. Structure of the Antithrombin-Binding Site in Heparin. *Proc. Natl. Acad. Sci. USA* **1979**, *76*, 3198–3202. [CrossRef] [PubMed]
17. Hansen, S.U.; Miller, G.J.; Cliff, M.J.; Jaysonc, G.C.; Gardiner, J.M. Making the Longest Sugars: A Chemical Synthesis of Heparin-Related [4](N) Oligosaccharides from 16-Mer to 40-Mer. *Chem. Sci.* **2015**, *6*, 6158–6164. [CrossRef]
18. Rosenberg, R.D. Actions and Interactions of Antithrombin and Heparin. *N. Engl. J. Med.* **1975**, *292*, 146–151. [PubMed]
19. Sahu, A.; Pangburn, M.K. Identification of Multiple Sites of Interaction between Heparin and the Complement-System. *Mol. Immunol.* **1993**, *30*, 679–684. [CrossRef]

20. Amara, U.; Flierl, M.A.; Rittirsch, D.; Klos, A.; Chen, H.; Acker, B.; Bruckner, U.B.; Nilsson, B.; Gebhard, F.; Lambris, J.D.; et al. Molecular Intercommunication between the Complement and Coagulation Systems. *J. Immunol.* **2010**, *185*, 5628–5636. [CrossRef] [PubMed]
21. Gandhi, N.S.; Mancera, R.L. The Structure of Glycosaminoglycans and Their Interactions with Proteins. *Chem. Biol. Drug Des.* **2008**, *72*, 455–482. [CrossRef] [PubMed]
22. Nelson, R.M.; Cecconi, O.; Roberts, W.G.; Aruffo, A.; Linhardt, R.J.; Bevilacqua, M.P. Heparin Oligosaccharides Bind L-Selectin and P-Selectin and Inhibit Acute-Inflammation. *Blood* **1993**, *82*, 3253–3258. [PubMed]
23. Joyce, J.G.; Tung, J.S.; Przysiecki, C.T.; Cook, J.C.; Lehman, E.D.; Sands, J.A.; Jansen, K.U.; Keller, P.M. The L1 Major Capsid Protein of Human Papillomavirus Type 11 Recombinant Virus-Like Particles Interacts with Heparin and Cell-Surface Glycosaminoglycans on Human Keratinocytes. *J. Biol. Chem.* **1999**, *274*, 5810–5822. [CrossRef] [PubMed]
24. Ascencio, F.; Fransson, L.A.; Wadstrom, T. Affinity of the Gastric Pathogen Helicobacter-Pylori for the N-Sulfated Glycosaminoglycan Heparan-Sulfate. *J. Med. Microbiol.* **1993**, *38*, 240–244. [CrossRef] [PubMed]
25. Spillmann, D.; Lindahl, U. Glycosaminoglycan Protein Interactions-a Question of Specificity. *Curr. Opin. Struct. Biol.* **1994**, *4*, 677–682. [CrossRef]
26. Lindahl, U. A Personal Voyage through the Proteoglycan Field. *Matrix Biol.* **2014**, *35*, 3–7. [CrossRef] [PubMed]
27. Hu, Y.P.; Zhong, Y.Q.; Chen, Z.G.; Chen, C.Y.; Shi, Z.; Zulueta, M.M.; Ku, C.C.; Lee, P.Y.; Wang, C.C.; Hung, S.C. Divergent Synthesis of 48 Heparan Sulfate-Based Disaccharides and Probing the Specific Sugar-Fibroblast Growth Factor-1 Interaction. *J. Am. Chem. Soc.* **2012**, *134*, 20722–20727. [CrossRef] [PubMed]
28. Foxall, C.; Holme, K.R.; Liang, W.H.; Wei, Z. An Enzyme-Linked-Immunosorbent-Assay Using Biotinylated Heparan-Sulfate to Evaluate the Interactions of Heparin-Like Molecules and Basic Fibroblast Growth-Factor. *Anal. Biochem.* **1995**, *231*, 366–373. [CrossRef] [PubMed]
29. Wang, L.C.; Brown, J.R.; Varki, A.; Esko, J.D. Heparin's Anti-Inflammatory Effects Require Glucosamine 6-*O*-Sulfation and Are Mediated by Blockade of L- and P-Selectins. *J. Clin. Investig.* **2002**, *110*, 127–136. [CrossRef] [PubMed]
30. Koenig, A.; Norgard-Sumnicht, K.; Linhardt, R.; Varki, A. Differential Interactions of Heparin and Heparan Sulfate Glycosaminoglycans with the Selectins-Implications for the Use of Unfractionated and Low Molecular Weight Heparins as Therapeutic Agents. *J. Clin Investig.* **1998**, *101*, 877–889. [CrossRef] [PubMed]
31. Skjåk-Bræk, G.; Donari, I.; Paoletti, S. Alginate Hydrogels: Properties and Applications. In *Polysaccharide Hydrogels*; Matricardi, P., Alhaique, F., Coviello, T., Eds.; Pan Stanford: Boca Raton, FL, USA, 2015.
32. Sarrazin, S.; Lamanna, W.C.; Esko, J.D. Heparan Sulfate Proteoglycans. *Cold Spring Harbor Perspect. Biol.* **2011**, *3*, 1–33. [CrossRef] [PubMed]
33. Stokke, B.T.; Smidsrød, O.; Bruheim, P.; Skjåk-Bræk, G. Distribution of Uronate Residues in Alginate Chains in Relation to Alginate Gelling Properties. *Macromolecules* **1991**, *24*, 4637–4645. [CrossRef]
34. Mørch, Y.A.; Donati, I.; Strand, B.L.; Skjåk-Bræk, G. Molecular Engineering as an Approach to Design New Functional Properties of Alginate. *Biomacromolecules* **2007**, *8*, 2809–2814. [CrossRef] [PubMed]
35. Høidal, H.K.; Ertesvåg, H.; Skjåk-Bræk, G.; Stokke, B.T.; Valla, S. The Recombinant Azotobacter Vinelandii Mannuronan C-5-Epimerase Alge4 Epimerizes Alginate by a Nonrandom Attack Mechanism. *J. Biol. Chem.* **1999**, *274*, 12316–12322. [CrossRef] [PubMed]
36. Pawar, S.N.; Edgar, K.J. Alginate Derivatization: A Review of Chemistry, Properties and Applications. *Biomaterials* **2012**, *33*, 3279–3305. [CrossRef] [PubMed]
37. Ertesvåg, H. Alginate-Modifying Enzymes: Biological Roles and Biotechnological Uses. *Front. Microbiol.* **2015**, *6*, 1–10.
38. Jacobs-Tulleneers-Thevissen, D.; Chintinne, M.; Ling, Z.; Gillard, P.; Schoonjans, L.; Delvaux, G.; Strand, B.L.; Gorus, F.; Keymeulen, B.; Pipeleers, D.; et al. Sustained Function of Alginate-Encapsulated Human Islet Cell Implants in the Peritoneal Cavity of Mice Leading to a Pilot Study in a Type 1 Diabetic Patient. *Diabetologia* **2013**, *56*, 1605–1614. [CrossRef] [PubMed]
39. Zhang, J.; Wang, Q.; Wang, A. In Situ Generation of Sodium Alginate/Hydroxyapatite Nanocomposite Beads as Drug-Controlled Release Matrices. *Acta Biomate.* **2010**, *6*, 445–454. [CrossRef] [PubMed]
40. Sandvig, I.; Karstensen, K.; Rokstad, A.M.; Aachmann, F.L.; Formo, K.; Sandvig, A.; Skjåk-Bræk, G.; Strand, B.L. Rgd-Peptide Modified Alginate by a Chemoenzymatic Strategy for Tissue Engineering Applications. *J. Biomed. Mater. Res. Part A* **2015**, *103*, 896–906. [CrossRef] [PubMed]

41. Markstedt, K.; Mantas, A.; Tournier, I.; Martinez, H.; Hägg, D.; Gatenholm, P. 3D Bioprinting Human Chondrocytes with Nanocellulose-Alginate Bioink for Cartilage Tissue Engineering Applications. *Biomacromolecules* **2015**, *16*, 1489–1496. [CrossRef] [PubMed]
42. Huang, R.H.; Du, Y.M.; Yang, J.H. Preparation and in Vitro Anticoagulant Activities of Alginate Sulfate and Its Quaterized Derivatives. *Carbohydr. Polym.* **2003**, *52*, 19–24.
43. Arlov, Ø.; Aachmann, F.L.; Feyzi, E.; Sundan, A.; Skjåk-Bræk, G. The Impact of Chain Length and Flexibility in the Interaction between Sulfated Alginates and Hgf and Fgf-2. *Biomacromolecules* **2015**, *16*, 3417–3424. [CrossRef] [PubMed]
44. Arlov, Ø.; Aachmann, F.L.; Sundan, A.; Espevik, T.; Skjåk-Bræk, G. Heparin-Like Properties of Sulfated Alginates with Defined Sequences and Sulfation Degrees. *Biomacromolecules* **2014**, *15*, 2744–2750. [CrossRef] [PubMed]
45. Miyaji, H.; Misaki, A. Distribution of Sulfate Groups in the Partially Sulfated Dextrans. *J. Biochem.* **1973**, *74*, 1131–1139. [CrossRef] [PubMed]
46. Mhanna, R.; Kashyap, A.; Palazzolo, G.; Vallmajo-Martin, Q.; Becher, J.; Möller, S.; Schnabelrauch, M.; Zenobi-Wong, M. Chondrocyte Culture in Three Dimensional Alginate Sulfate Hydrogels Promotes Proliferation While Maintaining Expression of Chondrogenic Markers. *Tissue Engl. Part A* **2014**, *20*, 1454–1464. [CrossRef] [PubMed]
47. Ma, L.; Cheng, C.; Nie, C.X.; He, C.; Deng, J.; Wang, L.R.; Xia, Y.; Zhao, C.S. Anticoagulant Sodium Alginate Sulfates and Their Mussel-Inspired Heparin-Mimetic Coatings. *J. Mater. Chem. B* **2016**, *4*, 203–215. [CrossRef]
48. Freeman, I.; Kedem, A.; Cohen, S. The Effect of Sulfation of Alginate Hydrogels on the Specific Binding and Controlled Release of Heparin-Binding Proteins. *Biomaterials* **2008**, *29*, 3260–3268. [CrossRef] [PubMed]
49. Fan, L.H.; Jiang, L.; Xu, Y.M.; Zhou, Y.; Shen, Y.A.; Xie, W.G.; Long, Z.H.; Zhou, J.P. Synthesis and Anticoagulant Activity of Sodium Alginate Sulfates. *Carbohydr. Polym.* **2011**, *83*, 1797–1803. [CrossRef]
50. Zhao, X.; Yu, G.L.; Guan, H.S.; Yue, N.; Zhang, Z.Q.; Li, H.H. Preparation of Low-Molecular-Weight Polyguluronate Sulfate and Its Anticoagulant and Anti-Inflammatory Activities. *Carbohydr. Polym.* **2007**, *69*, 272–279. [CrossRef]
51. Lindahl, U.; Kusche-Gullberg, M.; Kjellen, L. Regulated Diversity of Heparan Sulfate. *J. Biol. Chem.* **1998**, *273*, 24979–24982. [CrossRef] [PubMed]
52. Dodgson, K.S.; Price, R.G. A Note on the Determination of the Ester Sulphate Content of Sulphated Polysaccharides. *Biochem. J.* **1962**, *84*, 106–110. [CrossRef] [PubMed]
53. Yang, J.H.; Du, Y.M.; Huang, R.H.; Wan, Y.Y.; Wen, Y. The Structure-Anticoagulant Activity Relationships of Sulfated Lacquer Polysaccharide—Effect of Carboxyl Group and Position of Sulfation. *Int. J. Biol. Macromol.* **2005**, *36*, 9–15. [CrossRef] [PubMed]
54. Heymann, B.; Grubmuller, H. Chair-Boat′ Transitions and Side Groups Affect the Stiffness of Polysaccharides. *Chem. Phys. Lett.* **1999**, *305*, 202–208. [CrossRef]
55. Smidsrød, O.; Glover, R.M.; Whittington, S.G. The Relative Extension of Alginates Having Different Chemical Composition. *Carbohydr. Res.* **1973**, *27*, 107–118. [CrossRef]
56. Öztürk, E.; Arlov, Ø.; Aksel, S.; Li, L.; Ornitz, D.M.; Skjåk-Bræk, G.; Zenobi-Wong, M. Sulfated Hydrogel Matrices Direct Mitogenicity and Maintenance of Chondrocyte Phenotype through Activation of Fgf Signaling. *Adv. Funct. Mater.* **2016**, *26*, 3649–3662. [CrossRef]
57. Grant, G.T.; Morris, E.R.; Rees, D.A.; Smith, P.J.C.; Thom, D. Biological Interactions between Polysaccharides and Divalent Cations-Egg-Box Model. *Febs. Lett.* **1973**, *32*, 195–198. [CrossRef]
58. Arlov, Ø.; Steinwachs, M.; Skjåk-Bræk, G.; Zenobi-Wong, M. Biomimetic Sulphated Alginate Hydrogels Suppress Il-1beta-Induced Inflammatory Responses in Human Chondrocytes. *Eur. Cell. Mater.* **2017**, *33*, 76–89. [CrossRef] [PubMed]
59. Mørch, Ý.A.; Donati, I.; Strand, B.L.; Skjåk-Bræk, G. Effect of Ca^{2+}, Ba^{2+}, and Sr^{2+} on Alginate Microbeads. *Biomacromolecules* **2006**, *7*, 1471–1480. [CrossRef] [PubMed]
60. Draget, K.I.; Østgaard, K.; Smidsrød, O. Homogeneous Alginate Gels-a Technical Approach. *Carbohydr. Polym.* **1990**, *14*, 159–178. [CrossRef]
61. Li, Q.C.; Zeng, Y.Y.; Wang, L.L.; Guan, H.S.; Li, C.X.; Zhang, L.J. The Heparin-Like Activities of Negatively Charged Derivatives of Low-Molecular-Weight Polymannuronate and Polyguluronate. *Carbohydr. Polym.* **2017**, *155*, 313–320. [CrossRef] [PubMed]

62. Mousa, S.A.; Mohamed, S. Inhibition of Endothelial Cell Tube Formation by the Low Molecular Weight Heparin, Tinzaparin, Is Mediated by Tissue Factor Pathway Inhibitor. *Thromb. Haemost.* **2004**, *92*, 627–633. [CrossRef] [PubMed]
63. Ma, L.; Cheng, C.; He, C.; Nie, C.X.; Deng, J.; Sun, S.D.; Zhao, C.S. Substrate-Independent Robust and Heparin-Mimetic Hydrogel Thin Film Coating Via Combined Lbl Self-Assembly and Mussel-Inspired Post-Cross-Linking. *ACS Appl. Mater. Interfaces* **2015**, *7*, 26050–26062. [CrossRef] [PubMed]
64. Niimi, Y.; Ichinose, F.; Ishiguro, Y.; Terui, K.; Uezono, S.; Morita, S.; Yamane, S. The Effects of Heparin Coating of Oxygenator Fibers on Platelet Adhesion and Protein Adsorption. *Anesth. Analg.* **1999**, *89*, 573–579. [PubMed]
65. Arlov, Ø.; Skjåk-Bræk, G.; Rokstad, A.M. Sulfated Alginate Microspheres Associate with Factor H and Dampen the Inflammatory Cytokine Response. *Acta Biomater.* **2016**, *42*, 180–188. [CrossRef] [PubMed]
66. Weiler, J.M.; Edens, R.E.; Linhardt, R.J.; Kapelanski, D.P. Heparin and Modified Heparin Inhibit Complement Activation Invivo. *J. Immunol.* **1992**, *148*, 3210–3215. [PubMed]
67. Oikonomopoulou, K.; Ricklin, D.; Ward, P.A.; Lambris, J.D. Interactions between Coagulation and Complement-Their Role in Inflammation. *Semin. Immunopathol.* **2012**, *34*, 151–165. [CrossRef] [PubMed]
68. Spivak-Kroizman, T.; Lemmon, M.A.; Dikic, I.; Ladbury, J.E.; Pinchasi, D.; Huang, J.; Jaye, M.; Crumley, G.; Schlessinger, J.; Lax, I. Heparin-Induced Oligomerization of Fgf Molecules Is Responsible for Fgf Receptor Dimerization, Activation, and Cell-Proliferation. *Cell* **1994**, *79*, 1015–1024. [CrossRef]
69. Izaki, S.; Goldstein, S.M.; Fukuyama, K.; Epstein, W.L. Fibrin Deposition and Clearance in Chronic Granulomatous Inflammation: Correlation with T-Cell Function and Proteinase Inhibitor Activity in Tissue. *J. Investig. Dermatol.* **1979**, *73*, 561–565. [CrossRef] [PubMed]
70. Lukacs, N.W.; Chensue, S.W.; Strieter, R.M.; Warmington, K.; Kunkel, S.L. Inflammatory Granuloma-Formation Is Mediated by Tnf-Alpha-Inducible Intercellular-Adhesion Molecule-1. *J. Immunol.* **1994**, *152*, 5883–5889. [PubMed]
71. Ruvinov, E.; Leor, J.; Cohen, S. The Effects of Controlled Hgf Delivery from an Affinity-Binding Alginate Biomaterial on Angiogenesis and Blood Perfusion in a Hindlimb Ischemia Model. *Biomaterials* **2010**, *31*, 4573–4582. [CrossRef] [PubMed]
72. Freeman, I.; Cohen, S. The Influence of the Sequential Delivery of Angiogenic Factors from Affinity-Binding Alginate Scaffolds on Vascularization. *Biomaterials* **2009**, *30*, 2122–2131. [CrossRef] [PubMed]
73. Re'em, T.; Witte, F.; Willbold, E.; Ruvinov, E.; Cohen, S. Simultaneous Regeneration of Articular Cartilage and Subchondral Bone Induced by Spatially Presented Tgf-Beta and Bmp-4 in a Bilayer Affinity Binding System. *Acta Biomater.* **2012**, *8*, 3283–3293. [CrossRef] [PubMed]
74. Ruvinov, E.; Freeman, I.; Fredo, R.; Cohen, S. Spontaneous Coassembly of Biologically Active Nanoparticles Via Affinity Binding of Heparin-Binding Proteins to Alginate-Sulfate. *Nano Lett.* **2016**, *16*, 883–888. [CrossRef] [PubMed]
75. Müller, M.; Ece, Ö.; Øystein, A.; Paul, G.; Zenobi-Wong, M. Alginate Sulfate–Nanocellulose Bioinks for Cartilage Bioprinting Applications. *Annals Biomed. Eng.* **2016**, *45*, 210–223. [CrossRef] [PubMed]
76. Makris, E.A.; Gomoll, A.H.; Malizos, K.N.; Hu, J.C.; Athanasiou, K.A. Repair and Tissue Engineering Techniques for Articular Cartilage. *Nat. Rev. Rheumatol.* **2015**, *11*, 21–34. [CrossRef] [PubMed]
77. Duflo, S.; Thibeault, S.L.; Li, W.H.; Shu, X.Z.; Prestwich, G.D. Vocal Fold Tissue Repair in Vivo Using a Synthetic Extracellular Matrix. *Tissue Eng.* **2006**, *12*, 2171–2180. [CrossRef] [PubMed]
78. Hartmann, M.; Dentini, M.; Draget, K.I.; Skjåk-Bræk, G. Enzymatic Modification of Alginates with the Mannuronan C-5 Epimerase Alge4 Enhances Their Solubility at Low Ph. *Carbohydr. Poly.* **2006**, *63*, 257–262. [CrossRef]
79. Liu, H.Y.; Geng, M.Y.; Xin, X.L.; Li, F.C.; Zhang, Z.Q.; Li, J.; Ding, J. Multiple and Multivalent Interactions of Novel Anti-Aids Drug Candidates, Sulfated Polymannuronate (Spmg)-Derived Oligosaccharides, with Gp120 and Their Anti-Hiv Activities. *Glycobiology* **2005**, *15*, 501–510. [CrossRef] [PubMed]

14

A Fluorescent Probe for Glycosaminoglycans Applied to the Detection of Dermatan Sulfate by a Mix-and-Read Assay

Melissa Rappold, Ulrich Warttinger and Roland Krämer *

Inorganic Chemistry Institute, Heidelberg University, Im Neuenheimer Feld 270, 69120 Heidelberg, Germany; melissa.rappold@aci.uni-heidelberg.de (M.R.); ulrich.warttinger@aci.uni-heidelberg.de (U.W.)
* Correspondence: kraemer@aci.uni-heidelberg.de

Academic Editors: Giangiacomo Torri and Jawed Fareed

Abstract: Glycosaminoglycans are complex biomolecules of great biological and medical importance. The quantification of glycosaminoglycans, in particular in complex matrices, is challenging due to their inherent structural heterogeneity. Heparin Red, a polycationic, fluorescent perylene diimide derivative, has recently emerged as a commercial probe for the convenient detection of heparins by a mix-and-read fluorescence assay. The probe also detects glycosaminoglycans with a lower negative charge density than heparin, although with lower sensitivity. We describe here the synthesis and characterization of a structurally related molecular probe with a higher positive charge of +10 (vs. +8 of Heparin Red). The superior performance of this probe is exemplified by the quantification of low dermatan sulfate concentrations in an aqueous matrix (quantification limit 1 ng/mL) and the detection of dermatan sulfate in blood plasma in a clinically relevant concentration range. The potential applications of this probe include monitoring the blood levels of dermatan sulfate after administration as an antithrombotic drug in the absence of heparin and other glycosaminoglycans.

Keywords: perylene diimide dyes; dermatan sulfate; fluorescent probe; Heparin Red; assay; dermatan sulfate; human plasma

---

1. Introduction

Glycosaminoglycans are complex biomolecules of great biological and medical importance. They are composed of linear, polydisperse polysaccharides with a highly variable sulfation pattern (with the exception of hyaluronate, which is not sulfated). This structural heterogeneity makes the quantification of glycosaminoglycans challenging. There is a continuous search for more convenient, precise and sensitive quantification methods, in particular for complex biological matrices. Various molecular probes for the direct optical detection of glycosaminoglycans (mainly of heparin, a widely-used antithrombotic drug) have been described [1]. Such probes enable convenient detection by photometry or fluorimetry, although their performance in complex biological matrices is often limited by interference. The fluorescent probe **Heparin Red** has recently emerged as a component of commercially available assays for the quantification of heparins in various matrices [2–4]. It is implemented in several drug development projects for the pharmacokinetic monitoring of non-anticoagulant heparins, a promising class of drug candidates [5]. **Heparin Red** is a polyamine modified, red-emissive perylene diimide fluorophore (Scheme 1, right).

It forms a supramolecular aggregate with glycosaminoglycans, resulting in contact quenching of fluorescence (Scheme 2). The strong binding of the polycationic probe to polyanionic heparin appears to be controlled by both electrostatic and aromatic π-stacking interactions [6]. While electrostatic repulsion between dye molecules prevents spontaneous aggregation in the solution, the charge neutralization by polyanionic heparin favors the formation of π-stacked complexes between the hydrophobic chromophore moieties in the ground state, leading to efficient static quenching. **Heparin Red** has also been applied to the determination of polysaccharides, such as heparan sulfate [7] and fucoidan [8], that have a lower negative charge density than heparin, but the sensitivity in a plasma matrix is significantly lower. An ultrasensitive assay with a quantification limit in the pg/mL range for the highly sulfated polysaccharide dextran sulfate in an aqueous matrix has also been described [9].

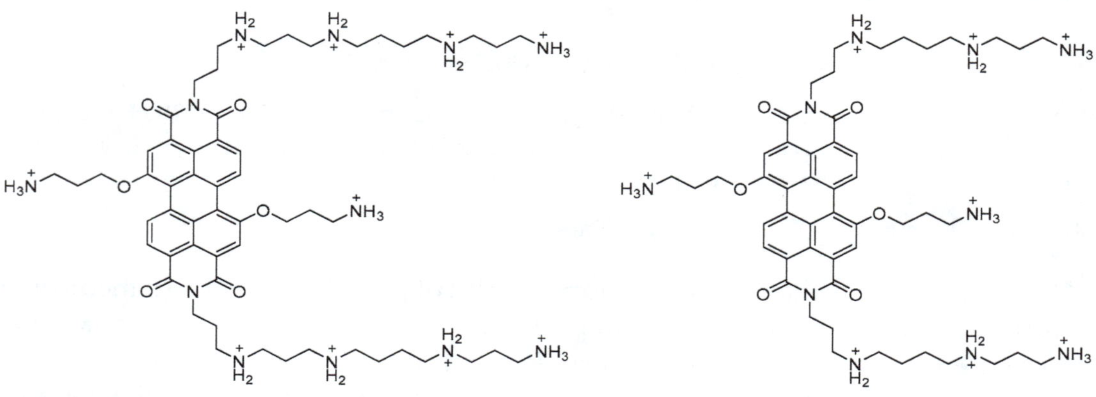

PDI-1 Heparin Red

Scheme 1. Molecular structures of the probes **PDI-1** and **Heparin Red** in their fully protonated state (charge +10 and +8, respectively).

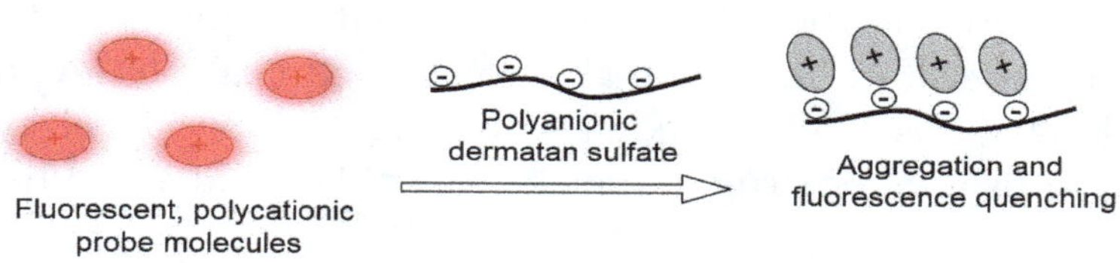

Scheme 2. Schematic representation of fluorescence quenching of polycationic probe molecules in the presence of dermatan sulfate due to the formation of non-fluorescent aggregates.

Dermatan sulfate is a linear, polydisperse sulfated polysaccharide belonging to the glycosaminoglycan family. It is built of a major repeating disaccharide unit consisting of iduronic acid and galactosamine (Scheme 3). The galactosamine may be 4-*O* or 6-*O*-sulfated and the iduronic acid is 2-*O*-sulfated. Typically, the average degree of sulfation is around one per disaccharide. Dermatan sulfate is the predominant glycosaminoglycan expressed in the skin and is released at high concentrations during wound repair. It is also implicated in other biological processes [10], such as development, growth, infection, tumorigenesis and coagulation [11]. Elevated dermatan sulfate levels in plasma or urine have been suggested as a biomarker for certain types of mucopolysaccharidosis [12]. Dermatan sulfate-based drug formulations have been launched for the prevention of venous thromboembolism in Italy (marketed as Mistral) [13] and Portugal (marketed as Venorix). It is also a component of Sulodexide, a more widely-used antithrombotic agent [14]. Dermatan sulfate is produced by extraction from animal tissues, including a complex multistep purification process. The structural heterogeneity makes the direct quantification of dermatan sulfate in complex matrices such as human plasma challenging. Disaccharide analysis [15] provides both quantification and valuable information on dermatan sulfate structure, but involves tedious multistep protocols with sample pretreatment. In clinical settings, dermatan sulfate blood levels are indirectly monitored by coagulation assays [16].

We describe here the direct determination of dermatan sulfate in aqueous and plasma matrices by a new fluorescent probe, **PDI-1** (Scheme 1). The latter is structurally related to **Heparin Red** but has a higher positive molecular charge (+10 vs. +8 for Heparin Red). The enhanced performance of this probe is demonstrated by the determination of dermatan sulfate at low concentrations and in a competitive human plasma matrix.

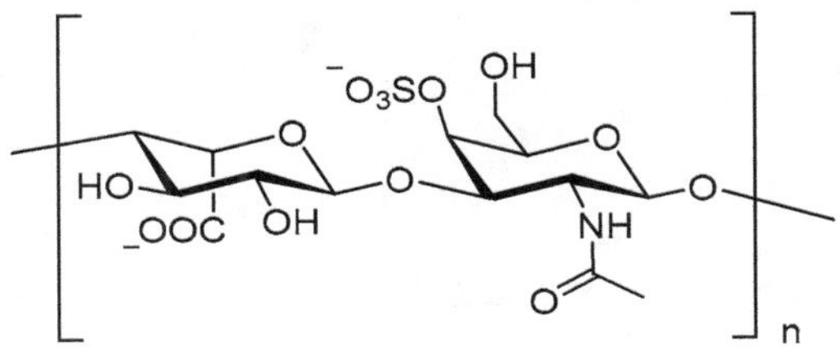

Scheme 3. Major iduronic acid-galactosamine repeating disaccharide unit of dermatan sulfate, mono-sulfated form. The sulfation pattern is variable; possible sites of sulfation are galactosamine 4-*O*, 6-*O* and iduronic acid 2-*O*. The disaccharide moiety may be unsulfated, mono- or disulfated.

2. Results and Discussion

2.1. Synthesis and Properties of the Polyamine-Functionalized Perylene Diimide Probe **PDI-1**

The synthesis of **PDI-1** is described by Scheme 4. A tetra-Boc-protected form of the pentaamine 1,5,9,14,18-pentaza-octadecane was prepared based on a procedure described in the literature [17], and combined with 1,7-dibromoperylene-3,4:9,10-tetracarboxylic acid dianhydride [18] in refluxing toluene to the perylene diimide derivative **PDI-3**. The latter was reacted further with 3-(*N*-Boc)-aminopropanol in tetrahydrofuran, using the base lithium diisopropylamide for the deprotonation of the OH-group; nucleophilic aromatic substitution of bromide led to the fully N-protected intermediate **PDI-4**. The deprotection of **PDI-4** in MeOH/HCl, purification by semi-preparative high-performance liquid chromatography (HPLC) using aqueous trifluoroacetic acid-acetonitrile as an eluent and exchange of the trifluoroacetate counterion with chloride by precipitation from acetonitrile gave the target compound [**PDI-1**]Cl_{10}. The probe was characterized by ^{1}H- and ^{13}C-NMR spectroscopy, electrospray mass spectrometry, UV-Vis spectroscopy, fluorimetry and analytical HPLC. The photophysical properties such as visible absorbance and fluorescence spectra ($\lambda_{max\,(Abs)}$ = 576 nm, ε (576 nm) = 35,300 M^{-1} cm^{-1}), λ_{max} = 615 nm, quantum yield ϕ_F = 0.17) in a buffered aqueous medium (pH 7) of **PDI-1** are very similar to those of **Heparin Red**.

2.2. Detection of Dermatan Sulfate in Aqueous Samples

The response of the probes to dermatan sulfate is controlled by the detection medium; while a high proportion of dimethyl sulfoxide (DMSO) suppresses any response [4], the assay becomes sensitive to dermatan sulfate at a high proportion of water. All detections were performed with spiked samples using commercially available dermatan sulfate sodium salt from porcine intestinal mucosa. A sulfation degree of 1.1 per disaccharide was calculated from the analytical data given in the certificate of the provider (S elemental analysis and water content), and refers to the repeating disaccharide unit given in Scheme 3. The resulting negative charge density per monosaccharide is −1.05, significantly lower in comparison to heparin (−1.7).

Figure 1 shows the titration of 1 μM solutions of the fluorescent probes **PDI-1** and **Heparin Red**, respectively, with dermatan sulfate in an aqueous buffer. A linear decrease of fluorescence intensity with increasing dermatan sulfate concentration was observed. To reach the endpoint of the titration, 19% more dermatan sulfate was needed in case of **PDI-1**. This is in line with the formation of charge neutral, fluorescence-quenched aggregates [6]. Since the charge of **PDI-1** in its fully protonated state is +10 but the fully protonated state of **Heparin Red** only +8, more dermatan sulfate is required for neutralization of the former. The experimental titration endpoints of 1.6 μg/mL for **Heparin Red** and 1.9 μg/mL for **PDI-1** were somewhat lower than the theoretical values of 1.7 and 2.2 μg/mL, respectively, due to the formation of charge-neutral aggregates. The probes may not be fully protonated in the aggregates under the specified conditions, since the proximity of the dye molecules (Scheme 1) could lower the pK_a value of the ammonium groups.

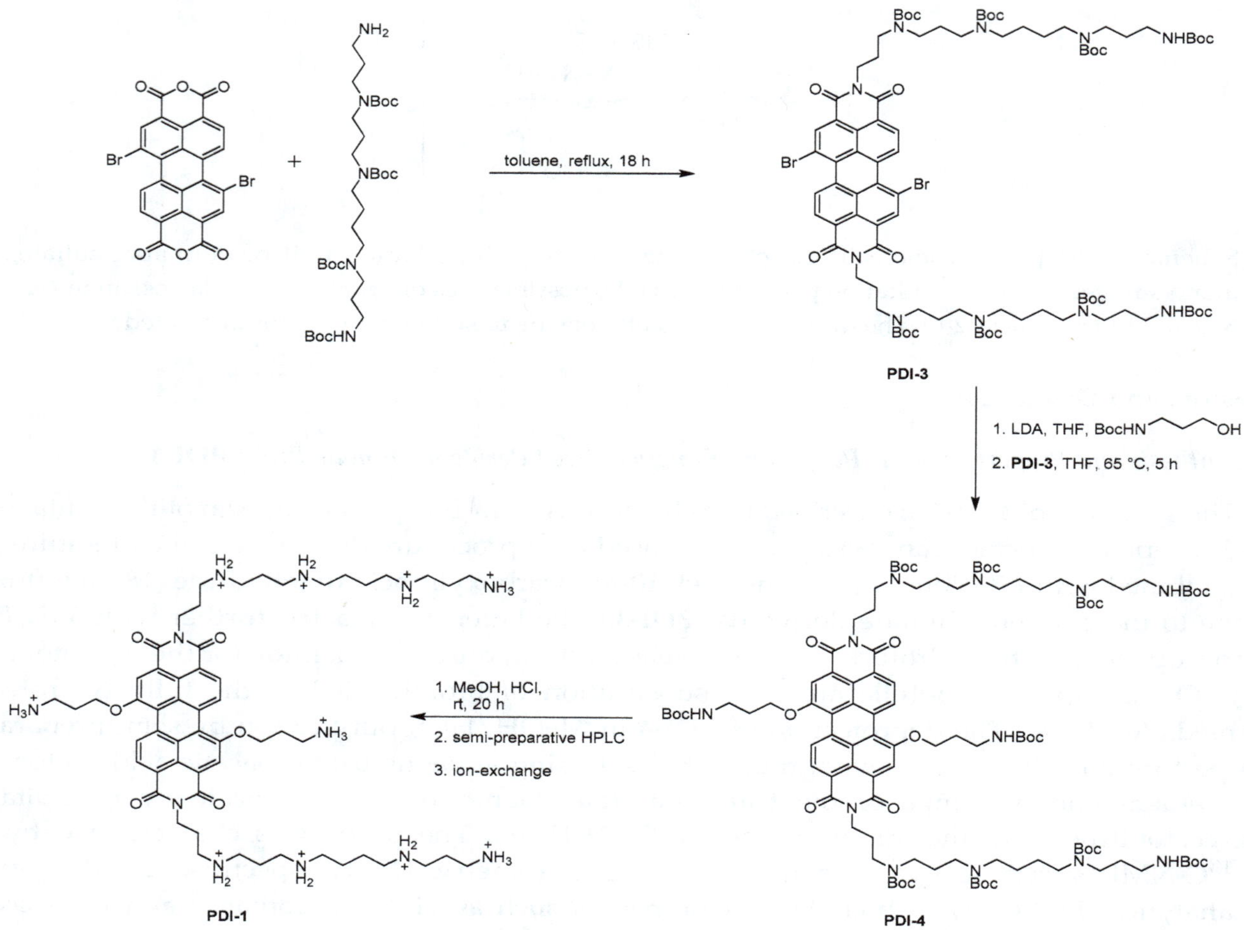

Scheme 4. Synthesis of probe **PDI-1**, chloride counterions not shown.

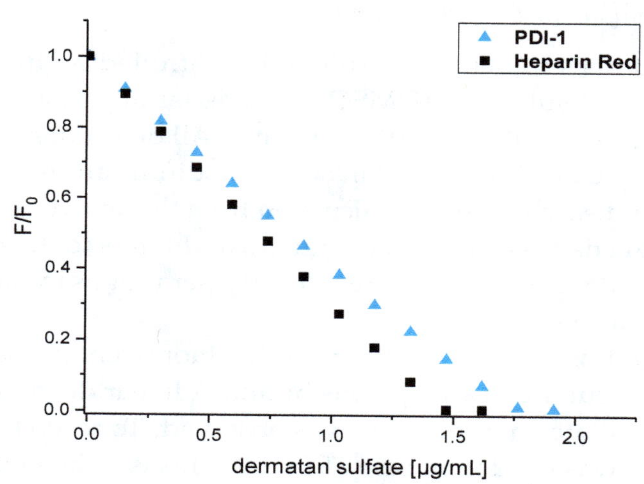

Figure 1. Normalized fluorescence response (F/F_0) of probes **PDI-1** and **Heparin Red** to dermatan sulfate. Excitation at 550 nm, fluorescence emission recorded at 610 nm. A solution of 1 μM probe in 10 mM MOPS pH 7 was placed into a polymethyl methacrylate (PMMA) cuvette and "titrated" with 10 μL aliquots of a 25 μg/mL dermatan sulfate solution.

We have recently described [9] a modified **Heparin Red** assay that enables the very sensitive quantification in the pg/mL range of the sulfated polysaccharide dextran sulfate in an aqueous matrix. The same protocol (see Materials and Methods for details) enables the highly sensitive detection of dermatan sulfate. Figure 2 compares the titration of a 1 nM solution of **PDI-1** and **Heparin Red**, respectively, with dermatan sulfate. Interestingly, less dermatan sulfate is required for the quenching of probe **PDI-1** under these conditions. The dermatan sulfate/**PDI-1** ratio at the titration endpoint is higher compared with the titration in Figure 1. Apparently, excess dermatan sulfate is needed to shift the equilibrium towards the aggregate at a low concentration of the components. This can only partly be interpreted with a protonation of the carboxylate groups of dermatan sulfate under the assay conditions (5 mM HCl), which may lead to a lower charge density of −0.5 per monosaccharide. Interestingly, even more dermatan sulfate is required for the quenching of **Heparin Red**. This, in contrast to the results in Figure 1, indicates a significantly higher stability of the **PDI-1**-dermatan sulfate aggregates.

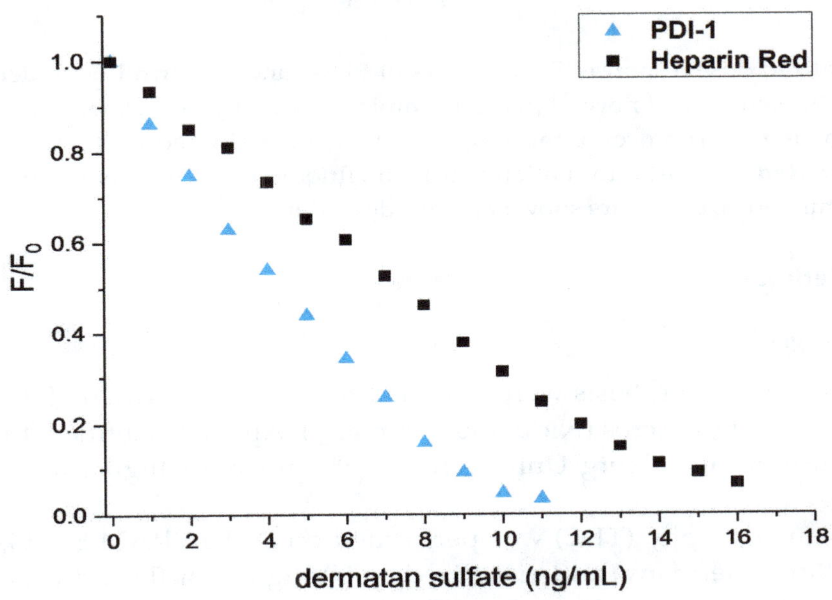

Figure 2. Normalized fluorescence response (F/F_0) of **PDI-1** and **Heparin Red** to dermatan sulfate. Excitation at 570 nm, fluorescence emission recorded at 610 nm. 2.5 mL water and 0.5 mL probe solution (6 nM in DMSO/30 mM HCl) were mixed in a polystyrene cuvette and the mixture was "titrated" with 5 μL aliquots of a 500 ng/mL dermatan sulfate solution. The indicated dermatan sulfate concentration does not correspond to the actual concentration in the reaction mixture (3 mL) but is related to the 2.5 mL aqueous portion.

Pooled normal plasma was spiked with dermatan sulfate and the standard protocol for heparin detection by the **Heparin Red** Kit was applied (Figure 3). Obviously, **PDI-1** responded more strongly than **Heparin Red** to the analyte, with about 50% fluorescence quenching at 10 μg/mL. At higher dermatan sulfate levels, the response curve flattens, possibly due to the partial, tight association of the probe with specific plasma components. Apparently, **PDI-1** forms stronger complexes with dermatan sulfate than **Heparin Red** in the human plasma matrix, and detects dermatan sulfate in the clinically relevant concentration range of 1–10 μg/mL. Like **Heparin Red, PDI-1** is not selective for dermatan sulfate but also responds strongly to heparin (data not shown), and interference by other glycosaminoglycans that have a similar or higher sulfation degree than dermatan sulfate is expected. A potential application of this probe is the monitoring of blood levels of dermatan sulfate after administration as an antithrombotic drug. Endogenous plasma levels of glycosaminoglycans are too low for significant interference. Only chondroitin sulfate may reach low μg/mL levels but, is present in an undersulfated form [19,20] that does not respond to **Heparin Red** in a plasma matrix.

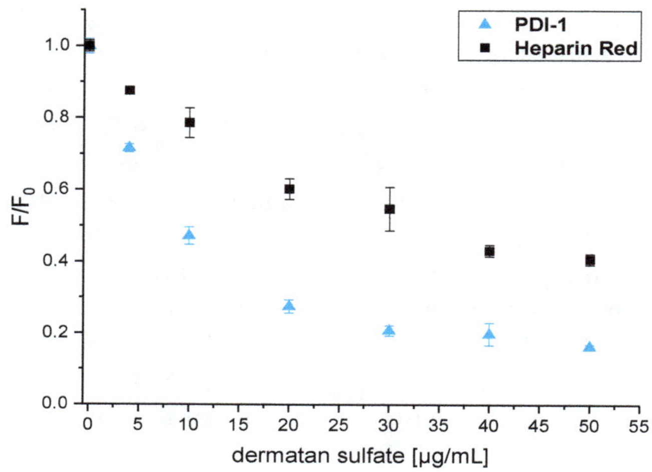

Figure 3. Normalized dose response (F/F_0) curves of **PDI-1** and **Heparin Red** to dermatan sulfate in human plasma. Spiked pooled normal plasma samples. Manually performed microplate assay was conducted, following the protocol of the supplier for the Heparin Red Kit (using 100-µM solutions of either **Heparin Red** or **PDI-1**). Excitation at 570 nm, fluorescence emission at 605 nm. Averages of duplicate determinations; error bars show standard deviation.

3. Materials and Methods

3.1. Chemicals and Reagents

Chemicals used for the synthesis were obtained from Sigma-Aldrich (Taufkirchen, Germany), Merck (Darmstadt, Germany), Acros (Nidderau, Germany), Apollo Scientific (Stockport, UK) or from the central warehouse of Heidelberg University in 95% purity or higher and were used without further purification.

Thin layer chromatography (TLC) was performed on POLYGRAM SIL G/UV$_{254}$ plates from Macherey-Nagel (Düren, Germany) and visualized by UV light. For flash chromatography, silica gel (40–63 µm, 60 Å pore size) from Macherey-Nagel (Düren, Germany) was used.

3.1.1. **Heparin Red** Kit

The **Heparin Red** Kit was a gift from Redprobes UG (Münster, Germany) [21]. Kit components included: **Heparin Red** solution (used for measurements shown in Figure 2), Product No. HR001, Lot 001-003, and Enhancer Solution, Product No. ES001, Lot 005. For the measurements shown in Figures 1 and 3, a solution of **Heparin Red**, synthesized as described in [22], was used.

3.1.2. Dermatan Sulfate

Dermatan sulfate sodium from porcine mucosa, product number C3788 (referred to as chondroitin sulfate B), batch SLBM9912V, was purchased from Sigma-Aldrich. According to the certificate of analysis of the provider, the batch contained 9% water, 6.5% S and 8.6% Na. Identity was confirmed by an ^{1}H-NMR spectrum in D_2O (see Supplementary Materials) and comparison with literature-reported spectra [23]. The lack of signals at >5 ppm indicates the absence of heparin and heparan sulfate. The *N*-Acetyl resonance and spiking experiments suggested that the sample may have contained minor impurities of chondroitin sulfate A and/or C [24].

3.1.3. Plasma

Pooled human normal plasma, applied as a matrix for the detections shown in Figure 3, was obtained from PrecisionBioLogic (Dartmouth, NS, Canada): Lot A1161, CRYOcheck. A 100 µg/mL stock solution of dermatan sulfate in plasma was prepared by mixing a 1 mg/mL aqueous dermatan sulfate solution with plasma in a volume ratio 1:9, followed by further dilution with plasma to the desired concentration. All samples were stored at −20 °C for at least one day and up to several months, and were thawed at room temperature and vortexed before use.

3.1.4. Other

All aqueous solutions were prepared with HPLC grade water purchased from VWR (Bruchsal, Germany), product No. 23595.328. DMSO, product number 34869, Lot # STBF6384V, and hydrochloric acid (1.0 M), product number 35328, Lot # SZBF2050V, were purchased from Sigma-Aldrich.

3.2. Instrumentation

3.2.1. Analytics

Nuclear magnetic resonance spectra were recorded on a Bruker Avance III (600 MHz) spectrometer (Bruker Corporation, Billercia, MA, USA). Chemical shifts δ are given in ppm and coupling constants *J* in Hz. All spectra were recorded at 295 K and calibrated using the residual ^{1}H- or ^{13}C-signals of the deuterated solvents [25]. The following abbreviations were used to describe the multiplicities of the signals: s (singlet), d (doublet), m (multiplet), b (broad). Signals were assigned using COSY, HSQC and HMBC spectra. Mass spectra were recorded on a Bruker ApexQe Hybrid 9.4 FT-ICR (Bruker Corporation, Billercia, MA, USA). Semi-preparative and analytical HPLCs were performed on a Shimadzu HPLC system at 20 °C using a SPD-10Avp detector (semi-preparative) or a SPD-M20A Photodiode Array Detector (analytical), respectively. Water with 0.1% trifluoracetic acid and acetonitrile were used as eluents and C18 columns were used as the stationary phase. UV/Vis spectra were recorded on a Varian Cary 100 Bio UV/Vis and fluorescence-spectra on a Varian Cary Eclipse spectrometer (Varian Inc., Palo Alto, CA, USA) using 4.5 mL PMMA-cuvettes purchased from Sigma-Aldrich.

3.2.2. Fluorescence Measurements

Fluorescence in microplates was measured with the reader Biotek Synergy Mx (Biotek Instruments, Winooski, VT, USA), with an excitation at 570 nm, emission recorded at 605 nm, spectral band width 13.5–17 nm, gain 90–110, read height of 8 mm. Fluorescence in cuvettes was measured with either (Figure 1) Trilogy Laboratory Fluorimeter (Trilogy Modul RWT/PE, GUI Selection Green, excitation at 550 nm, emission recorded at 610 nm) or (Figure 2) the benchtop fluorimeter FluoroLog-3 (Horiba Scientific, Kyoto, Japan), with an excitation at 570 nm, emission recorded at 590–650 nm, integration time 0.4 s, average of 3 scans, and spectral band width Ex/Em 7 nm.

3.2.3. Microplates, Cuvettes, Pipettes

For fluorescence measurements, 96-well microplates, polystyrene, Item No. 655076, were purchased from Greiner Bio-One GmbH (Frickenhausen, Germany). Disposable PMMA cuvettes were used for absorbance or fluorescence measurements in aqueous medium. Disposable polystyrene fluorescence cuvettes were used for measurements in water/DMSO medium. Transferpette 0.5–10 μL, Transferpette-8 20–200 μL and Transferpette-12 20–200 μL, purchased from Brand GmbH (Wertheim, Germany). Rainin Pipettes 100–1000 μL, 20–200 μL, and 2–20 μL purchased from Mettler Toledo (Columbus, OH, USA).

3.3. Synthesis

To improve comprehensibility, simplified names were used for some synthesized compounds rather than using exact IUPAC names. 1,7-dibromoperylene-3,4:9,10-tetracarboxylic acid dianhydride [18], N^1,N^4,N^9,N^{13}-Tetra-*tert*-butyloxycarbonyl-1,16-diamino-4,9,13-triazahexadecane [17] and *N*,*N*′-Bis-(1-amino-4,9-diiazadodecyl)-1,7-di-(1-amino-3-hydroxypropyl)-perylene-3,4:9,10-tetracarboxydiimide

(**Heparin Red**) [2,26] were prepared according to literature-reported methods which were slightly modified [22].

3.3.1. Synthesis of *N*,*N*′-Bis-(N^1,N^4,N^9,N^{13}-tetra-*tert*-butyloxycarbonyl-1-amino-4,9,13- triazahexadecyl)-1,7-dibromperylene-3,4:9,10-tetracarboxylic acid bisimide **PDI-3**

N^1,N^4,N^9,N^{13}-Tetra-*tert*-butyloxycarbonyl-1,16-diamino-4,9,13-triazahexadecane (600 mg, 909 μmol) was dissolved in anhydrous toluene (20 mL) prior to the addition of 1,7-dibromoperylene-3,4:9,10-tetracarboxylic acid dianhydride (227 mg, 413 μmol). The reaction mixture was stirred under reflux for 18 h. Insoluble residues were removed by filtration. The filtrate was evaporated to dryness and the crude product was purified by column chromatography (SiO_2, CH_2Cl_2:MeOH—98:2). Compound **PDI-3** was isolated as a red powder (302 mg, 165 μmol, 40%). R_f (CH_2Cl_2:MeOH—95:5) 0.50; ^{1}H-NMR (600.13 MHz, $CDCl_3$): δ (ppm) = 9.50 (d, $^3J_{H-H}$ = 8.17 Hz, 2H, perylene-H), 8.92 (s, 2H, perylene-H), 8.71 (d, $^3J_{H-H}$ = 8.17 Hz, 2H, perylene-H), 4.17–4.27 (m, 4H, CH_2), 3.31–3.40 (m, 4H, CH_2), 3.07–3.26 (m, 24H, CH_2), 1.95–2.03 (m, 4H, CH_2), 1.73–1.83 (m, 4H, CH_2), 1.62–1.69 (m, 4H, CH_2), 1.50–1.53 (m, 8H, CH_2), 1.41–1.46 (m, 72H, Boc-H); ^{13}C{^{1}H}-NMR (150.91 MHz, $CDCl_3$): δ (ppm) = 138.0, 130.2, 128.6, 46.6, 44.8, 43.8, 38.6, 37.5, 28.5, 28.4, 27.6, 27.0, 25.8; MS (HR-ESI$^+$): *m*/*z* = 1853.7890 [M + Na]$^+$, calculated for $C_{90}H_{132}{}^{79}Br_2N_{10}NaO_{20}{}^+$: 1853.7878, *m*/*z* = 1831.8037 [M + H]$^+$, calculated for $C_{90}H_{133}{}^{79}Br_2N_{10}O_{20}{}^+$: 1831.8059.

3.3.2. Synthesis of *N*,*N*′-Bis-(1-amino-4,9,13-triazahexadecyl)-1,7-di-(1-amino-3-hydroxypropyl)-perylene-3,4:9,10-tetracarboxydiimide **PDI-1**

Compound **PDI-3** (20.0 mg, 19.9 μmol) was dissolved in anhydrous tetrahydrofurane (THF, 2 mL). In another flask, 3-(*N*-(*tert*-butyloxycarbonyl)-amino)1-propanol (191 mg, 1.09 mmol) was dissolved in anhydrous THF (2 mL) prior to the addition of lithium diisopropylamide (2.0 M solution in THF, 500 μL). This mixture was then added to the first flask and stirred for 5 h at 65 °C. The cooled reaction mixture was diluted with an excess of ethyl acetate. The organic layer was washed with brine and water, dried with anhydrous Na_2SO_4, and concentrated under reduced pressure. The crude product (**PDI-4**) was purified by column chromatography (SiO_2, CH_2Cl_2:MeOH—98:2) to afford a violet solid, which was used without further purification. R_f (CH_2Cl_2:MeOH—95:5) 0.28; MS (HR-ESI$^+$): *m*/*z* = 2045.1841 [M + Na]$^+$ calculated for $C_{106}H_{164}N_{12}NaO_{26}{}^+$: 2045.1850, *m*/*z* = 1034.0868 [M + 2Na]$^{2+}$ calculated for $C_{106}H_{164}N_{12}Na_2O_{26}{}^{2+}$: 1034.0849.

The crude product (**PDI-4**) was dissolved in methanol (10 mL), and concentrated HCl (1 mL) was added to remove the Boc-protecting groups. This reaction mixture was stirred for 20 h at room temperature. The solvent was removed under reduced pressure. Purification by semi-preparative HPLC (Macherey-Nagel C18 (250 mm × 10 mm), H_2O with 0.1% trifluoroacetic acid (TFA)/MeCN, 4 mL/min, 0–5 min—0% MeCN, 15 min—12% MeCN, 30–35 min—24% MeCN, 55 min—90% MeCN) and subsequent lyophilization yielded the TFA salt of **PDI-1** (1.53 mg, 1.50 μmol, 8%) as a violet solid.

The trifluoroacetate counterions were exchanged by dissolving the product in 0.6 M HCl followed by precipitation from acetonitrile. After washing with acetonitrile, re-dissolution in water and subsequent lyophilization, the target compound [**PDI-1**]Cl_{10} was ready to use. ^{1}H-NMR (600.13 MHz, MeOD): δ (ppm) = 9.48–9.58 (m, 2H, perylene-H), 8.63 (d, $^3J_{H-H}$ = 8.28 Hz, 2H, perylene-H), 8.45 (bs, 2H, perylene-H), 4.58–4.71 (m, 4H, CH_2), 4.32–4.40 (m, 4H, CH_2), 3.32–3.35 (m, 4H, CH_2, superimposed by MeOD), 3.03–3.23 (m, 32H, CH_2, N–H), 2.47–2.53 (m, 4H, CH_2), 2.14–2.26 (m, 8H, CH_2), 2.05–2.11 (m, 4H, CH_2), 1.79–1.83 (m, 8H, CH_2); ^{13}C{^{1}H}-NMR (150.90 MHz, MeOD): δ (ppm) = 130.0, 129.5, 68.8, 48.3, 47.0, 45.7, 46.0, 38.4, 38.0, 37.9, 28.2, 25.9, 25.1, 24.0, 23.9; MS (HR-ESI$^+$): *m*/*z* = 1021.6722 [M + H]$^+$ calculated for $C_{56}H_{85}N_{12}O_6{}^+$: 1021.6710 *m*/*z* = 511.3395 [M + 2H]$^{2+}$, calculated for $C_{56}H_{86}N_{12}O_6{}^{2+}$: 511.3391; UV/Vis ($H_2O$, 10 mM MOPS, pH 7): $\lambda_{max\,(Abs)}$ (ε [M^{-1} cm^{-1}]) = 402 nm (5,900), 542 nm (24,100), 576 nm (35,300); Fluorescence (H_2O, 10 mM MOPS, pH 7): λ_{Ex} = 530 nm, $\lambda_{Abs(Em)}$ = 615 nm, ϕ_F = 0.17; Analytical HPLC: (Macherey-Nagel C18 (250 mm × 4.6 mm), H_2O with 0.1% TFA/MeCN, 1 mL/min, 0–5 min—0% MeCN, 15 min—12% MeCN, 30–35 min—24% MeCN, 55 min—90% MeCN) t_R = 31.6 min.

3.4. Assays

Dermatan Sulfate Assay in Aqueous and Plasma Matrix

For titrations of probe solutions with dermatan sulfate, the solutions described in the legends of Figures 1 and 2 of **PDI-1** and **Heparin Red**, respectively, were prepared using 100 μM aqueous stock solutions of the probes. Then, 6-nM probe solutions in DMSO/30 mM HCl (Figure 2) were prepared as described in detail in [9] for **Heparin Red**. Dermatan sulfate in spiked plasma samples was detected as described for heparin, following the protocol of the provider of the **Heparin Red** Kit for a 96-well microplate, using either a 100-μM aqueous solution of **Heparin Red** or of **PDI-1**. In brief, the 100-μM solution of **PDI-1** or **Heparin Red** was freshly mixed with Enhancer solution at a volume ratio of 1:90. Subsequently, 20 μL of the dermatan sulfate spiked plasma sample was pipetted into a microplate well, followed by 80 μL of the probe—Enhancer mixture. For sample numbers >10, a 12-channel pipette was used for the addition of the probe—Enhancer solution. The microplate was introduced in the fluorescence reader and mixing was performed using the plate shaking function of the microplate reader (setting "high," 3 min). Immediately after mixing, fluorescence was recorded within 1 min.

4. Conclusions

This contribution describes the synthesis and properties of the new fluorescent probe **PDI-1**, a polyamine-functionalized perylene diimide. **PDI-1** is structurally related to the commercial probe **Heparin Red**, but has in its protonated form a higher molecular charge of +10, compared to +8 for **Heparin Red**. The superior performance of **PDI-1** for sensing of a glycosaminoglycan with low negative charge density is exemplified by the detection of dermatan sulfate at a low concentration or in a competitive blood plasma matrix. A potential application of this probe is the direct monitoring of the antithrombotic drug dermatan sulfate in plasma in the absence of administered heparin and other glycosaminoglycans.

Acknowledgments: This research was supported by Heidelberg University. We thank C. Giese for preparing the plasma spikes and Redprobes UG for a gift of the Heparin Red Kit.

Author Contributions: M.R. conceived, designed and performed the experiments, analyzed the data and wrote parts of the paper. U.W. performed the titrations in Figure 2 and analyzed the data. R.K. contributed reagents, materials and analysis tools, and wrote parts of the paper.

References

1. Bromfield, S.M.; Wilde, E.; Smith, D.K. Heparin sensing and binding—Taking supramolecular chemistry towards clinical applications. *Chem. Soc. Rev.* **2013**, *42*, 9184–9195. [CrossRef] [PubMed]
2. Szelke, H.; Schübel, S.; Harenberg, J.; Krämer, R. A fluorescent probe for the quantification of heparin in clinical samples with minimal matrix interference. *Chem. Commun.* **2010**, *46*, 1667–1669. [CrossRef] [PubMed]
3. Warttinger, U.; Giese, C.; Harenberg, J.; Holmer, E.; Krämer, R. A fluorescent probe assay (Heparin Red) for direct detection of heparins in human plasma. *Anal. Bioanal. Chem.* **2016**, *408*, 8241–8251. [CrossRef] [PubMed]
4. Warttinger, U.; Krämer, R. Quantification of heparin in complex matrices (including urine) using a mix-and-read fluorescence assay. *arXiv* **2016**, arXiv:1611.02482.
5. Galli, M.; Magen, H.; Einsele, H.; Chatterjee, M.; Grasso, M.; Specchia, G.; Barbieri, P.; Paoletti, D.; Pace, S.; Sanderson, R.D.; et al. Roneparstat (SST0001), an Innovative Heparanase (HPSE) Inhibitor for Multiple Myeloma (MM) Therapy: First in Man Study. *Blood* **2015**, *126*, 3246.
6. Szelke, H.; Schübel, S.; Harenberg, J.; Krämer, R. Interaction of heparin with cationic molecular probes: Probe charge is a major determinant of binding stoichiometry and affinity. *Bioorg. Med. Chem. Lett.* **2010**, *20*, 1445–1447. [CrossRef] [PubMed]

7. Warttinger, U.; Krämer, R. Instant determination of the potential biomarker heparan sulfate in human plasma by a mix-and-read fluorescence assay. *arXiv* **2017**, arXiv:1702.05288.
8. Warttinger, U.; Giese, C.; Harenberg, J.; Krämer, R. Direct quantification of brown algae-derived fucoidans in human plasma by a fluorescent probe assay. *arXiv* **2016**, arXiv:1608.00108.
9. Groß, N.; Arian, D.; Warttinger, U.; Krämer, R. Ultrasensitive quantification of dextran sulfate by a mix-and-read fluorescent probe assay. *arXiv* **2017**, arXiv:1703.08663.
10. Trowbridge, J.M.; Gallo, R.L. Dermatan sulfate: New functions from an old glycosaminoglycan. *Glycobiology* **2002**, *12*, 117R–125R. [CrossRef] [PubMed]
11. Benito, C.; Marco, G.; Giangiacomo, T. Structural and Conformational Aspects of the Anticoagulant and Antithrombotic Activity of Heparin and Dermatan Sulfate. *Curr. Pharm. Des.* **2004**, *10*, 939–949.
12. Mashima, R.; Sakai, E.; Tanaka, M.; Kosuga, M.; Okuyama, T. The levels of urinary glycosaminoglycans of patients with attenuated and severe type of mucopolysaccharidosis II determined by liquid chromatography-tandem mass spectrometry. *Mol. Genet. Metab. Rep.* **2016**, *7*, 87–91. [CrossRef] [PubMed]
13. Saivin, S.; Cambus, J.-P.; Thalamus, C.; Lau, G.; Boneu, B.; Houin, G.; Gianese, F. Pharmacokinetics and Pharmacodynamics of Intramuscular Dermatan Sulfate Revisited. *Clin. Drug Investig.* **2003**, *23*, 533–543. [CrossRef] [PubMed]
14. Coccheri, S.; Mannello, F. Development and use of sulodexide in vascular diseases: Implications for treatment. *Drug Des. Dev. Ther.* **2014**, *8*, 49–65. [CrossRef] [PubMed]
15. Auray-Blais, C.; Lavoie, P.; Tomatsu, S.; Valayannopoulos, V.; Mitchell, J.J.; Raiman, J.; Beaudoin, M.; Maranda, B.; Clarke, J.T.R. UPLC-MS/MS detection of disaccharides derived from glycosaminoglycans as biomarkers of mucopolysaccharidoses. *Anal. Chim. Acta* **2016**, *936*, 139–148. [CrossRef] [PubMed]
16. Vitale, C.; Berutti, S.; Bagnis, C.; Soragna, G.; Gabella, P.; Fruttero, C.; Marangella, M. Dermatan sulfate: An alternative to unfractionated heparin for anticoagulation in hemodialysis patients. *J. Nephrol.* **2013**, *26*, 158–163. [CrossRef] [PubMed]
17. Geall, A.J.; Blagbrough, I.S. Homologation of Polyamines in the Rapid Synthesis of Lipospermine Conjugates and Related Lipoplexes. *Tetrahedron* **2000**, *56*, 2449–2460. [CrossRef]
18. Boehm, A.; Arms, H.; Henning, G.; Blaschka, P. 1,7-Disubstituierte Perylen-3,4,9-10-tetracarbonsäuren, deren Dianhydride und Diimide. BASF AG Germany, Patent DE19547210A1, 19 June 1997.
19. Volpi, N.; Maccari, F. Microdetermination of chondroitin sulfate in normal human plasma by fluorophore-assisted carbohydrate electrophoresis (FACE). *Clin. Chim. Acta* **2005**, *356*, 125–133. [CrossRef] [PubMed]
20. Zinellu, E.; Lepedda, A.J.; Cigliano, A.; Pisanu, S.; Zinellu, A.; Carru, C.; Bacciu, P.P.; Piredda, F.; Guarino, A.; Spirito, R.; et al. Association between Human Plasma Chondroitin Sulfate Isomers and Carotid Atherosclerotic Plaques. *Biochem. Res. Int.* **2012**, *2012*, 281284. [CrossRef] [PubMed]
21. Mix-and-Read Assays for Heparins. Available online: www.redprobes.com (accessed on 05 May 2017).
22. Rappold, M. Perylendiimid-Basierte Fluoreszenzfarbstoffe: Synthese, Detektion von Glykosaminoglykanen und Photoinduzierte Zyklisierungsreaktionen. Ph.D. Thesis, Heidelberg University, Heidelberg, Germany, 2016.
23. Guerrini, M.; Zhang, Z.; Shriver, Z.; Naggi, A.; Masuko, S.; Langer, R.; Casu, B.; Linhardt, R.J.; Torri, G.; Sasisekharan, R. Orthogonal analytical approaches to detect potential contaminants in heparin. *Proc. Natl. Acad. Sci. USA* **2009**, *106*, 16956–16961. [CrossRef] [PubMed]
24. Carnachan, S.M.; Hinkley, S.F.R. Heparan Sulfate Identification and Characterisation: Method I. Heparan Sulfate Identification by NMR Analysis. *Bio-Protocol* **2017**, *7*, e2196. [CrossRef]
25. Fulmer, G.R.; Miller, A.J.M.; Sherden, N.H.; Gottlieb, H.E.; Nudelman, A.; Stoltz, B.M.; Bercaw, J.E.; Goldberg, K.I. NMR Chemical Shifts of Trace Impurities: Common Laboratory Solvents, Organics, and Gases in Deuterated Solvents Relevant to the Organometallic Chemist. *Organometallics* **2010**, *29*, 2176–2179. [CrossRef]
26. Poeck, A. Ionische Fluoreszenzsonden zur Heparinbestimmung: Synthese und Anwendung. Ph.D. Thesis, Heidelberg University, Heidelberg, Germany, 2013.

15

New Insights in Thrombin Inhibition Structure–Activity Relationships by Characterization of Octadecasaccharides from Low Molecular Weight Heparin†

Pierre A. J. Mourier, Olivier Y. Guichard, Fréderic Herman, Philippe Sizun and Christian Viskov *

Sanofi, 13 Quai Jules Guesde, 94403 Vitry sur Seine, France; pierre.mourier@sanofi.com (P.A.J.M.); olivier.guichard@sanofi.com (O.Y.G.); frederic.herman@sanofi.com (F.H.); philippe.sizun@sanofi.com (P.S.)

* Correspondence: christian.viskov@sanofi.com

† *In Memoriam*: The authors would like to respectfully dedicate this article to Pr. B. Casu, a brilliant pioneer in glycosaminoglycan chemistry and analysis, who passed away on 11 November 2016.

Academic Editors: Giangiacomo Torri and Jawed Fareed

Abstract: Low Molecular Weight Heparins (LMWH) are complex anticoagulant drugs that mainly inhibit the blood coagulation cascade through indirect interaction with antithrombin. While inhibition of the factor Xa is well described, little is known about the polysaccharide structure inhibiting thrombin. In fact, a minimal chain length of 18 saccharides units, including an antithrombin (AT) binding pentasaccharide, is mandatory to form the active ternary complex for LMWH obtained by alkaline β-elimination (e.g., enoxaparin). However, the relationship between structure of octadecasaccharides and their thrombin inhibition has not been yet assessed on natural compounds due to technical hurdles to isolate sufficiently pure material. We report the preparation of five octadecasaccharides by using orthogonal separation methods including size exclusion, AT affinity, ion pairing and strong anion exchange chromatography. Each of these octadecasaccharides possesses two AT binding pentasaccharide sequences located at various positions. After structural elucidation using enzymatic sequencing and NMR, in vitro aFXa and aFIIa were determined. The biological activities reveal the critical role of each pentasaccharide sequence position within the octadecasaccharides and structural requirements to inhibit thrombin. Significant differences in potency, such as the twenty-fold magnitude difference observed between two regioisomers, further highlights the importance of depolymerisation process conditions on LMWH biological activity.

Keywords: thrombin inhibition; LMWH; antithrombin; heparin oligosaccharides; ternary complex

---

1. Introduction

Low Molecular Weight Heparins (LMWH) are lifesaving anticoagulant drugs which have been used for several decades in the prevention and treatment of venous and arterial thromboembolism [1]. LMWH are industrially derived from the starting material heparin, a complex mixture of mammalian polysaccharides extracted from porcine mucosa. The centenary of the discovery of heparin has been widely celebrated around the world and many symposia, such as the 24th Glycosaminoglycans Symposium, held in September 2016 (Villa Vigoni, Loveno di Menaggio—Italy, the first symposia of these series was initiated by Pr Casu), were dedicated to this endeavor. Even with state of the art analytical methods, this "ever young life-saving drug" [2] is also one of the most complex products to analyze, as direct characterization of the polysaccharidic chains is still not feasible. Heparin is a mixture of heteropolymeric chains having a mean molecular weight around 15,000 Dalton. It consists of alternating units of 2-deoxy-2-sulfamido-α-D-glucopyranose (possibly *O*-sulfated,

N-sulfated or *N*-acetylated) and *O*-sulfated uronic acids (α-L-iduronic acid or β-D-glucuronic acid). The specific structure of each polysaccharidic chain, built up of these alternating motifs, is governed by enzymatic machinery of the host mast cells where it is stored [3]. Heparin interacts with about one hundred proteins [4] but its anticoagulant activity is mainly mediated indirectly through activation of antithrombin, a serine protease inhibitor, member of the serpin family [5]. The activation of antithrombin induces a protein conformational change and dramatically accelerates the inhibition of the Stuart factor (FXa) [6]. The discovery of the antithrombin (AT) binding pentasaccharide was the hallmark of a new era of understanding of the structure activity of this complex medicine [7,8], and the so-called AGA*IA sequence (GlcN$_{NAc/NS,6S}$-GlcA-GlcN$_{NS,3S,6S}$-IdoUA$_{2S}$GlcN$_{NS,6S}$) was identified as the specific binding sequence of heparin [7]. Then, several variants of the consensus pentasaccharide sequence were discovered and reported a posteriori [9–11]. The evolution of analytical methodologies has also permitted the identification of longer AT binding oligosaccharides from LMWH [12]. Structure-activity studies on octa to octadecasaccharides have demonstrated that interaction with antithrombin is more complex than initially envisioned and that flanking saccharide units play an important role in the modulation of the AGA*IA affinity (the synthetic version of AGA*IA, drug substance commercially known as fondaparinux was used as reference) [13]. They may affect the Kd variation by three orders of magnitude when compared to fondaparinux (Kd = 21 nM) [14], either strengthening or destabilizing this complex.

Furthermore, semuloparin an experimental drug for which development was stopped in 2012 was designed with a depolymerisation process which preserves the AT binding region from β-eliminative cleavage and increases their concentration in this particular LMWH [15]. Therefore, it allowed the isolation of unexpected multiple of two and three consecutive AGA*IA sequences in the dodecasaccharide ΔIIa-II$\underline{s}$-Is-IIa-II$\underline{s}$-Is [16] and the octadecasaccharide **1** ΔIIa-II$\underline{s}$-Is-IIa-II$\underline{s}$-Is-IIa-II$\underline{s}$-Is [17], respectively (structural symbols are listed in Table 1; previous studies had concluded the possible presence of two AT binding sites on a single heparin chain without isolation and structural elucidation [18]). This compositional specificity is directly due to the depolymerisation selectivity with the sterically hindered phosphazene bases. Therefore, semuloparin appears as a particularly interesting tool compound to gather new insights on structure-activity relationships.

Table 1. Structural symbols.

Structural Symbols		
ΔIVa = ΔU-GlcNAc	-IVa$_{id}$- = -IdoA-GlcNAc-	-IVa$_{glu}$- = -GlcA-GlcNAc-
ΔIVs = ΔU-GlcNS		-IVs$_{glu}$- = -GlcA-GlcNS-
Δ$\underline{IVs}$ = ΔU-GlcNS,3S		-$\underline{IVs_{glu}}$- = -GlcA-GlcNS,3S-
ΔIIa = ΔU-GlcNAc,6S	-IIa$_{id}$- = -IdoA-GlcNAc,6S-	
ΔIIIa = ΔU2S-GlcNAc	-IIIa$_{id}$- = -IdoA2S-GlcNAc-	
ΔIIs = ΔU-GlcNS,6S		-IIs$_{glu}$- = -GlcA-GlcNS,6S-
Δ$\underline{IIs}$ = ΔU-GlcNS,3S,6S		-$\underline{IIs_{glu}}$-= -GcA-GlcNS,3S,6S-
ΔIIIs = ΔU2S-GlcNS	-IIIs$_{id}$- = -IdoA2S-GlcNS-	
ΔIa = ΔU2S-GlcNAc,6S	-Ia$_{id}$- = -IdoA2S-GlcNAc,6S-	
ΔIs = ΔU2S-GlcNS,6S	-Is$_{id}$- = -IdoA2S-GlcNS,6S-	
Δ$\underline{Is}$ = ΔU2S-GlcNS,3S,6S	-$\underline{Is_{id}}$- = -IdoA2S-GlcNS,3S,6S-	

It is noteworthy that we have previously observed that Kd affinity and molar anti FXa activity of the dodecasaccharide was twice that of fondaparinux, suggesting a dynamic equilibrium with two antithrombin proteins, which may potentiate the anticoagulant activity of such compound series.

Although thrombin is one of the key coagulation proteases for heparin and LMWHs, structure-activity data are not available due to the challenge of isolating polysaccharides that are able to form the ternary complex with antithrombin and thrombin. In fact, until the isolation of octadecasaccharide **1** (Figure 1) [17], there was no structural data on pure natural compounds that were responsible for this important mechanism of action. Interestingly, the only structure-activity relationship evidence that existed were generated on synthetic compounds [19–21] and showed that the inhibition may be potent starting from hexadecasaccharides.

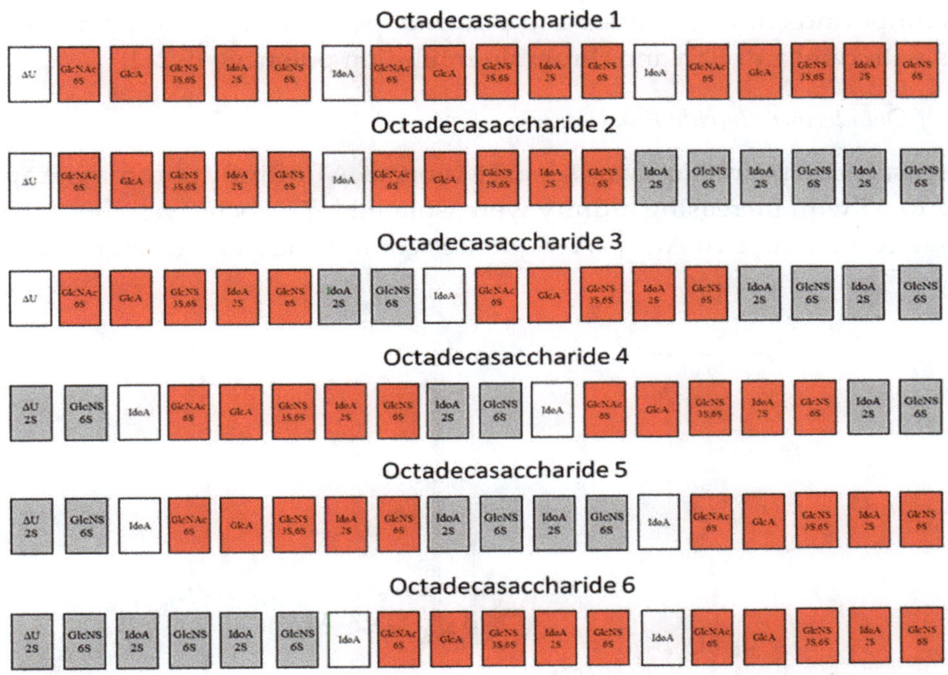

Figure 1. Studied octadecasaccharides (in red saccharide units from AGA*IA sequence). In grey, flanking saccharide units are represented. In white, additional uronic acid present in the minimal natural sequence.

With the octadecasaccharide **1**, a suitable chain length was reached so that the inhibition of the thrombin (FIIa) became possible in the case of LMWH products (no significant activity assayed on hexadecasaccharides), and activities of aFXa = 562 IU/mg and aFIIa = 8.8 IU/mg were found. Nevertheless, with respect to the whole fraction from which it was isolated (aFIIa ~20 UI/mg), the aFIIa for 1 was significantly lower than expected.

It was therefore critical to further evaluate new octadecasaccharides to increase our understanding of the electrostatic interactions with thrombin and compare them to the synthetic compounds from Petitou et al. [19–21].

For this endeavor, by using orthogonal chromatographic techniques, we have isolated five compounds from the octadecasaccharide AT affine fraction of semuloparin. Each of these compounds contain two AGA*IA sequences located at different positions within the polysaccharide chain (Figure 1). Their structure has been fully elucidated by enzymatic sequencing and NMR analysis and their anticoagulant activity was evaluated both for inhibition of factor Xa and IIa.

2. Results and Discussion

In our previous work [17], we reported the isolation from semuloparin of the first natural octadecasaccharide having AT binding affinity and able to inhibit both aFXa and aFIIa. This compound had the peculiarity to bear three consecutive AGA*IA sequences. Surprisingly, the activation of thrombin was weak (only 8.8 IU/mg; USP Heparin is about 180 IU/mg) despite the fact that it was isolated from an octadecasaccharide fraction with a specific aFIIa activity of ~20 UI/mg. All the criteria for activity were there, i.e., size of the chain, presence of AGA*IA sequences, and high anti FXa (about three times more than USP heparin) activity, but the low thrombin inhibition raised new questions. Front running hypotheses to explain low thrombin inhibition included: a lack of charge density to stabilize the ternary complex with the protein, or a dynamic equilibrium between antithrombin with all three AGA*IA sequences, which might generate in turn a steric hindrance for thrombin complexation. The later hypothesis could also explain the twofold molar aFXa activity of the compound with respect to the pentasaccharide [17]. To shed light on the origin of such biological properties, it was critical to study more compounds of these series and put in perspective the work performed on synthetic polysaccharides with dual anti FXa and thrombin inhibition potency [19,21].

2.1. Purification of Octadecasaccharide Fraction F3

The octadecasaccharide fraction was separated on an AT affinity chromatography column and five fractions F1 to F5 with increasing affinity were isolated [17]. Focus was concentrated on fraction F3, where isomers containing two AGA*IA sequences could be identified (Figure 2).

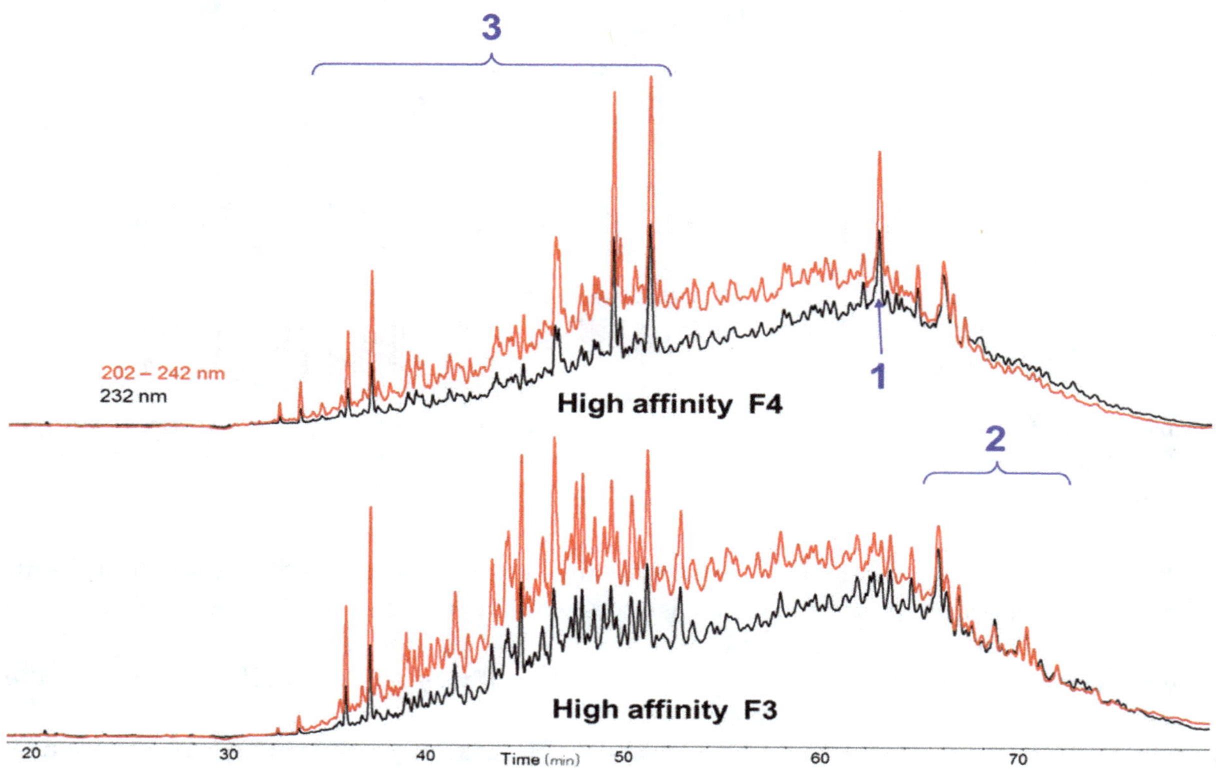

Figure 2. Cetyltrimethylammonium strong anion exchange (CTA-SAX) chromatograms of octadecasaccharide fractions F3 and F4: 1-triple site, 2-double sites, 3-glycoserine octadecasaccharides.

The overall activity was in the same order of magnitude than fraction 4 from which octadecasaccharide **1** was isolated (aFXa: F3 401 IU/mg; F4 422 IU/mg; aFIIa: F3 18.1 IU/mg; F4 19.8 IU/mg). The modest aFIIa activity may be partly related to the presence of glycoserine oligosaccharides. These oligosaccharides contain an oxidized glycoserine sequence (-GlcA-Gal-Gal-Xyl-CH_2-COOH) at their reducing end [22]. These compounds are eluted in the less retained part of the chromatogram (Figure 2) and represent more than 50% of the affine fractions. None of the glycoserine octadecasaccharides isolated in this study (not described here) had any measurable aFIIa activity while having aFXa. Compared to the separation of the octadecasaccharide **1**, the isolation of five regioisomers containing two AGA*IA sequences was more complex and the resolution power of ion pair chromatography was critical to enable the separation. From the key step of cetyltrimethylammonium strong anion exchange (CTA-SAX) separation (Figure 3), reconstructed ion mass LC/MS chromatograms corresponding to Mw 4957 Da (Figure 4) were used to select the fractions to be gathered. Molecular weights deduced from LC/MS analysis were sufficient to deduce the sulfate group number, *N*-acetyl number and presence or not of characteristic glycoserine moieties. These pieces of information were helpful to guide us in the last purification steps.

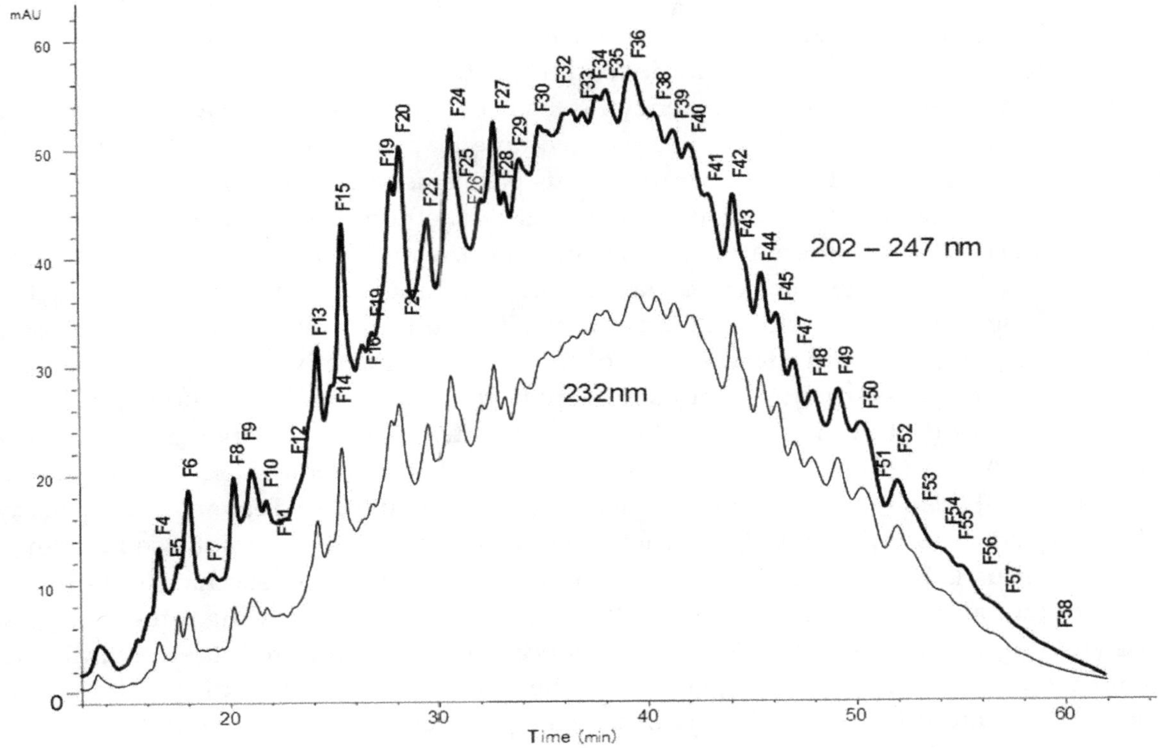

Figure 3. Preparative CTA-SAX chromatography of fraction F3.

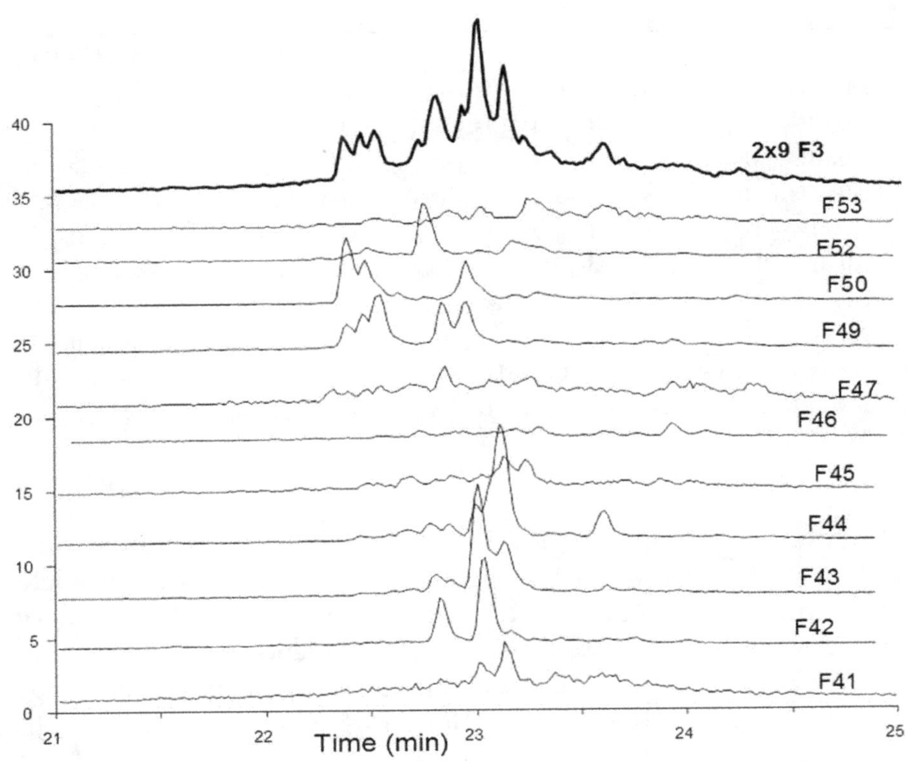

Figure 4. LC/MS reconstructed ion mass chromatograms of initial fraction F3 and sub fractions of interest corresponding to MW 4957 Da (m/z 2430.2: $(4957 + 23 \times \text{HXA} + 2\text{H})^{3+}$).

2.2. *Enzymatic Sequencing*

Sequencing methods based on partial or selective depolymerisation with enzymes from *Flavobacterium heparinum* and particularly heparinases have been already developed [23,24]. Monitoring of digestion and fragment analysis were done by MALDI-MS and capillary electrophoresis. Another efficient technique using a preliminary radiolabeling of the substrate, followed by partial nitrous depolymerisation and sequencing with exoenzymes has been proposed [25]. However, this method is long and most exoenzymes used in the study are not commercially available. In fact, the key element for any sequencing method is an efficient separation. This part is usually time consuming and, as already stated, requires use of many consecutive chromatographic methods with orthogonal specificities.

For long heparin-like oligosaccharides, heparinase I is the most convenient choice for sequencing experiments. Heparinase II is less selective than heparinase I and, as an exolithic enzyme, it does not generate many long fragments in detectable amounts. The full exploitation of the digestion process by heparinase I requires a good understanding of the enzyme's selectivity and behavior. Basic rules for selectivity [26] are necessary but are not sufficient to this endeavor. Know-how in that field is all the more important as current literature data may give only partially the heparinase I mechanism of digestion [27]. As a matter of fact, much evidence exists that heparinase I is not exolithic but rather endolithic [28] (also reflected in our sequencing experiments), all cleavable sites present in the chain being cleaved simultaneously. The structural determination by enzymatic sequencing of long oligosaccharides is usually a challenging experiment due to the number of saccharides bound together and to their potential arrangement. The fact that there are two AT binding sites –IIa_{id}-IIs_{glu}-Is_{id}- distributed with three –Is_{id}- disaccharides in an octadecasaccharide simplifies its structural elucidation. Consequently, only 10 theoretical arrangements can be found (Table 2). In addition, the UV spectrum can be used [17] to determine the beginning of the chain (either ΔIIa-$\underline{IIs_{glu}}$-Is_{id}- or ΔIs-), allowing the separation into two types of octadecasaccharides.

Table 2. Heparinase 1 cleaving sites ($\downarrow$ major sites; $\downarrow$ minor sites).

	Structure	Heparinase I Cleaving Sites
Octadeca. 2	ΔIIa-$\underline{IIs_{glu}}$-Is_{id}-IIa_{id}-$\underline{IIs_{glu}}$-Is_{id}-Is_{id}-Is_{id}-Is_{id}	ΔIIa-$\underline{IIs_{glu}}\downarrow Is_{id}$-$IIa_{id}$-$\underline{IIs_{glu}}\downarrow Is_{id}\downarrow Is_{id}\downarrow Is_{id}$-$Is_{id}{}^{red}$
Octadeca. 3	ΔIIa-$\underline{IIs_{glu}}$-Is_{id}-Is_{id}-IIa_{id}-$\underline{IIs_{glu}}$-Is_{id}-Is_{id}-Is_{id}	ΔIIa-$\underline{IIs_{glu}}\downarrow Is_{id}\downarrow Is_{id}$-$IIa_{id}$-$\underline{IIs_{glu}}\downarrow Is_{id}\downarrow Is_{id}$-$Is_{id}{}^{red}$
	ΔIIa-$\underline{IIs_{glu}}$-Is_{id}-Is_{id}-Is_{id}-IIa_{id}-$\underline{IIs_{glu}}$-Is_{id}-Is_{id}	ΔIIa-$\underline{IIs_{glu}}\downarrow Is_{id}\downarrow Is_{id}\downarrow Is_{id}$-$IIa_{id}$-$\underline{IIs_{glu}}\downarrow Is_{id}$-$Is_{id}{}^{red}$
	ΔIIa-$\underline{IIs_{glu}}$-Is_{id}-Is_{id}-Is_{id}-Is_{id}-IIa_{id}-$\underline{IIs_{glu}}$-Is_{id}	ΔIIa-$\underline{IIs_{glu}}\downarrow Is_{id}\downarrow Is_{id}\downarrow Is_{id}\downarrow Is_{id}$-$IIa_{id}$-$\underline{IIs_{glu}}$-$Is_{id}{}^{red}$
	ΔIs-IIa_{id}-$\underline{IIs_{glu}}$-Is_{id}-IIa_{id}-$\underline{IIs_{glu}}$-Is_{id}-Is_{id}-Is_{id}	ΔIIs-IIa_{id}-$\underline{IIs_{glu}}\downarrow Is_{id}$-$IIa_{id}$-$\underline{IIs_{glu}}\downarrow Is_{id}\downarrow Is_{id}$-$Is_{id}{}^{red}$
Octadeca. 4	ΔIs-IIa_{id}-$\underline{IIs_{glu}}$-Is_{id}-Is_{id}-IIa_{id}-$\underline{IIs_{glu}}$-Is_{id}-Is_{id}	ΔIIs-IIa_{id}-$\underline{IIs_{glu}}\downarrow Is_{id}\downarrow Is_{id}$-$IIa_{id}$-$\underline{IIs_{glu}}\downarrow Is_{id}$-$Is_{id}{}^{red}$
Octadeca. 5	ΔIs-IIa_{id}-$\underline{IIs_{glu}}$-Is_{id}-Is_{id}-Is_{id}-IIa_{id}-$\underline{IIs_{glu}}$-Is_{id}	ΔIIs-IIa_{id}-$\underline{IIs_{glu}}\downarrow Is_{id}\downarrow Is_{id}\downarrow Is_{id}$-$IIa_{id}$-$\underline{IIs_{glu}}$-$Is_{id}{}^{red}$
	ΔIs-Is_{id}-IIa_{id}-$\underline{IIs_{glu}}$-Is_{id}-IIa_{id}-$\underline{IIs_{glu}}$-Is_{id}-Is_{id}	ΔIIs$\downarrow Is_{id}$-IIa_{id}-$\underline{IIs_{glu}}\downarrow Is_{id}$-$IIa_{id}$-$\underline{IIs_{glu}}\downarrow Is_{id}$-$Is_{id}{}^{red}$
	ΔIs-Is_{id}-IIa_{id}-$\underline{IIs_{glu}}$-Is_{id}-Is_{id}-IIa_{id}-$\underline{IIs_{glu}}$-Is_{id}	ΔIIs$\downarrow Is_{id}$-IIa_{id}-$\underline{IIs_{glu}}\downarrow Is_{id}\downarrow Is_{id}$-$IIa_{id}$-$\underline{IIs_{glu}}$-$Is_{id}{}^{red}$
Octadeca. 6	ΔIs-Is_{id}-Is_{id}-IIa_{id}-$\underline{IIs_{glu}}$-Is_{id}-IIa_{id}-$\underline{IIs_{glu}}$-Is_{id}	ΔIIs$\downarrow Is_{id}\downarrow Is_{id}$-$IIa_{id}$-$\underline{IIs_{glu}}\downarrow Is_{id}$-$IIa_{id}$-$\underline{IIs_{glu}}$-$Is_{id}{}^{red}$

2.2.1. Type I Octadecasaccharides

In this case of Type I octadecasaccharides, the position of the first binding site is known and the remaining question is the position of the second one. Key elements for such sequencing were described [17] for structural determination of triple site ΔIIa-$\underline{IIs_{glu}}$-Is_{id}-IIa_{id}-$\underline{IIs_{glu}}$-Is_{id}-IIa_{id}-$\underline{IIs_{glu}}$-Is_{id}. $NaBH_4$ preliminary reduction was used to label the reducing end.

Putative structures are listed in Table 2 as well as the heparinase I cleavage sites of the four possible isomers. Heparinase I cleaves preferentially highly sulfated moieties like -$\underline{IIs_{glu}}\downarrow Is_{id}$ and $Is_{id}\downarrow Is_{id}$-$Is_{id}{}^{red}$ and its action on other cleavable sites like $Is_{id}\downarrow Is_{id}{}^{red}$ is less pronounced.

Table 3 gathers key fragments for type I octadecasaccharides. The resistance of these fragments to the action of heparinase I mainly depends on the number of cleaving sites, so that the order of increasing resistance is the following: ΔIIa-$\underline{IIs_{glu}}$-Is_{id}-Is_{id}-Is_{id}-IIa_{id}-$\underline{IIs_{glu}}$ $<$

$\Delta\mathrm{IIa}\text{-}\underline{\mathrm{IIs}_{glu}}\text{-}\mathrm{Is}_{id}\text{-}\mathrm{Is}_{id}\text{-}\mathrm{IIa}_{id}\text{-}\underline{\mathrm{IIs}_{glu}} < \Delta\mathrm{IIa}\text{-}\underline{\mathrm{IIs}_{glu}}\text{-}\mathrm{Is}_{id}\text{-}\mathrm{IIa}_{id}\text{-}\underline{\mathrm{IIs}_{glu}} << \Delta\mathrm{Is}\text{-}\mathrm{IIa}_{id}\text{-}\underline{\mathrm{IIs}_{glu}}\text{-}\mathrm{Is}_{id}{}^{red}$. The sequencing details for octadecasaccharide **2** and **3** are reported in supplementary data.

Table 3. Key fragments for octadecasaccharides.

	Key Fragments for Type I Octadecasaccharides
Octadecasaccharide **2**	$\Delta\mathrm{IIa}\text{-}\underline{\mathrm{IIs}_{glu}}\text{-}\mathrm{Is}_{id}\text{-}\mathrm{IIa}_{id}\text{-}\underline{\mathrm{IIs}_{glu}}$; $\Delta\mathrm{Is}\text{-}\mathrm{Is}_{id}{}^{red}$
Octadecasaccharide **3**	$\Delta\mathrm{IIa}\text{-}\underline{\mathrm{IIs}_{glu}}\text{-}\mathrm{Is}_{id}\text{-}\mathrm{Is}_{id}\text{-}\mathrm{IIa}_{id}\text{-}\underline{\mathrm{IIs}_{glu}}$; $\Delta\mathrm{Is}\text{-}\mathrm{Is}_{id}{}^{red}$
	Key Fragments for Type II Octadecasaccharides
Octadecasaccharide **4**	$\Delta\mathrm{IIs}\text{-}\mathrm{IIa}_{id}\text{-}\underline{\mathrm{IIs}_{glu}}$; $\Delta\mathrm{IIs}\text{-}\mathrm{IIa}_{id}\text{-}\underline{\mathrm{IIs}_{glu}}\text{-}\mathrm{Is}_{id}\text{-}\mathrm{Is}_{id}\text{-}\mathrm{IIa}_{id}\text{-}\underline{\mathrm{IIs}_{glu}}$; $\Delta\mathrm{Is}\text{-}\mathrm{Is}_{id}{}^{red}$
Octadecasaccharide **5**	$\Delta\mathrm{IIs}\text{-}\mathrm{IIa}_{id}\text{-}\underline{\mathrm{IIs}_{glu}}$; $\Delta\mathrm{Is}\text{-}\mathrm{IIa}_{id}\text{-}\underline{\mathrm{IIs}_{glu}}\text{-}\mathrm{Is}_{id}{}^{red}$
Octadecasaccharide **6**	$\Delta\mathrm{IIs}$; $\Delta\mathrm{IIs}\text{-}\mathrm{Is}_{id}$; $\Delta\mathrm{IIs}\text{-}\mathrm{Is}_{id}\text{-}\mathrm{Is}_{id}\text{-}\mathrm{IIa}_{id}\text{-}\underline{\mathrm{IIs}_{glu}}$; $\Delta\mathrm{Is}\text{-}\mathrm{IIa}_{id}\text{-}\underline{\mathrm{IIs}_{glu}}\text{-}\mathrm{Is}_{id}{}^{red}$

2.2.2. Type II Octadecasaccharides

The sequencing of type II octadecasaccharides is more challenging than that of type I. In this case, the position of the two binding sites has to be determined. Preliminary 2-O desulfatation of unsaturated acid by $\Delta^{4,5}$-glucuronate-2-sulfatase is crucial to differentiate the first AT binding site from the second one. This reaction is achieved before $NaBH_4$ reduction and heparinase I addition. It appears that the activity of the sulfatase is highly dependent on the structure and more especially on the number of disaccharide Is at the non-reducing end. Octadecasaccharides **4** and **5** are entirely transformed after one addition of sulfatase. For compound **6**, the desulfatation is very slow, and the quantity of sulfatase necessary to the transformation exceeds all other cases. The activity of *O*-sulfatase is found to be dependent on the substrate structure. The following order is observed: $\Delta\mathrm{Is}\text{-}\mathrm{IIa}_{id}\text{-}\underline{\mathrm{IIs}_{glu}}\text{-} > \Delta\mathrm{Is}\text{-}\mathrm{Is}_{id}\text{-}\mathrm{IIa}_{id}\text{-}\underline{\mathrm{IIs}_{glu}}\text{-} > \Delta\mathrm{Is}\text{-}\mathrm{Is}_{id}\text{-}\mathrm{Is}_{id}\text{-}\mathrm{IIa}_{id}\text{-}\underline{\mathrm{IIs}_{glu}}\text{-}$. This enzyme has already been cloned and its selectivity studied [29,30] but the selectivity observed above was not heretofore mentioned. Table 3 gathers key fragments generated subsequently after heparinase I treatment for type II octadecasaccharides. Full details of sequencing experiments of octadecasaccharides **4**, **5** and **6** are described in the Supplementary Data.

2.3. NMR

The ^{1}H-NMR spectrum of the octasaccharide **6** is shown in Figure 5. Proton and carbon resonances of each residue were assigned using COSY (correlation spectroscopy), TOCSY (total correlation spectroscopy) and HSQC (heteronuclear single quantum coherence spectroscopy) pulse sequences (Table 4) (octadecasaccharides **2**, **3**, **4** and **5** structural assignments are reported in the Supplementary Data).

A total of 18 proton signals were observed in the anomeric region between 5.55 and 4.55 ppm, indicating that the polysaccharide is an octadecasaccharide, with only 13 different chemical shifts. As a consequence, the proton spectrum did not appear as complex as might be expected for an octadecasaccharide. This feature indicated the presence of two repeating units in the sequence of the octadecasaccharide, with many resonance superimpositions. Chemical shift analysis was compatible with a composition including nine α-D-glucosamines, six α-L-iduronic acids, two β-D-glucuronic acids (anomeric proton resonance observed between 5.53 and 5,34 ppm, 5.22 and 5.01 ppm and at 4.60 ppm, respectively), and one 4,5-unsaturated uronic acid. Two central acetyl signals are visible at 2.05 ppm. The C_i-H1 to $C_{(i+1)}$-H4 connectivity, observed in the nuclear Overhauser spectroscopy (NOESY) experiment, were used for monosaccharides sequence determination (Figure 6). The well-resolved resonance of H4-ΔU uronic acid was used as the assignment starting point. The presence of *N*-sulfate or *N*-acetyl on α-D-glucosamine residues, and the presence or absence of *O*-sulfate groups, was deduced from ^{1}H and ^{13}C chemical shifts.

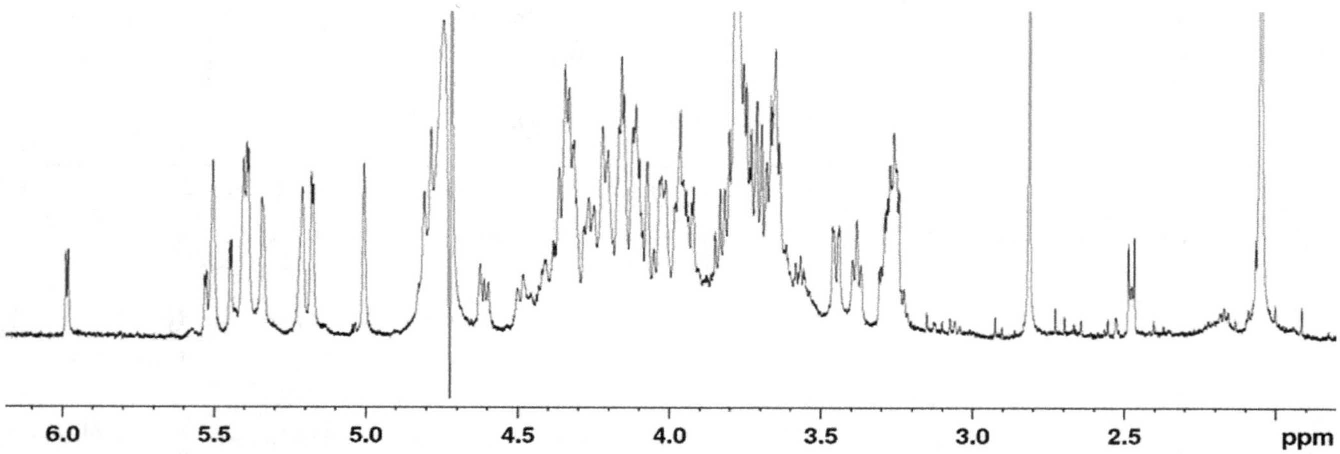

Figure 5. ^{1}H-NMR spectrum of octadecasaccharide **6** (D_2O, 30 °C, 600 MHz).

Table 4. Proton and carbon chemical shifts of the two pentasaccharide sequences identified inside octadecasaccharide **6**.

	ΔIs		Is_{id}		Is_{id}	
	ΔU_{2S}	$A_{NS,6S}$	I_{2S}	$A_{NS,6S}$	I_{2S}	$A_{NS,6S}$
1	5.51/98.4	5.40/98.1	5.21/100.4	5.41/97.8	5.22/100.4	5.34/96.6
2	4.62/75.7	3.30/58.9	4.34/76.9	3.27/59.0	4.35/76.9	3.26/59.0
3	4.31/64.0	3.65/70.8	4.22/70.2	3.66/70.8	4.20/70.4	3.65/70.8
4	5.98/107.1	3.84/79.3	4.10/77.5	3.76/77.1	4.11/77.1	3.78/77.2
5		4.03/70.0	4.81/70.5	4.02/70.3	4.81/70.5	3.96/70.4
6,6′		4.36/4.26 67.4		4.40/4.27 67.5		4.41/4.26 67.5
CH_3						
	Pentasaccharide 1					
	IIa_{id}		IIs_{glu}		Is_{id}	
	I	$A_{NAc,6S}$	G	$A_{NS,3S,6S}$	I_{2S}	$A_{NS,6S}$
1	5.01/103.1	5.39/98.1	4.60/102.2	5.51/97.2	5.18/100.6	5.34/96.6
2	3.78/69.8	3.93/55.0	3.38/74.6	3.45/57.8	4.32/78.1	3.26/59.0
3	4.12/68.9	3.77/70.7	3.70/77.5	4.37/77.4	4.17/71.6	3.66/70.8
4	4.08/75.8	3.73/78.5	3.80/77.8	3.97/74.1	4.14/77.1	3.79/77.7
5	4.79/69.8	4.02/70.4	3.76/78.3	4.16/70.7	4.79/71.2	3.96/70.4
6,6′		4.34/4.21 67.4		4.49/4.26 67.1		4.46/4.23 67.4
CH_3		2.05/23.2				
	Pentasaccharide 2					
	IIa_{id}		IIs_{glu}		Is_{id}	
	I	$A_{NAc,6S}$	G	$A_{NS,3S,6S}$	I_{2S}	$A_{NS,6S}$
1	5.01/103.1	5.39/98.1	4.60/102.2	5.53/97.1	5.18/100.6	4.45/92.2
2	3.78/69.8	3.93/55.0	3.39/74.6	3.45/57.8	4.31/78.1	3.27/59.0
3	4.12/68.9	3.77/70.7	3.70/77.5	4.36/77.4	4.17/71.6	3.70/70.6
4	4.08/75.8	3.73/78.5	3.80/77.8	3.97/74.1	4.16/77.2	3.78/77.6
5	4.79/69.8	4.02/70.4	3.76/78.3	4.17/70.7	4.74/71.5	4.13/69.7
6,6′		4.34/4.21 67.4		4.49/4.26 67.1		4.43/4.30 68.0
CH_3		2.05/23.2				

Note: Listed as H/C in ppm.

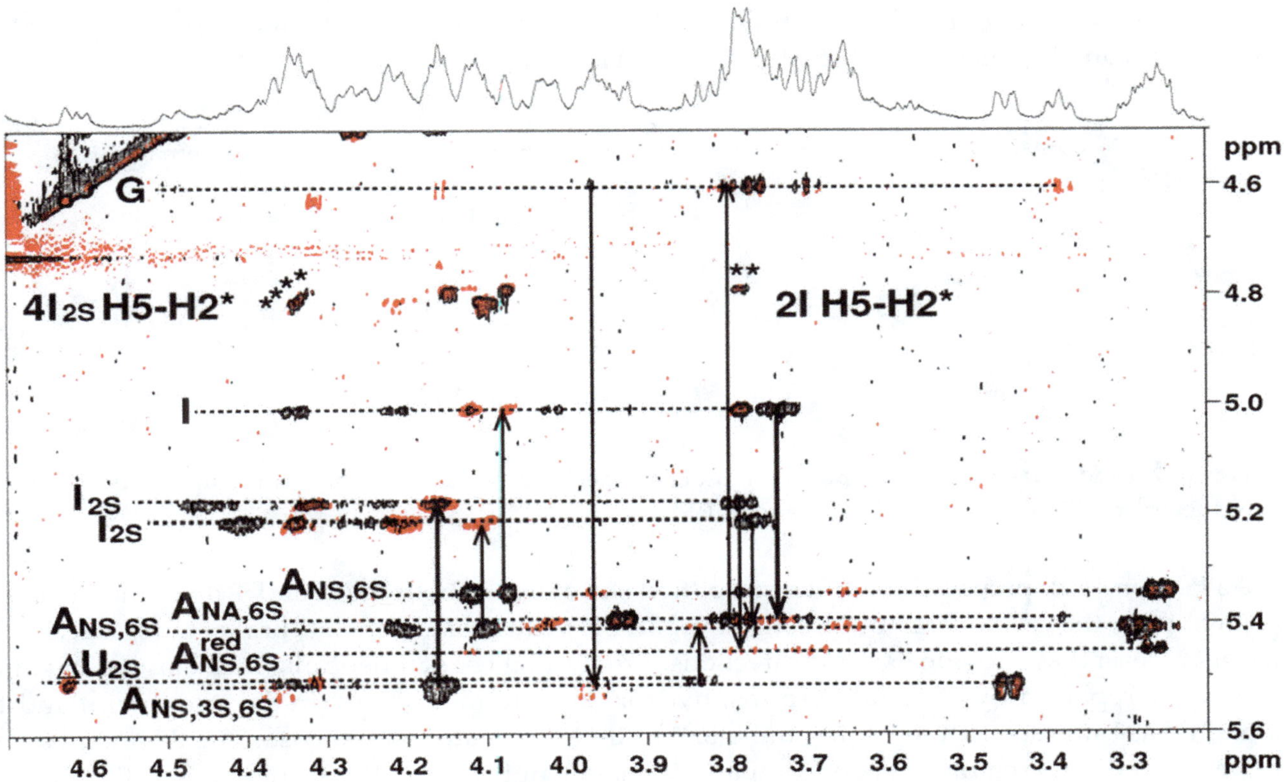

Figure 6. Superimposition of 2D nuclear Overhauser spectroscopy (NOESY) (black) and total correlation spectroscopy (TOCSY) (red) spectra for octadecasaccharide **6**: Correlations of anomeric protons. The dark lines show at start C_i-H1 to $C_{(i+1)}$-H4 connectivities on the NOESY experiment and at the arrows the C_i-H1 to C_i-H4 connectivities on the TOCSY experiment. The H5-H2 characteristic connectivity of $^2S_0$ conformation of each Iduronic acids is indicated by (*) on the NOESY experiment.

In spite of the ^{1}H signal broadness and many resonance superimpositions, it was possible to determine the main coupling constant for vicinal protons of pyranose rings in the well resolved COSY experiment. For glucosamines and glucuronic acids all $^3J_{H1\text{-}H2}$ coupling constants were superior to 8 Hz, except for the $^3J_{H1\text{-}H2}$ of glucosamines between 3and 4 Hz. Consequently, the conformational status of glucosamines and glucuronic acids was in the pure $^4C_1$ conformation. All iduronic acids signals showed small coupling constant for vicinal protons, except for the $^3J_{H2\text{-}H3}$ around 7 to 8 Hz. Besides weak-medium intensities were observed for the H5-H2 connectivities in the NOESY experiment (Figure 6). This information taken together suggested a $^1C_4 \leftrightarrow {}^2S0$ equilibrium for all iduronic acids [31].

The full proton and carbon chemical shift assignments, along with all sets of inter-residue correlations observed on the 2D NOESY spectrum, fully supported the structural determination of octadecasaccharide **6** with two pentasaccharide sequences as demonstrated by the enzymatic sequencing methodology. The two AGA*IA sequences are respectively located in the middle and at the reducing end of the octadecasaccharide. The NMR assignment tables for the octadecasaccharides **2**, **3**, **4** and **5** are reported in the Supplementary Data.

2.4. aFXa and aFIIa Activities

In their previous work [19,21], Petitou et al. introduced the concepts of A domain (AT binding domain AGA*IA) and thrombin binding domain (T domain) for their synthetic heparin mimetics. At that time, pure natural structures were not available and therefore, hypotheses had to be made to figure out the AGA*IA flanking oligosaccharides, which might constitute the T domain. Their structure-activity studies showed that the T domain should be highly sulfated in order to interact with the positively charged domain of thrombin [19]. Because heparin has some highly sulfated regular regions with repetitive units of trisulfated Is disaccharides, it was therefore presumed that the T domain was an oligomer of this structural motif (Figure 7).

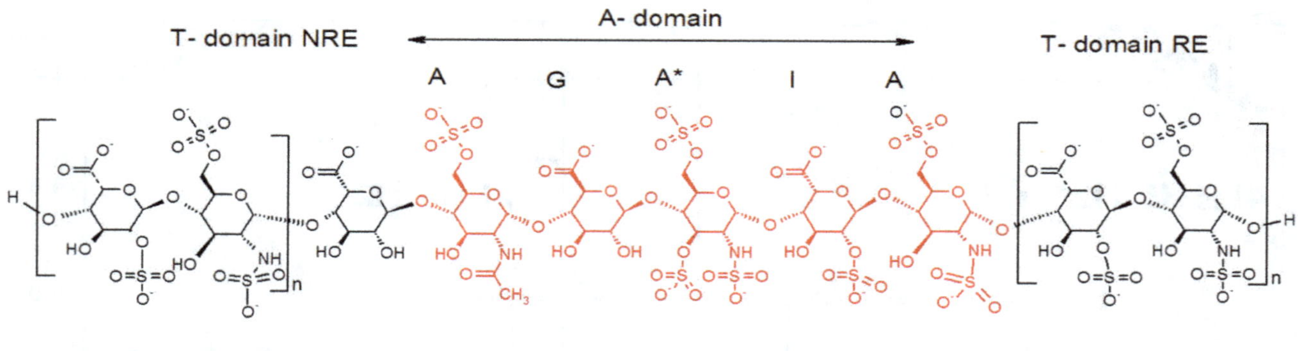

Figure 7. Model described for heparin oligosaccharides with Is disaccharide T domain extensions at reducing end (RE) and non-reducing end (NRE).

As Petitou et al. prepared modified simplified structures of both the A and T domain to generate biological data, the results are not directly comparable with those of the natural octadecasaccharide series but at least they provide us some directions. Briefly, in these synthetic oligosaccharides, *N*-sulfate groups were replaced by *O*-sulfate groups, hydroxyls were methylated in the A domain, and the T domain was built up with repeating units of 2,6-di-*O*-sulfonato β-D-glucose. The thrombin assays were performed with regioisomers of comparable chain length. When the T domain is at the reducing end, it was established that the thrombin inhibition is about 30 times less potent than when it is located at the non-reducing end (IC_{50} = 164 vs. 5 ng/mL, comparison made respectively with an octadecasaccharide and a heptadecasaccharide).

While heparin does contain sequences such as described in Figure 7, the overall picture of polysaccharide structures able to inhibit thrombin is more diverse, and the richness of activity of this collection of biosynthetic macromolecules is certainly not uniquely explained by such structures. As a matter of fact, the chromatographic complexity of the octadecasaccharide fractions speak to the diversity (Figure 2), just as well as the unexpected series of double AT binding octadecasaccharides regioisomers studied herein (Figure 1). For these, the aFXa and aFIIa were assayed by chromogenic assay and are reported in the Table 5.

Table 5. aFXa and aFIIa activities of isolated octadecasaccharides.

	Structure	aFXa Activity (IU/mg)	aFXa Activity (IU/μmol)	aFIIa Activity (IU/mg)
Octadecasaccharide 1	ΔIIa-IIs_{glu}-Is_{id}-IIa_{id}-IIs_{glu}-Is_{id}-IIa_{id}-IIs_{glu}-Is_{id}	562	3090	8.8
Octadecasaccharide 2	ΔIIa-IIs_{glu}-Is_{id}-IIa_{id}-IIs_{glu}-Is_{id}-Is_{id}-Is_{id}-Is_{id}	371	2100	5.9
Octadecasaccharide 3	ΔIIa-IIs_{glu}-Is_{id}-Is_{id}-IIa_{id}-IIs_{glu}-Is_{id}-Is_{id}-Is_{id}	442	2502	9
Octadecasaccharide 4	ΔIs-IIa_{id}-IIs_{glu}-Is_{id}-Is_{id}-IIa_{id}-IIs_{glu}-Is_{id}-Is_{id}	540	3057	22.6
Octadecasaccharide 5	ΔIs-IIa_{id}-IIs_{glu}-Is_{id}-Is_{id}-Is_{id}-IIa_{id}-IIs_{glu}-Is_{id}	517	2927	81.5
Octadecasaccharide 6	ΔIs-Is_{id}-Is_{id}-IIa_{id}-IIs_{glu}-Is_{id}-IIa_{id}-IIs_{glu}-Is_{id}	705	3991	119.3

Regarding aFXa inhibitory potency, these series are on molar basis 1.5 to 2.6 times more potent than the fondaparinux reference (1480 UI/μmol). This is in agreement with previous studies performed on dodecasaccharides and tetradecasaccharides where the same phenomenon was observed [32]. As a consequence, this further emphasizes that the double-site oligosaccharides are able, through a dynamic equilibrium, to engage both AGA*IA sites with antithrombin and to increase by about twofold the molar aFXa activity. At this stage however, more subtle interpretation of their ranking is difficult to assess as it is established that several parameters, either synergistic or antagonistic, might influence their potency. Among them, we could highlight the spacer length between two AGA*IA sequences, the nature of AGA*IA flanking oligosaccharides as well as their location either at RE or NRE.

Regarding thrombin activity, when the T-Domain flanking units are located at the reducing end, the potency is between 5 and 9 IU/mg. This is very low when compared to the NLT 180 IU/mg of USP Heparin. However, when T-domain flanking units are at the NRE, the thrombin activity is increasingly noteworthy. Interestingly, the octadecasaccharides **4** and **5** have the same T domain (ΔIs-IdoA) followed by an AGA*IA at the NRE but the aFIIa activities are respectively 22.6 and 81.5 IU/mg. In this case, the location of the reducing end AGA*IA plays an important role. For compound **4**, the RE pentasaccharide is not completely at the end of the chain, whereas for **5**, it is fully located at the reducing end of the octadecasaccharide. This sequence configuration provides the opportunity to maximize the chain length between at least one AGA*IA and the T-domain, which in turn strengthens the ternary complex with antithrombin and thrombin.

The octadecasaccharide **6** possesses three consecutive Is disaccharides at the NRE and one AGA*IA at the RE. This configuration maximizes both the anionic charge density for the T-domain and the spacer chain length with the reducing end AGA*IA pentasaccharide. As a consequence, the thrombin inhibition is the highest one observed in these series, with a value of 119.3 IU/mg. We conclude that between the regioisomers **2** and **6**, the thrombin inhibition potency increases by about 20 times, which is in good alignment with the results obtained on synthetic compounds. However, there are still some open questions remaining, especially when octadecasaccharide **1** is compared with octadecasaccharides **5** and **6**. For these three octadecasaccharides, there is one AGA*IA sequence fully located at the reducing end. Their differences lie in the T domain. The last two disaccharides could be considered to interact with thrombin and stabilize the complex according to Petitou et al. [19]. For octadecasaccharides **1**, **5** and **6**, there is respectively four, four and six sulfate groups. The charge density influence on thrombin inhibition could be expected for octadecasaccharides **5** and **6** but does not correlate for octadecasaccharide **1**, which is at least 10 times less potent than **5** and **6**. If we take into account that the T-domain is also an AGA*IA sequence, antithrombin could compete with thrombin and disfavor the ternary complex formation, which in turn might explain the very low potency of octadecasaccharide **1**.

3. Materials and Methods

3.1. Materials and Chemicals

Semuloparin was obtained from Sanofi (Vitry sur Seine, France). This product was prepared according to Example 2 described in a U.S. patent [33]. All other reagents and chemicals were of the highest quality available. Water was purified with a Millipore Milli-Q purification system. *Flavobacterium heparinum* heparinase I (EC 4.2.2.7) and $\Delta^{4,5}$-Glucuronate-2-sulfatase were obtained from Grampian Enzymes (Aberdeen, UK). AT used for the determination of biological activities was freeze-dried material of human origin (Instrumentation Laboratory, Le Pre Saint Gervais, France). FXa (71-nKat flask) was freeze-dried material of bovine origin (Instrument Laboratory). FIIa was freeze-dried material of human origin (Stago, Asnières sur Seine, France). FXa (S2765, Instrumentation Laboratory) and FIIa (S2238, Instrumentation Laboratory) substrates were freeze-dried materials.

3.2. Chromatographic Methods

Following the method in reference [12,17], 150 mm × 2.1 mm columns filled with Kinetex C_{18} 2.6 μm particles (Phenomenex, Le Pecq, France) were used after the CTA dynamic coating. A linear concentration gradient (0–2 M) of aqueous ammonium methane sulfonate, pH 2.5 was applied.

For the analytical control of collected fractions or chromatographic separations, a Carbopack AS11 column (250 mm × 2.1 mm) (Thermo Scientific Dionex, Courtaboeuf, France) was used with aqueous $NaClO_4$ mobile phase.

LC/MS with an ion-pairing chromatographic system (Acquity UPLC BEH C_{18} column, 2.1 mm × 150 mm, 1.7 μm, Waters, Saint-Quentin-en-Yvelines, France) was the third orthogonal method applied for deciphering the complex mixture [14,17]. The method initially described in [34] and adapted in [14] was broadened [17] to determine the number of ion-pair adducts included in the molecular ions. Briefly, each separation was duplicated, one using pentylamine (PTA) as ion pairing reagent and the second one using hexylamine (HXA). The number of adducts could be deduced from the mass shift in ion peaks obtained in parallel with both conditions. Partial degradation of 3-O sulfated glucosamines located at the reducing end was detected when working at 40 °C, and therefore, the operating column temperature was lowered to 30 °C for sequencing experiments.

3.3. Procedure for Isolation of Octadecasaccharides

The octadecasaccharide fraction was purified by gel permeation chromatography (GPC) from semuloparin as previously described [17]. 1.85 g of semuloparin were directly injected on a system equipped with two columns (100 × 5 cm (I.D.) connected in series, packed with polyacrylamide gel (Bio Gel P-30, Fine, Bio Rad, Marnes-la-Coquette, France)), and circulated at 1.7 mL/min with $NaClO_4$ 0.2 M. UV detection was used at 232 nm. 600 g of semuloparin were injected in fractions over about 350 runs. Selected fractions were first concentrated, desalted on Sephadex G10 columns (100 × 7 cm) and then lyophilized. Finally, 10 g of octadecasaccharides were obtained.

3.3.1. Fractionation on AT Affinity Chromatography

The octadecasaccharide fractionated by chromatography on an AT Sepharose column (30 cm × 7 cm) as previously described [17]. The column was prepared by coupling human AT (2 g) as described by Hoök et al. [35]. Octadecasaccharides (80 to 150 mg) were injected in each run. The low-affinity fraction was eluted from the column with a 0.25 M NaCl solution buffered at pH 7.4 with 1 mM Tris/HCl at 12 mL/min. The five high-affinity octasaccharide fractions were eluted with a five step gradient of NaCl (0.74 M, 1.23 M, 1.71 M, 2.2 M and 3.5 M NaCl and 1 mM Tris-HCl, pH 7.4). All fractions were desalted on Sephadex–G10. After 100 injections on AT-affinity chromatography, 4.2 g were collected for the low-affinity fraction, 800 mg for F1, 1.57 g for F2, 1.02 g for F3, 616 mg for F4 and 385 mg for F5.

3.3.2. Purification of Octadecasaccharide Fraction F3

Focus was given to the separation of octadecasaccharides regioisomers with 2 AGA*IA sequences positioned differently within the chain (Figure 1). These are the components of major interest in the affine fraction F3 (Figure 2). The five octadecasaccharide series were purified by combining three chromatographic methods with orthogonal selectivities following the previously described procedure [17] namely, CTA-SAX, AS11 and ion pairing chromatography. We distinguish herein two distinct types of octadecasaccharides to guide the separation strategy. Type I octadecasaccharides (**2** and **3**) are devoid of 2-O sulfation at the non-reducing end's uronic acid whereas Type II compounds (**4**, **5** and **6**) are 2-O sulfated (Figure 1). The 2-O sulfation influences the maximum of the UV spectrum and the retention behavior in CTA-SAX and AS11 chromatography. The details of the procedure are reported in the Supplementary Data.

3.4. Structural Characterization by Enzymatic Sequencing

The sequencing of octadecasaccharides (10 to 20 μg) was done by controlled depolymerisation with heparinase 1 from *Flavobacterium heparinum* following the described procedure [12,17]. The first step for Type I oligosaccharides was reduction by $NaBH_4$, used to selectively label the reducing end disaccharide [17]. For Type II octadecasaccharides, $\Delta^{4,5}$-glucuronate-2-sulfatase was initially applied to differentiate the non-reducing end, before the $NaBH_4$ reduction. The reaction was initiated by the addition of 10 μL of a 0.5 UI/mL solution of sulfatase diluted in KH_2PO_4 10 mM pH 7 and added in combination with 2 mg/mL of bovine serum albumin (BSA). The advancement of the 2-O desulfatation was followed by analytical CTA-SAX chromatography. At the end of the reaction, the residual enzyme was destroyed by a 2 min boiling step before performing $NaBH_4$ reduction. After vacuum evaporation, reduced octadecasaccharide was diluted in a 1.7 mL HPLC vial and the pH was adjusted to 7 by addition of diluted ammonia or hydrochloric acid. Heparinase I was added (2 µL of a 0.5 UI/mL solution) and depolymerisation was performed at 16 °C. The monitoring of the fragmentation was done by injection on CTA-SAX and AS11 analytical columns. Injection in LC/MS was also performed to confirm the structure of fragments.

3.5. Mass Spectrometry Conditions

ESI mass spectra were obtained using a Waters Xevo Q-Tof mass spectrometer. The electrospray interface was set in positive ion mode with a capillary voltage of 2000 V and a sampling cone voltage of 20 V. The source and the desolvation temperatures were respectively 120 and 400 °C. Nitrogen was used as desolvation (750 L/min) and cone gas (25 L/min). The mass range used was 200–2000 Da (scan rate 0.5 s).

3.6. NMR Spectroscopy

The octadecasaccharide sample (1 mg) was dissolved in D_2O, freeze-dried with a final dissolution in D_2O (99.96% Euriso-Top, Saint-Aubin, France) and transferred into a 3-mm nuclear magnetic resonance (NMR) sample tube. One-dimensional and two-dimensional (2D) NMR (^1H-^1H and ^1H-^{13}C) spectra were recorded on a 600 MHz AVANCE II spectrometer (Bruker, Wissembourg, France) operating at 599.80 MHz using a 5-mm TXI cryoprobe with standard pulse sequences and a probe temperature of 30 °C. Proton spectra were recorded in 256 scans with a 2 s presaturation and a full recycle time of 6.5 s. The resolution prior zero filling was 0.2 Hz/pt. 2D-COSY and 2D-TOCSY with a mixing time value of 120 ms were acquired using 64 scans per series of 4 K × 512 W with a resolution of 1.16 Hz/pt before zero filling (4 K × 2 K) and appropriate apodization was applied prior to Fourier transformation. The 2D-nuclear Overhauser enhancement spectroscopy (NOESY) was performed in similar way with a mixing time value of 300 ms. The 2D-HSQC was performed using 64 scans per series of 1.5 K × 512 W with a resolution of 3.28 Hz/pt before zero filling (2 K × 1 K). Spectrum calibration was achieved by setting as external standard reference trimethylsilyl 2,2′3,3′-tetradeuteropropionoic acid (TSP-D_4) signal to 0 ppm.

3.7. Anti-Factor IIa Activity and Anti-Factor Xa Activity

AT solution of 1 IU/mL were prepared in pH 7.4 PEG 6000 buffer (0.1% PEG 6000 in pH 7.4 buffer [50 mM Tris and 150 mM NaCl adjusted by HCl to pH 7.4]). FXa was prepared to 1.8 nkat/mL in pH 7.4 PEG6000 buffer. FIIa was prepared to 5 IU/mL in pH 7.4 PEG6000 buffer. The chromogenic substrate solution for FXa and FIIa was prepared to a final concentration of 0.5 mM in pH 8.4 buffer (50 mM Tris, 175 mM NaCl, and 7.5 mM edetate disodium adjusted by HCl to pH 8.4). Semuloparin biological standard (3000ET with assigned potencies of 101.4 IU/mL for anti-FXa and 1.8 IU/mL for anti-FIIa), calibrated against the second LMWH international standard (NIBSC, code 01/608), was used for calibration.

For anti-FXa titration, the semuloparin standard solution was diluted with pH 7.4 buffer to obtain target concentrations of 0.04, 0.05, 0.06, and 0.07 IU/mL. Each concentration was assessed in duplicate (two wells filled with the same diluted solution), and two independent experiments (independent dispensing and dilutions) were conducted.

For anti-FIIa titration, the semuloparin standard solution was diluted with pH 7.4 buffer to obtain target concentrations of 0.007, 0.008, 0.010, and 0.012 IU/mL. Each concentration was assessed in duplicate (two wells filled with the same diluted solution), and three independent experiments (independent dispensing and dilutions) were conducted.

Octadecasaccharide solution was prepared to a final concentration with activities in IU/mL close to the semuloparin standard. The solution was then diluted and dispensed as for the standards.

Plates were heated at 37 °C. Solutions for analysis (20 μL) were pipetted into a 96-well plate, and 20 μL of AT solution was added. Samples were then mixed and left for 60 s before 40 μL of the FXa (or FIIa) solution were added, and the solutions were mixed and left for a further 60 s. Next, 100 μL of chromogenic substrate solution were added, mixed, and left for 240 s. Finally, 100 μL of 42% acetic acid solution were added, mixed, and left for 60 s before the optical density at 405 nm was read.

The internally developed software "Parallel", running on the Statistical Analysis System (SAS version 9.1, SAS France, Grégy-sur-Yerres, France)), was used for statistical analysis according to the European Pharmacopoeia Ph. Eur. § 5.3 for parallel-line models. Each assay result was the mean average of the independent valid tests.

4. Conclusions

The results of this study, while confirming the structure-activity relationship on synthetic compounds, also demonstrate that the overall picture for thrombin inhibition compounds may be much more complex in natural heparin sequences as well as for LMWH products. We have demonstrated that for octadecasaccharide regioisomers, built up from the same AGA*IA sequences and Is flanking disaccharides, thrombin inhibition potency may dramatically differ. Indeed, when the AGA*IA sequences are located at the reducing end vs. the non-reducing end, the octadecasaccharide becomes 20 times more potent in aFIIa activity (compound **6** vs. **2**). This is in agreement with the previous findings reported on synthetic compounds by Petitou et al. [19–21]. However, even if an AGA*IA sequence is borne at the reducing end, the presence of another one at the non-reducing end (compound **1**) obviously destabilize the complex with thrombin and decrease the potency by one log of magnitude order. The anionic charge density of T-domain is an important factor for thrombin binding but its ability to interact strongly with other proteins should be taken into consideration to improve our prediction of structure activity relationships. The findings developed in this paper pointed out that for octadecasaccharides regioisomers the sequence arrangement is critical for interaction with proteins regulating the coagulation cascade. This is emphasizing the role and the potential impact of the selectivity of the heparin depolymerization process on the overall biological properties of LMWH.

Acknowledgments: The authors warmly thank Nathalie Karst, Andrew Van-Sickle and Marco Guerrini for their thoughtful review and recommendations to improve the manuscript as well as Min Zhang for her active contribution in the chromatographic purification of octadecasaccharides. We would like to thank also Celine Martinez for her appreciated input in the redaction of the experimental biological section, Brigitte Bordier and Monique Cherel for performing aFXa and aFIIa assay.

Author Contributions: Pierre Mourier and Christian Viskov designed the study. Pierre Mourier isolated, purified and characterized the octadecasaccharides by enzymatic sequencing. Olivier Guichard performed the mass spectrometry experiments. Philippe Sizun and Frederic Herman characterized the octadecasaccharides by NMR. Christian Viskov, Pierre Mourier, Philippe Sizun analyzed the data and reviewed the data before submission. Christian Viskov and Pierre Mourier wrote the paper.

Abbreviations

AT, antithrombin; FXa, factor Xa; FIIa, factor IIa or thrombin; SAX, strong anion exchange; CTA-SAX, cetyltrimethylammonium strong anion exchange; LMWH, low-molecular-weight heparin; GPC, gel permeation chromatography; PTA, pentylamine; HXA, hexylamine; HFIP, 1,1,1,3,3,3-hexafluoro-2-propanol; LC/MS, liquid chromatography–mass spectrometry; DQF-COSY, double-quantum-filter correlation spectroscopy; 2D-NOESY, nuclear Overhauser enhancement spectroscopy; HSQC, heteronuclear single-quantum coherence; TOCSY, total correlated spectroscopy; Glc_{Nac}; *N*-acetyl-α-D-glucosamine; $Glc_{NAc,6S}$, *N*-acetylated, 6-*O*-sulfated GlcN; $Glc_{NS,6S}$, *N*,6-*O*-disulfated GlcN; $Glc_{NS,3,6S}$, *N*,3,6-*O*-trisulfated GlcN; IdoA, α-L-iduronic acid; $IdoA_{2S}$, 2-*O*-sulfated IdoA; AGA∗IA, pentasaccharide sequence of $Glc_{NAc,6S}$-GlcA-$Glc_{NS,3,6S}$-$IdoA_{2S}$-$Glc_{NS,6S}$; ΔU, 4,5-unsaturated uronic acid; ΔU_{2S}, 2-*O*-sulfated, 4,5-unsaturated uronic acid.

References

1. Choay, J.; Lormeau, J.-C.; Petitou, M.; Sinaÿ, P.; Casu, B.; Oreste, P.; Torri, G.; Gatti, G. Anti-Xa active heparin oligosaccharides. *Thromb. Res.* **1980**, *18*, 573–578. [CrossRef]
2. Torri, G.; Naggi, A. Heparin centenary—An ever-young live-saving drug. *Int. J. Cardiol.* **2016**, *212*, S1–S4. [CrossRef]
3. Nader, H.B.; Dietrich, C.P. Natural occurrence, and possible biological role of heparin. In *Heparin: Chemical and Biological Properties, Clinical Applications*; Lane, D.A., Lindahl, U., Eds.; CRC Press Inc.: Boca Raton, FL, USA, 1989; pp. 81–96.
4. Conrad, H.E. *Heparin Binding Proteins*; Academic Press: Millbrae, CA, USA, 1998.
5. Bock, S.C. Antithrombin and heparin cofactor II. In *Hemostasis and Thrombosis: Basic Principles and Clinical Practice*; Lippincott Williams and Wilkins: Philadelphia, PA, USA, 2006; pp. 235–248.
6. Danielsson, A.; Raub, E.; Lindahl, U.; Björk, I. Role of Ternary Complexes, in Which Heparin Binds Both Antithrombin and Proteinase, in the Acceleration of the Reactions between Antithrombin and Thrombin or Factor Xa. *J. Biol. Chem.* **1986**, *261*, 15467–15473. [PubMed]
7. Petitou, M.; Casu, B.; Lindahl, U. 1976–1983, a critical period in the history of heparin: The discovery of the antithrombin binding site. *Biochimie* **2003**, *85*, 83–89. [CrossRef]
8. Hricovini, M.; Guerrini, M.; Bisio, A.; Torri, G.; Petitou, M.; Casu, B. Conformation of heparin pentasaccharide bound to antithrombin III. *Biochem. J.* **2001**, *359*, 265–272. [CrossRef] [PubMed]
9. Loganathan, D.H.; Wang, M.; Mallis, L.M.; Linhardt, R.J. Structural variation in the antithrombin III binding site region and its occurrence in heparin from different sources. *Biochemistry* **1990**, *29*, 4362–4368. [CrossRef] [PubMed]
10. Lindahl, U.; Thunberg, L.; Bäckstrőm, G.; Riesenfeld, J.; Nordling, K.; Bjork, I. Extension and structural variability of the antithrombin binding sequence in heparin. *J. Biol. Chem.* **1984**, *259*, 12368–12376. [PubMed]
11. Guerrini, M.; Elli, S.; Mourier, P.; Rudd, T.R.; Gaudesi, D.; Casu, B.; Boudier, C.; Torri, G.; Viskov, C. An unusual antithrombin-binding heparin octasaccharide with an additional 3-*O*-sulfated glucosamine in the active pentasaccharide sequence. *Biochem. J.* **2013**, *449*, 343–351. [CrossRef] [PubMed]
12. Mourier, P.A.J.; Viskov, C. Chromatographic analysis and sequencing approach of heparin oligosaccharides using cetyltrimethylammonium dynamically coated stationary phases. *Anal. Biochem.* **2004**, *332*, 299–313. [CrossRef] [PubMed]
13. Guerrini, M.; Mourier, P.A.J.; Torri, J.; Viskov, C. Antithrombin-binding oligosaccharides: Structural diversities in a unique function? *Glycoconj. J.* **2014**, *31*, 409–416. [CrossRef] [PubMed]
14. Guerrini, M.; Guglieri, S.; Casu, B.; Torri, G.; Mourier, P.; Boudier, C.; Viskov, C. Antithrombin-binding octasaccharides and role of extensions of the active pentasaccharide sequence in the specificity and strength of interaction: Evidence for very high affinity induced by an unusual glucuronic acid residue. *J. Biol. Chem.* **2008**, *283*, 26662–26675. [CrossRef] [PubMed]
15. Viskov, C.; Just, M.; Laux, V.; Mourier, P.; Lorenz, M. Description of the chemical and pharmacological characteristics of a new hemisynthetic ultra-low-molecular-weight heparin, AVE5026. *J. Thromb. Haemost.* **2009**, *7*, 1143–1151. [CrossRef] [PubMed]
16. Viskov, C.; Elli, S.; Urso, E.; Gaudesi, D.; Mourier, P.; Herman, F.; Boudier, C.; Casu, B.; Torri, G.; Guerrini, M. Heparin dodecasaccharide containing two antithrombin binding pentasaccharides. Structural features and biological properties. *J. Biol. Chem.* **2013**, *288*, 25895–25907. [CrossRef] [PubMed]
17. Mourier, P.A.; Guichard, O.Y.; Herman, F.; Viskov, C. Isolation of a pure octadecasaccharide with antithrombin activity from an ultra-low-molecular-weight heparin. *Anal. Biochem.* **2014**, *453*, 7–15. [CrossRef] [PubMed]
18. Jordan, R.E.; Favreau, L.V.; Braswell, E.H.; Rosenberg, R.D. Heparin with Two Binding Sites for Antithrombin or Platelet Factor 4. *J. Biol. Chem.* **1982**, *257*, 400–406. [PubMed]
19. Petitou, M.; Van Boeckel, C.A. A synthetic antithrombin III binding pentasaccharide is now a drug! What comes next? *Angew. Chem. Int. Ed. Engl.* **2004**, *43*, 3118–3133. [CrossRef] [PubMed]
20. Petitou, M.; Hérault, J.M.; Bernat, A.; Driguez, P.A.; Duchaussoy, P.; Lormeau, J.C.; Herbert, J.M. Synthesis of thrombin-inhibiting heparin mimetics without side effects. *Nature* **1999**, *398*, 417–422. [PubMed]
21. Petitou, M.; Imberty, A.; Duchaussoy, P.; Driguez, P.A.; Ceccato, M.L.; Gourvenec, F.; Sizun, P.; Hérault, J.P.; Pérez, S.; Herbert, J.M. Experimental Proof for the structure of a Thrombin-inhibiting heparin molecule. *Chem. Eur. J.* **2001**, *7*, 858–873. [CrossRef]

22. Mourier, P.; Anger, P.; Martinez, C.; Herman, F.; Viskov, C. Quantitative compositional analysis of heparin using exhaustive heparinase digestion and strong anion exchange chromatography. *Anal. Chem. Res.* **2015**, *3*, 46–53. [CrossRef]
23. Venkataraman, G.; Shriver, Z.; Raman, R.; Sasisekharan, R. Sequencing complex polysaccharides. *Science* **1999**, *286*, 537–542. [CrossRef] [PubMed]
24. Keiseri, N.; Venkataraman, G.; Shriver, Z.; Sasisekharan, R. Direct isolation and sequencing of specific protein-binding glycosaminoglycans. *Nat. Med.* **2001**, *7*, 123–128.
25. Stringer, S.E.; Kandola, B.S.; Pye, D.A.; Gallagher, J.T. Heparin sequencing. *Glycobiology* **2003**, *13*, 97–107. [CrossRef] [PubMed]
26. Desai, U.R.; Wang, H.; Linhardt, R.J. Substrate specificity of the heparin lyases from *Flavobacterium heparinum*. *Arch. Biochem. Biophys.* **1993**, *306*, 461–468. [CrossRef] [PubMed]
27. Ernst, S.; Rhomberg, A.J.; Bieman, K.; Sasisekharan, R. Direct evidence for a predominantly exolytic processive mechanism for depolymerization of heparin-like glycosaminoglycans by heparinase I. *Proc. Natl. Acad. Sci. USA* **1998**, *95*, 4182–4187. [CrossRef] [PubMed]
28. Xiao, Z.; Zhao, W.; Yang, B.; Zhang, Z.; Guan, H.; Linhardt, R.J. Heparinase I selectivity for the 3,6-di-*O*-sulfo-2-deoxy-2-sulfamido-α-D-glucopyranose (1,4) 2-*O*-sulfo-α-L-idopyranosyluronic acid (GlcNS3S6S-IdoA2S) linkages. *Glycobiology* **2011**, *21*, 13–22. [CrossRef] [PubMed]
29. Myette, J.R.; Shriver, Z.; Claycamp, C.; McLean, M.W.; Venkatarama, G.; Sasisekharan, R. The Heparin/Heparan Sulfate 2-*O*-Sulfatase from *Flavobacterium heparinum*. Molecular cloning, recombinant expression, and biochemical characterization. *J. Biol. Chem.* **2003**, *278*, 12157–12166. [CrossRef] [PubMed]
30. Raman, R.; Myette, J.R.; Shriver, Z.; Pojasek, K.; Venkataraman, G.; Sasisekharan, R. The Heparin/Heparan Sulfate 2-*O*-Sulfatase from *Flavobacterium heparinum*. A structural and biochemical study of the enzyme active site and saccharide substrate specificity. *J. Biol. Chem.* **2003**, *278*, 12167–12174. [CrossRef] [PubMed]
31. Ferro, D.R.; Provasoli, A.; Ragazzi, M.; Torri, G.; Casu, B.; Gatti, G.; Jacquinet, J.-C.; Sinaÿ, P.; Petitou, M.; Choay, J. Evidence for conformational equilibrium of the sulfated L-iduronate residue in heparin and in synthetic heparin mono- and oligo-saccharides: NMR and force-field studies. *J. Am. Chem. Soc.* **1986**, *108*, 6773–6778. [CrossRef]
32. Mourier, P.; Viskov, C. Polysaccharides Comprising Two Antithrombin III-Binding Sites, Preparation Thereof and Use Thereof as Antithrombin Medicaments. U.S. Patent 9,346,894 B2, 18 October 2016.
33. Biberovic, V.; Grondard, L.; Mourier, P.; Viskov, C. Mixture of Sulfated Oligosaccharides. U.S. Patents 8,003,623 B2 and 8,071,570 B2, 23 August 2011.
34. Doneanu, C.E.; Chen, W.; Gebler, J.C. Analysis of oligosaccharides derived from heparin by Ion-Pair Reversed-Phase Chromatography/Mass Spectrometry. *Anal. Chem.* **2009**, *81*, 3485–3499. [CrossRef] [PubMed]
35. Höök, M.; Björk, I.; Hopwood, J.; Lindahl, U. Anticoagulant activity of heparin: Separation of high-activity and low-activity heparin species by affinity chromatography on immobilized antithrombin. *FEBS Lett.* **1976**, *66*, 90–93. [CrossRef]

Permissions

All chapters in this book were first published by MDPI; hereby published with permission under the Creative Commons Attribution License or equivalent. Every chapter published in this book has been scrutinized by our experts. Their significance has been extensively debated. The topics covered herein carry significant findings which will fuel the growth of the discipline. They may even be implemented as practical applications or may be referred to as a beginning point for another development.

The contributors of this book come from diverse backgrounds, making this book a truly international effort. This book will bring forth new frontiers with its revolutionizing research information and detailed analysis of the nascent developments around the world.

We would like to thank all the contributing authors for lending their expertise to make the book truly unique. They have played a crucial role in the development of this book. Without their invaluable contributions this book wouldn't have been possible. They have made vital efforts to compile up to date information on the varied aspects of this subject to make this book a valuable addition to the collection of many professionals and students.

This book was conceptualized with the vision of imparting up-to-date information and advanced data in this field. To ensure the same, a matchless editorial board was set up. Every individual on the board went through rigorous rounds of assessment to prove their worth. After which they invested a large part of their time researching and compiling the most relevant data for our readers.

The editorial board has been involved in producing this book since its inception. They have spent rigorous hours researching and exploring the diverse topics which have resulted in the successful publishing of this book. They have passed on their knowledge of decades through this book. To expedite this challenging task, the publisher supported the team at every step. A small team of assistant editors was also appointed to further simplify the editing procedure and attain best results for the readers.

Apart from the editorial board, the designing team has also invested a significant amount of their time in understanding the subject and creating the most relevant covers. They scrutinized every image to scout for the most suitable representation of the subject and create an appropriate cover for the book.

The publishing team has been an ardent support to the editorial, designing and production team. Their endless efforts to recruit the best for this project, has resulted in the accomplishment of this book. They are a veteran in the field of academics and their pool of knowledge is as vast as their experience in printing. Their expertise and guidance has proved useful at every step. Their uncompromising quality standards have made this book an exceptional effort. Their encouragement from time to time has been an inspiration for everyone.

The publisher and the editorial board hope that this book will prove to be a valuable piece of knowledge for researchers, students, practitioners and scholars across the globe.

List of Contributors

Zheng Cai, Mark I. Greene, Zhiqiang Zhu and Hongtao Zhang
Departments of Pathology and Laboratory Medicine, Perelman School of Medicine, University of Pennsylvania, Philadelphia, PA 19301, USA

Lina Ma, Jiawei Wu, Ying Zheng, Zimei Shu, Zhenquan Wei and Aiwu Zhou
Department of Pathophysiology, Shanghai Jiao Tong University School of Medicine, Shanghai 200025, China

Yinbiao Sun
Randall Division of Cell & Molecular Biophysics, Faculty of Life Sciences & Medicine, King's College London, New Hunt's House, Guy's Campus, London SE1 1UL, UK

Robin W. Carrell
Department of Haematology, University of Cambridge, Cambridge CB2 0XY, UK

Noemi Veraldi
Division of Clinical Pathology, Department of Diagnostics, Geneva University Hospitals, 1211 Geneva 14, Switzerland

Nawel Zouggari
Department of Biochemistry, Faculty of Science and Department of Pathology and Immunology, School of Medicine, University of Geneva, 1211 Geneva 14, Switzerland

Ariane de Agostini
Department of Pathology and Immunology, School of Medicine, University of Geneva and Division of Clinical Pathology, Department of Diagnostics, Geneva University Hospitals, 1211 Geneva 14, Switzerland

Jung-Min Lee, Ah-Young Kim, Sang Hyun Park, Jae-Seok Kim, Jung-Won Park, Jong-Hyeon Park and Young-Joon Ko
Animal and Plant Quarantine Agency, 177 Hyeoksin-8-ro, Gimcheon-si 39660, Gyeongsangbuk-do, Korea

Choi-Kyu Park
Animal Disease Intervention Center, College of Veterinary Medicine, Kyungpook National University, Daegu 41566, Gyeongsangbuk-do, Korea

Sun Young Park and Hyejin Kim
Animal and Plant Quarantine Agency, 177 Hyeoksin-8-ro, Gimcheon-si 39660, Gyeongsangbuk-do, Korea
Animal Disease Intervention Center, College of Veterinary Medicine, Kyungpook National University, Daegu 41566, Gyeongsangbuk-do, Korea

Cristina Gardini
Centro Alta Tecnologia Istituto di Ricerche Chimiche e Biochimiche G. Ronzoni S.r.l., via G. Colombo 81, 20133 Milan, Italy

René van Herpen
Aspen Oss B.V., Kloosterstraat 6, 5349 AB Oss, The Netherlands

Lucio Mauri, Maria Marinozzi, Giulia Mazzini and Marco Guerrini
Institute for Chemical and Biochemical Research G. Ronzoni, via G. Colombo 81, 20133 Milan, Italy

Richard E. Kolinski, Michael Karfunkle and David A. Keire
Division of Pharmaceutical Analysis, Office of Testing and Research, Center for Drug Evaluation and Research, U.S. Food and Drug Administration, 645 S. Newstead Ave., St. Louis, MO 63110, USA

Marcelo Lima and Edwin Yates
Department of Biochemistry, Federal University of São Paulo (UNIFESP), Vila Clementino, São Paulo, S.P. 04044-020, Brazil
Department of Biochemistry, Institute of Integrative Biology, University of Liverpool, Crown Street, Liverpool L69 7ZB, UK

Timothy Rudd
Department of Biochemistry, Institute of Integrative Biology, University of Liverpool, Crown Street, Liverpool L69 7ZB, UK
National Institute of Biological Standards and Controls (NIBSC), Blanche Lane, Potters Bar, Herts EN6 3QG, UK

Ha Na Kim, John M. Whitelock and Megan S. Lord
Graduate School of Biomedical Engineering, University of New SouthWales, Sydney, NSW 2052, Australia

Elena Vismara, Chiara Bongio, Alessia Coletti and Andrea Serafini
Department of Chemistry, Materials and Chemical Engineering "G. Natta", Politecnico di Milano, 20131 Milano, Italy

Ravit Edelman and Yoav D. Livney
Biotechnology and Food Engineering Department, Technion-Israel Institute of Technology, Haifa 3200000, Israel

Michele Mauri and Roberto Simonutti
Department of Materials Science, University of Milan Bicocca, 20125 Milano, Italy

Yehuda G. Assaraf
Biology Department, Technion-Israel Institute of Technology, Haifa 3200000, Israel

William de Wildt, Carel Funke, Bülent Üstün, Afranina Leika, Maarten Lunenburg and Frans Kaspersen
DTS Aspen Oss B.V., 5223BB Oss, The Netherlands

Huub Kooijman
Bijvoet Center for Biomolecular Research, Crystal and Structural Chemistry, Faculty of Science, Utrecht University, Padualaan 8, 3584 CH Utrecht, The Netherlands

Jan-Ytzen van der Meer, Edwin Kellenbach and Leendert J. van den Bos
Development and Technical Support Aspen Oss, Kloosterstraat 6, 5340 AB Oss, The Netherlands

Antonella Bisio, Elena Urso, Giangiacomo Torri, Annamaria Naggi and Sabrina Bertini
Istituto di Ricerche Chimiche e Biochimiche G. Ronzoni S.r.l., via G. Colombo 81, 20133 Milan, Italy

Pauline de Wit
Istituto di Ricerche Chimiche e Biochimiche G. Ronzoni, 20133 Milan, Italy
Department of Cell and Applied Biology, Faculty of Science, Radboud University Nijmegen, 6525 HP Nijmegen, The Netherlands

Øystein Arlov
Department of Biotechnology and Nanomedicine, SINTEF Materials and Chemistry, Richard Birkelands vei 3B, 7034 Trondheim, Norway

Gudmund Skjåk-Bræk
Department of Biotechnology, Norwegian University of Science and Technology, Sem Sælands vei 6/8, 7034 Trondheim, Norway

Melissa Rappold, Ulrich Warttinger and Roland Krämer
Inorganic Chemistry Institute, Heidelberg University, Im Neuenheimer Feld 270, 69120 Heidelberg, Germany

Pierre A. J. Mourier, Olivier Y. Guichard, Fréderic Herman, Philippe Sizun and Christian Viskov
Sanofi, 13 Quai Jules Guesde, 94403 Vitry sur Seine, France

Index

Printed in the USA
CPSIA information can be obtained
at www.ICGtesting.com
LVHW080046211023
761596LV00010BA/1940